KEY TOPICS IN

CARDIAC SURGERY

The KEY TOPICS Series

Advisors:

TM Craft *Department of Anaesthesia and Intensive Care, Royal United Hospital, Bath, UK*
CS Garrard *Intensive Therapy Unit, John Radcliffe Hospital, Oxford, UK*
PM Upton *Department of Anaesthesia, Royal Cornwall Hospital, Treliske, Truro, UK*

Accident and Emergency Medicine, Second Edition
Anaesthesia; Clinical Aspects, Third Edition
Cardiovascular Medicine
Chronic Pain, Second Edition
Critical Care
Evidence-Based Medicine
Gastroenterology
General Surgery
Neonatology
Neurology
Obstetrics and Gynaecology, Second Edition
Oncology
Ophthalmology, Second Edition
Oral and Maxillofacial Surgery
Orthopaedic Surgery
Orthopaedic Trauma Surgery
Otolaryngology, Second Edition
Paediatrics, Second Edition
Psychiatry
Renal Medicine
Respiratory Medicine
Thoracic Surgery
Trauma

Forthcoming titles include:

Critical Care, Second Edition
Neonatology, Second Edition
Plastic and Reconstructive Surgery
Sexual Health

KEY TOPICS IN
CARDIAC SURGERY

Sunil K Ohri
MD FRCS(Eng, Ed & C-Th) FESC
Consultant Cardiac Surgeon
Wessex Cardiothoracic Centre
Southampton General Hospital
and
Honorary Senior Lecturer
University of Southampton
Southampton, UK

Augustine Tang
BMedSc(Hon) DM FRCS(Ed & C-Th) FETCS
Consultant Cardiothoracic Surgeon
Blackpool Victoria Hospital
Whiney Heys Road
Blackpool, UK

Larry W Stephenson
MD FACC FCCP FACS
Professor of Surgery and Chief,
Division of Cardiothoracic Surgery
Harper University Hospital
Detroit, MI
USA

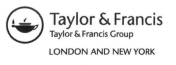
Taylor & Francis
Taylor & Francis Group

LONDON AND NEW YORK

A MARTIN DUNITZ BOOK

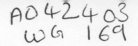

© 2005 Taylor & Francis, an imprint of the Taylor & Francis Group

First published in the United Kingdom in 2005
by Taylor & Francis, an imprint of the Taylor & Francis Group, 2 Park Square, Milton Park, Abingdon, Oxon OX14 4RN.

Tel: +44 (0)20 7017 6000
Fax: +44 (0)20 7017 6699
E-mail: info@dunitz.co.uk
Website: http://www.dunitz.co.uk

Although every effort has been made to ensure that all owners of copyright material have been acknowledged in this publication, we would be glad to acknowledge in subsequent reprints or editions any omissions brought to our attention.

A CIP record for this book is available from the British Library.

Library of Congress Cataloging-in-Publication Data

Data available on application

ISBN 1 85996 033 2

Distributed in North and South America by
Taylor & Francis
2000 NW Corporate Blvd
Boca Raton, FL 33431, USA

Within Continental USA
Tel.: 800 272 7737; Fax.: 800 374 3401
Outside Continental USA
Tel.: 561 994 0555; Fax.: 561 361 6018
E-mail: orders@crcpress.com

Distributed in the rest of the world by
Thomson Publishing Services
Cheriton House
North Way
Andover, Hampshire SP10 5BE, UK
Tel.: +44 (0)1264 332424
E-mail: salesorder.tandf@thomsonpublishingservices.co.uk

Composition by Wearset Ltd, Boldon, Tyne and Wear

Printed and bound in Great Britain by TJ International Ltd, Padstow, Cornwall

CONTENTS

LIST OF CONTRIBUTORS

USA

Frank A Baciewicz
Wayne State University,
Harper Hospital, Detroit,
USA

Carl L Backer
Children's Memorial
Hospital, Chicago, USA

Vinay Badhwar
University of Michigan
Hospital, Ann Arbor,
Michigan, USA

William Baumgartner
Johns Hopkins Hospital,
Baltimore, Maryland, USA

Jennifer A Berry
University of Michigan
Hospital, Ann Arbor,
Michigan, USA

Steven F Bolling
University of Michigan
Hospital, Ann Arbor,
Michigan, USA

Charles R Bridges
Division of Cardiothoracic
Surgery, Pennysylvania
Hospital, Philadelphia, USA

David G Cable
Mayo Clinic, Rochester,
Minnesota, USA

Rachel H Cohn
Division of Cardiothoracic
Surgery, Evanston Hospital,
Illinois, USA

Lori D Conklin
Baylor College of Medicine,
Houston, USA

Delos M Cosgrove
Cleveland Clinic
Foundation, Cleveland,
Ohio, USA

Wilson J Couto
Texas Heart Institute,
Houston, USA

Joseph S Coselli
Baylor College of Medicine,
Houston, USA

Richard C Daly
Mayo Clinic, Rochester,
Minnesota, USA

Ralph E Delius
Children's Hospital of
Michigan, Detroit, USA

Carlos Duran
International Heart Institute
of Montana, Missoula, USA

O Howard Frazier
Texas Heart Institute,
Houston, USA

A Marc Gillinov
Cleveland Clinic
Foundation, Cleveland,
Ohio, USA

Igor D Gregoric
Texas Heart Institute,
Housaton, USA

Daniel N Gwan-Nulla
Wayne State University,
Harper Hospital, Detroit,
USA

Frank L Hanley
Stanford University School
of Medicine, California,
USA

Stuart W Jamieson
UCSD Medical Center, San
Diego, USA

Scott A LeMaire
Baylor College of Medicine,
Houston, USA

Constantine Mavroudis
Children's Memorial
Hospital, Chicago, USA

Derlis Martino
Wayne State University,
Harper Hospital, Detroit,
USA

Alberto Pochettino
University of Pennsylvania
Medical Center,
Philadelphia, USA

V Mohan Reddy
Stanford University School
of Medicine, California,
USA

Mark D Rodefeld
James Whitcomb Riley
Hospital for Children,
Indianapolis, USA

Todd K Rosengart
Division of Cardiothoracic
Surgery, Evanston Hospital,
Illinois, USA

Irving Shen
Doernbecher Children's
Hospital, Oregon Health
Sciences University, USA

Larry W Stephenson
Wayne State University,
Harper Hospital, Detroit,
USA

R Scott Stuart
Mid America Thoracic and
Cardiovascular Surgery,
Kansas City, Missouri, USA

James G Tyburski
Wayne State University,
Detroit Receiving Hospital,
Detroit, USA

Ross M Ungerleider
Doernbecher Children's
Hospital, Oregon Health
Sciences University, USA

Henry L Walters III
Children's Hospital of
Michigan, Detroit, USA

Robert F Wilson
Wayne State University,
Detroit Receiving Hospital,
Detroit, USA

UK and Europe
Kyriakos Anastasiadis
Oxford Heart Centre, John
Radcliffe Hospital, UK

Robert H Anderson
Institute of Child Health,
University College London,
UK

Gianni D Angelini
Bristol Heart Institute,
University of Bristol, Bristol
Royal Infirmary, UK

Ani C Anyanwu
Harefield Hospital, London,
UK

Raimondo Ascione
Bristol Heart Institute,
University of Bristol, Bristol
Royal Infirmary, UK

George Asimakopoulos
Imperial School of
Medicine, Hammersmith
Hospital, London, UK

Emma J Birks
Harefield Hospital, London,
UK

Robert S Bonser
Department of Cardiac
Surgery, Queen Elizabeth
Medical Centre,
Birmingham, UK

William Brawn
Department of Cardiac
Surgery, Diana Princess
of Wales Children's
Hospital, Birmingham,
UK

Gareth Charlton
Department of Anaethesia,
Southampton, General
Hospital, UK

Gordon A Cohen
Great Ormond Street
Hospital, London, UK

Andrew Cook
Institute of Child Health,
University College London,
UK

Malcolm Dalrymple-Hay
Plymouth Hospitals NHS
Trust, Derriford Hospital,
UK

Keith D Dawkins
Department of Cardiology,
Southampton, General
Hospital, UK

Charles D Deakin
Department of Anaesthesia,
Southampton, General
Hospital, UK

David Delany
Department of Radiology,
Southampton General
Hospital, UK

Anthony C de Souza
Department of Cardiac
Surgery, Royal Brompton
Hospital, London, UK

Vincent M Dor
Cardio Thoracic Center,
Monte Carlo, Monaco

Martin J Elliott
Great Ormond Street
Hospital, London, UK

A Fisher
Imperial School of
Medicine, Hammersmith
Hospital, London, UK

Ravi Gill
Department of Anaesthesia,
Southampton General
Hospital, UK

Terry Gourlay
Imperial School of
Medicine, Hammersmith
Hospital, London, UK

Huon Gray
Department of Cardiology,
Southampton General
Hospital, UK

Mark Hanson
Division of Fetal Origins of
Adult Disease, University of
Southampton, UK

Marcus M Haw
Department of Cardiac
Surgery, Southampton
General Hospital, UK

Michael Herbertson
Department of Anaesthesia,
Southampton General
Hospital, UK

David A Hett
Department of Anaesthesia,
Southampton General
Hospital, UK

Vibeke E Hjortdal
Department of Thoracic and
Cardiovascular Surgery,
Skejby Hospital, University
Hospital of Aarhus,
Denmark

Sir Bruce E Keogh
Department of Cardiac
Surgery, Queen Elizabeth
Hospital, Birmingham,
UK

Asghar Khaghani
Harefield Hospital, London,
UK

Robin Kinsman
Dendrite Clinical Systems,
Henley-on-Thames, UK

Stephen M Langley
Department of Cardiac
Surgery, Southampton
General Hospital, UK

Eric Lim
Department of
Cardiothoracic Surgery,
Papworth Hospital,
Cambridge, UK

Steven A Livesey
Department of Cardiac
Surgery, Southampton
General Hospital, UK

Neil McGill
Department of Anaesthesia,
Southampton General
Hospital, UK

Adrian Mellor
Department of Anaesthesia,
Southampton General
Hospital, UK

John Morgan
Department of Cardiology,
Southampton General
Hospital, UK

James L Monro
Department of Cardiac
Surgery, Southampton
General Hospital, UK

Sunil K Ohri
Department of Cardiac
Surgery, Southampton
General Hospital, UK

Ravi Pillai
Oxford Heart Centre, John
Radcliffe Hospital, UK

M Pitt
Department of Cardiology,
Queen Elizabeth Medical
Centre, Birmingham, UK

Paul Roberts
Department of Cardiology,
Southampton General
Hospital, UK

David Royston
Department of Anaesthesia,
Harefield Hospital, London,
UK

Iain A Simpson
Department of Cardiology,
Southampton General
Hospital, UK

Michael Stewart
Queen Alexandra Hospital,
Portsmouth, UK

Augustine TM Tang
Department of Cardiac
Surgery, Blackpool Victoria
Hospital, UK

Kenneth M Taylor
Imperial School of
Medicine, Hammersmith
Hospital, London, UK

Richard Thomas
Department of Anaesthesia,
Southampton, General
Hospital, UK

Geoffrey M Tsang
Department of Cardiac
Surgery, Southampton
General Hospital, UK

Victor T Tsang
Cardiothoracic Unit, Great
Ormond Street Hospital,
London, UK

Crispin Weidemann
Department of Anaesthesia,
Southampton General
Hospital, UK

Francis Wells
Department of Cardiac
Surgery, Papworth Hospital,
Cambridge, UK

Douglas G West
Department of Cardiac
Surgery, Royal Brompton
Hospital, London, UK

Rest of the World
Michael A Borger
Division of Cardiovascular
Surgery, Toronto General
Hospital, Canada

Brian F Buxton
Austin Hospital,
Melbourne, Victoria,
Australia

Shafie Fazel
Division of Cardiovascular
Surgery, Toronto General
Hospital, Canada

Christopher M Feindel
Division of Cardiovascular
Surgery, Toronto General
Hospital, Canada

Jai Raman
Austin Hospital, Melbourne,
Victoria, Australia

Vivek Rao
Division of Cardiovascular
Surgery, Toronto General
Hospital, Canada

Heather J Ross
Division of Cardiology,
Toronto General Hospital,
Canada

Hisayoshi Suma
Hayama Heart Center,
Hayama, Kanagawa
Prefecture, Japan

GLOSSARY OF ABBREVIATIONS

ACE	angiotensin-converting enzyme	MI	myocardial infarction
AICD	automatic implantable cardiac defibrillator	MIDCAB	minimally invasive direct coronary artery bypass grafting
ASD	atrial septal defect	MRI	magnetic resonance imaging
ATP	adenosine triphosphate	NSAID	nonsteroidal anti-inflammatory drug
AVN	atrioventricular node		
AVSD	atrioventricular septal defect	OPCAB	off-pump coronary artery bypass grafting
BSA	body surface area		
CABG	coronary artery bypass grafting	PA	pulmonary artery
CCF	congestive cardiac failure	PAP	pulmonary artery pressure
CI	cardiac index	PDA	posterior descending coronary artery; patent ductus arteriosus
CO	cardiac output		
CPB	cardiopulmonary bypass	PFO	patent foramen ovale
CT	computed tomography	PVR	pulmonary vascular resistance
CVA	cerebrovascular accident	PAWP	pulmonary artery wedge pressure
CVP	central venous pressure		
CVS	cardiovascular system	RA	right atrium
CXR	chest x ray	RBBB	right bundle branch block
DORV	double outlet right ventricle	RCA	right coronary artery
EF	ejection fraction	RV	right ventricle
EKG	electrocardiogram	RVOT	right ventricular outflow tract
IABP	intra-aortic balloon pump	SR	sinus rhythm
INR	International Normalized Ratio	SVC	superior vena cava
ITA	internal thoracic artery	SVG	saphenous vein graft
IVC	inferior vena cava	SVR	systemic vascular resistance
JVP	jugular venous pressure	TEE	transesophageal echocardiography
LA	left atrium		
LAD	left anterior descending coronary artery	TOF	tetralogy of fallot
		TTE	transthoracic echocardiography
LAST	left anterior small thoracotomy	VATS	video-assisted thoracoscopic surgery
LV	left ventricle		
LVH	left ventricular hypertrophy	VSD	ventricular septal defect
LVOT	left ventricular outflow tract		

PREFACE

Tremendous surgical and technological advances have occurred within the specialist area of cardiac surgery in the past decade. Minimally invasive approaches, 'beating heart' coronary revascularization and non-transplant heart failure surgery are among many aspects of our practice which have gained prominence in recent times. For surgical trainees learning the art of cardiac surgery, the process of gathering useful information can often be haphazard. Large multi-volume reference tomes are available and the mainstream journals offer a myriad of topics. However, there is an overwhelming need for all essential materials to be presented in a succinct and easily digestible manner.

In this book we have endeavored to include every current key topic central to the modern practice of cardiac surgery. Essential information on each topic is summarized on several pages and presented as a succinct chapter with cross-references. A bibliography of important reading materials is also included in each chapter. This book should be used as a 'first-stop' pocket reference in conjunction with more comprehensive and specialist texts where further details on any key topic are required. The systematic and structured format of this book makes it an ideal revision aid for postgraduate trainees in cardiac surgery preparing for certification and fellowship examination. To ensure that the materials included are tailored to their needs, each topic has been carefully reviewed by cardiac surgical trainees and the editors. Furthermore, other personnel involved in the care of cardiac surgical patients, particularly those in cardiac anesthesia, cardiac intensive care, cardiology and paramedical disciplines, including perfusionists, nurses and physiotherapists, will also find this concise reference source invaluable.

SK Ohri, ATM Tang, and LW Stephenson

PART A   FUNDAMENTALS

1 Cardiac surgical anatomy

1.1 Heart valves

Andrew Cook, Robert H Anderson

Position

The cardiac valves are intimately related: their juxtaposition and proximity is best appreciated in the short-axis view at the level of the atrioventricular (AV) junctions. The pulmonary valve is the most superior, whilst the tricuspid and mitral valves guard the diaphragmatic border. Cradled by these structures is the aortic valve whose central location underpins the understanding of cardiac surgical anatomy.

Fibrous skeleton

Although the cardiac valves are closely related, there is no evidence that they are connected to one another via a well-structured and continuous fibrous skeleton. The best formed parts of the skeleton are at either ends of the area of fibrous continuity, between the leaflets of the aortic and mitral valves – left and right fibrous trigones. The right trigone blends with the membranous septum, and together they form the central fibrous body. Here, leaflets of the tricuspid, mitral and aortic valves adjoin each other. The pulmonary valve is encircled by free-standing muscle, the infundibulum; therefore its leaflets are detached from other cardiac valves. Furthermore, along most of the tricuspid annulus and the mural leaflet of the mitral valve, the atria and ventricles are separated by loose fibro-fatty tissue rather than a defined fibrous annulus.

The atrioventricular valves

The tricuspid and mitral valves are the inlet valves of the ventricular pumps. Each AV valve possesses four components: a hinge, valvar leaflets, tendinous cords and papillary muscles all acting in harmony (Figure 1). Disease or surgery to any one component can affect valvar function. The tricuspid valve has three leaflets, positioned septally, antero-superiorly and inferiorly (murally). The mitral valve is bi-leaflet, possessing mural (posterior) and aortic (anterior) leaflets. The number of leaflets and commissures is a matter of considerable debate. The pattern of valvar closure permits the assessment of the zones of apposition along the entire skirt of leaflet tissue. On this basis the normal mitral valve has a solitary zone of apposition between its primary components whilst the tricuspid valve closes in trifoliate fashion.

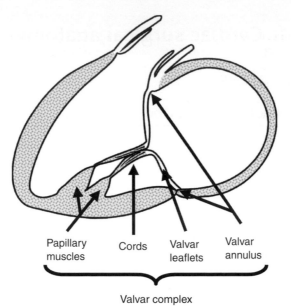

Papillary | Cords | Valvar | Valvar
muscles | | leaflets | annulus

Valvar complex

Figure 1 Since the closed atrioventricular valves must withstand the full force of ventricular systole during ejection through the open arterial valve, they have a complex arrangement made up of annulus, leaflets, tendinous cords, and papillary muscles. All these components must work in harmony for the valve to remain competent.

Hinge points

Each AV valve hinges from the AV junction either directly, involving the muscular sandwich, or from the fibrous AV septum. Together, the hinge points form a true mitral and a true tricuspid valvar annulus. Disease or surgery that crosses outside the annulus of the AV valves, therefore, can affect adjacent structures.

Tricuspid valve

The septal leaflet of the tricuspid valve, as the name suggests, is hinged along the length of the septal aspect of the right ventricular inlet. The inferior and and antero-superior leaflets are hinged directly from the parietal AV junction. The inferior leaflet is hinged along the anterior and diaphragmatic surfaces of the heart, starting from the junction of the right ventricle (RV) with the ventricular septum and running to the acute margin of the heart. The antero-superior leaflet continues from the acute margin to the anteroseptal commissure close to the aortic valve. Since the right coronary artery (RCA) courses within the epicardial fat surrounding this part of the AV junction, it is jeopardized by surgery to the hinge of the antero-superior or the inferior leaflets. In contrast, the septal leaflet hinges directly from an infolded region of the AV junction that forms part of the 'AV septum' – in reality, a muscular sandwich. The sandwich extends from the cardiac crux and comprises atrial myocardium, epicardial fat and ventricular myocardium. Running into this sandwich is the artery supplying the AV node. Surgery or disease to this region, therefore, risks perforating the heart inferiorly and damaging blood supply to the AV node.

Mitral valve

The hinge of the mural, or posterior, leaflet is subtended from the parietal AV junction. Disrupting this border will expose the left AV groove and its contents (circumflex coronary artery, great cardiac vein/coronary sinus). Crossing the hinge of the aortic, or anterior leaflet will reveal the left ventricle (LV) outflow tract. The fibrous continuity between the aortic and mitral valves means that this maneuver risks damage to the non-coronary and left coronary leaflets of the aortic valve. More extensive incisions across the area of fibrous continuity may reach the transverse pericardial sinus.

Valvar leaflets

Each valvar leaflet consists of a spongy atrial layer and a fibrous ventricular layer. It is best to think of the AV valvar leaflets, as well as their cordal attachments, as a continual hierarchy of division. The best example is illustrated in the mitral valve: the mural leaflet occupies two-thirds of the AV junction and is shorter while the aortic leaflet is longer but guards only one-third of the left AV junction. The two leaflets meet together along a single primary zone of apposition, with the ends of this line of closure within the AV junction defined as dual commissures. The leaflets appose at a point one-third of the distance between the annulus and free edge. Since the left AV junction is kidney-shaped, it is necessary for the leaflets to contain a number of slits in order to create a hemodynamically effective seal. For the mitral valve, these slits are mainly contained within the mural leaflet, but are extremely variable in their number and depth. They are supported by cords that can be fan-shaped. Within each compartment delineated by the slits, there are further divisions that allow the slits themselves to sit correctly together, and so on. Major subdivisions of the mitral leaflets are often used clinically to describe precisely areas of dysfunction and surgical repair (e.g. P2 prolapse). For the tricuspid valve with three major leaflets, there are three zones of apposition and hence three commissures.

Cords and papillary muscles

To withstand the full pumping force during ventricular systole, AV valves are supported by the tension apparatus – a system of cords and papillary muscles. Like the valvar leaflets, the anatomy of cords is hierarchical. Three major types of cord are defined by their relationship to the valvar leaflet:

- free edge cords – multiple and run from the free edge of each leaflet
- strut cords – run from a roughened zone on the ventricular surface of each leaflet
- basal cords – situated close to the AV junction.

Disease of free edge and strut cords is most likely to affect valvar function.

For the tricuspid valve, the number and size of cords and papillary muscles are particularly variable. Commonly, an anterior papillary muscle arises from the moderator band and supports the antero-superior leaflet. The medial papillary muscle is more variable in size and marks the site of the right bundle branch. The inferior papillary muscles support the inferior leaflet. A characteristic feature is the multiple cordal attachments of its septal leaflet to the ventricular septum. In contrast, the mitral valve is supported by two major papillary muscle groups that are attached to the parietal ventricular walls rather than the septum.

The arterial valves

Valvar competence requires that the various components of the valvar complex (junctions, sinuses and leaflets) work in harmony. Although there is no evidence that the hemodynamic junction of either the aortic or pulmonary valve consists of an annulus, such a structure is widely accepted by surgeons. Within each arterial root there are three ring-like structures:

- sinu-tubular junction (STJ) between the distal part of the sinuses and the proximal portion of the arterial trunk
- anatomic ventriculo-arterial junction between the ventricular myocardium and the arterial sinuses
- basal ring that can be drawn joining the proximal parts of the valvar leaflets (Figure 2).

The hemodynamic border between each corresponding ventricle and its artery is formed not by rings, but by the attachments of the valvar leaflets within the arterial root. This junction is crown-shaped, since the line of attachment of each of the three valvar leaflets is semilunar. For each leaflet, the line of attachment starts at the level of the STJ, runs down the arterial root to a nadir at the level of the basal ring and returns to the level of the STJ, so forming each valvar sinus. The hinge point of each valvar leaflet crosses the anatomic ventriculo-arterial junction leaving triangles of arterial wall on the ventricular aspect of the valvar attachment and crescents of ventricular myocardium with the arterial sinus. In the pulmonary position, the three interleaflet triangles and sinusal crescents interdigitate around the entire circumference of the sub-pulmonary infundibulum. In the aortic root, the appearance is much the same except in the region of the aortomitral continuity where the sinusal crescent is formed, not of myocardium, but of fibrous tissue. Consequently, part of the distal outflow tract at the apex of the interleaflet triangles will be made up of arterial wall. Disease or resection of the interleaflet triangles will lead from the respective ventricle outside the heart.

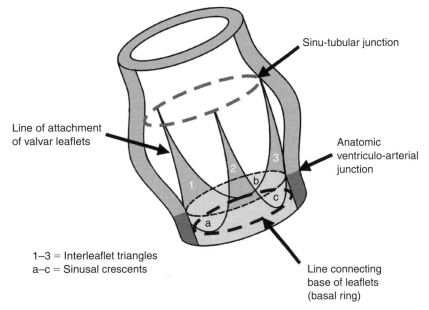

Figure 2 The three ring-like structures of the arterial root.

Sinuses

The three dilations of the arterial roots, the sinuses, arranged in clover-leaf fashion at their base, allow the valvar leaflets to fall back during ventricular systole. The column of blood is then able to pass unobstructed from ventricle to arterial root. In the normal heart, four of the six sinuses face one another. In the aortic position, it is from these facing sinuses that the coronary arteries usually arise. Consequently, it is easy to designate the aortic sinuses as non-coronary, right coronary, and left coronary. The junction between each sinus and the tubular portion of the arterial trunk also plays an important part in the function of the valvar complex. This is most evident in 'supravalvar' aortic stenosis, where constriction at the STJ distorts the entrance into the arterial sinuses, producing a narrowing between the arterial wall and free edge of the valvar leaflets.

Valvar leaflets

These are pockets of fibrous tissue lined by endothelium. When closed, their shape and attachments enable them to withstand diastolic blood pressure. The three valvar leaflets have three zones of apposition, and hence three commissures. The attachment of each leaflet is semilunar. The leaflets do not meet at their free edges; their points of contact are along the ventricular margin of each leaflet. The center of each leaflet becomes thickened with age, producing the nodules of Arantius.

Further reading

1. Anderson RH. Clinical anatomy of the aortic root. *Heart* 2000; **84**: 670–3.
2. Anderson RH. The structure of the aortic root. *J Thorac Cardiovasc Surg* 1997; **114**: 870–1.
3. Sutton JP III, Ho SY, Anderson RH. The forgotten interleaflet triangles: a review of the surgical anatomy of the aortic valve. *Ann Thorac Surg* 1995; **59**: 419–27.
4. Wilcox BR, Anderson RH. *Surgical Anatomy of the Heart. 2nd Edn.* Gower Medical Publishing: London, 1992.

1.2 Coronary circulation

Andrew Cook, Robert H Anderson

The coronary circulation consists of the coronary arteries, veins, and the lymphatics. Of these, it is the coronary arteries, and to a lesser extent the veins, that have the most surgical relevance. The pattern of coronary circulation, in particular the veins, may differ markedly between patients. The following describes characteristics in the majority of individuals.

Coronary arteries

Emerging as first branches from the aorta, the two arteries arise from the aortic sinuses adjacent to the pulmonary trunk (facing sinuses) and become epicardial. Considerable variations exist in the position of the coronary ostia within the sinus, the number of orifices, and their epicardial course. Either the left or right coronary artery can arise ectopically above the level of the sinu-tubular junction. Multiple orifices are found most frequently in the right coronary sinus with separate origins of infundibular branches and the sinus node artery. Rarely, a coronary artery will originate in one sinus and run within the wall of the aorta, crossing the commissure between sinuses. These intra-mural coronary arteries are prone to compression if they run between the two arterial trunks. They can be difficult surgically to relocate.

Naming of the coronary sinuses has remained controversial. In the normal heart the right-sided and left-sided sinuses, facing the pulmonary trunk, give rise to the right and left coronary arteries, respectively. In congenitally malformed hearts the sinuses can malrotate into unusual positions concomitant with abnormal relations of the great arterial trunks. Consequently, the best nomenclature was conceived by the Leiden group, specifically identifying the sinuses as #1 and #2. In this convention, an imaginary observer is visualized standing in the non-facing sinus of the aorta. Sinus #1 is then designated as the sinus to the right hand, while sinus #2 is to the left hand (Figure 1).

Epicardial course

The main stem left coronary artery passes behind the pulmonary trunk and then divides into the circumflex artery, superior (anterior) interventricular artery and frequently an additional major branch supplying the obtuse margin of the heart (intermediate). A variable number of diagonal branches spring from the superior interventricular artery (clinically known as the left anterior descending artery) to supply the anterior and posterior walls of the left ventricle. The right coronary artery usually passes directly into the right AV groove. A number of branches along the acute margin of the heart supply the antero-lateral surface of the right ventricle. In 90% of individuals (right dominance) it will also supply the diaphragmatic surface of the heart via the inferior interventricular coronary artery (clinically known as the posterior descending artery) at the crux of the heart. In 90% of cases the artery continues beyond the crux to supply the diaphragmatic surface of the LV by the inferior LV branches.

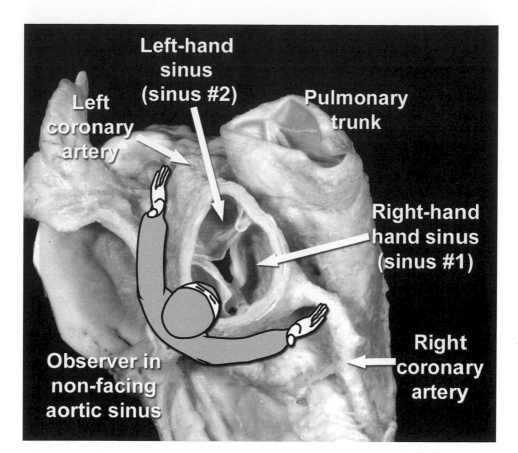

Figure 1 The diagram illustrates the most widely accepted methodology for naming the aortic sinuses, termed the Leiden convention. An observer is imagined standing within the non-facing aortic sinus, looking towards the pulmonary trunk. One aortic sinus is to the observer's left hand and is designated sinus #2, while the other is to the right hand, sinus #1.

In the other 10% of individuals (left dominance) this area is supplied by the circumflex artery via the inferior interventricular artery.

Major branches of the coronary arteries carry important surgical significance. The superior interventricular artery gives rise to the first septal perforating artery which supplies the superior portions and sometimes also the inferior parts of the ventricular bundle branches. Being the first major branch of the superior interventricular artery, it tunnels perpendicularly into the ventricular septum towards the medial papillary muscle of the tricuspid valve (Figure 2). Since it lies immediately beneath the free-standing muscular sleeve that forms the sub-pulmonary infundibulum, it is at risk during operative procedures involving this structure, particularly during harvest of the pulmonary autograft in the Ross procedure. In 90% of individuals, the right coronary artery will give rise to the AV node artery. In the remainder, left dominant pattern, the AV node artery originates from the circumflex artery. This vessel runs within the fibro-fatty sandwich that forms part of the atrioventricular 'septum'. It supplies the AV node and also, in some patients, parts of the branching bundles. The origin and course of the sinus node artery are variable: in 55% of patients, it will arise from the right

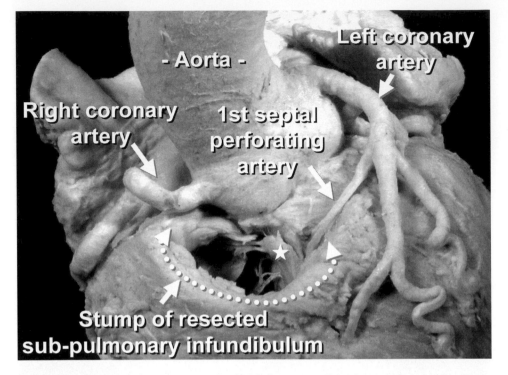

Figure 2 The specimen has been prepared to show the course of the first septal perforating artery which supplies the anterior portion of the conduction system. In this specimen, the muscular sleeve that supports the pulmonary valve, its infundibulum, has been removed as is often reproduced in the Ross procedure. The artery lies just beneath this sleeve, branches perpendicularly from the left coronary artery and passes obliquely into the ventricular septum towards the medial papillary muscle (denoted by star).

coronary artery and in the remainder, from the circumflex. Often it will arise close to the origin of the respective artery but sometimes more distally. It will then take a more lengthy course either across the right atrium (RA) appendage or across the dome of the left atrium (LA). The artery can then approach the sinus node from the front (60% of patients), from behind (33% of patients), or completely surround the cavo-atrial junction, in the remainder.

The coronary veins

Although their complex and frequent variations have been known since the early 1900s, coronary venous anatomy receives little attention. Some generalizations can be made: the majority of the coronary veins drain to the coronary sinus situated within the left AV groove and draining to the RA. Additionally, several minor Thebesian veins and somewhat larger anterior veins can open directly to the RA, bypassing the coronary sinus. The major veins consist of the small cardiac vein, which runs anteriorly around the right AV junction and is of variable size; the middle cardiac vein, which runs within the inferior interventricular groove next to the inferior interventricular coronary artery; and the great cardiac vein, which runs around the left AV junction to the superior surface of the heart to mirror the course of the superior interventricular artery. The great cardiac vein is a direct continuation of the coronary sinus. The exact point at which one becomes the other has been a matter of debate, some supporting the notion that the valve of Vieussens marks the border, while others consider the origin of the oblique vein of the left atrium as the delimiting boundary.

Recent work has demonstrated that the coronary sinus itself, like the great cardiac vein, possesses its own discrete walls, rather than being part of the wall of the left atrium, as was often thought. In diagnostic terms, the coronary sinus can still be considered as a left atrial structure, since it runs within the left AV groove. Its presence can be used to infer the presence of a morphologically left atrium. Consequently, in congenitally malformed hearts with bilateral right atrial appendages (asplenia syndrome or right isomerism), there is complete absence of the coronary sinus. In this setting, alternative patterns of coronary venous drainage exists directly into the atrial chambers.

Further reading

1. Cook AC, Anderson RH. Attitudinally correct nomenclature. *Heart* 2002; **87**: 503–6.
2. Anderson KR, Ho SY, Anderson RH. The location and vascular supply of the sinus node in the human heart. *Br Heart J* 1979: **41**: 28–32.
3. Anderson RH. Anatomy. In: *Paediatric Cardiology. 2nd Edn.* Anderson RH, Baker EJ, Macartney FJ et al (eds). Churchill Livingstone: London, 2002: pp 19–36.
4. Wilcox BR, Anderson RH. *Surgical Anatomy of the Heart. 2nd Edn.* Gower Medical Publishing: London, 1992.
5. James TN. *Anatomy of the Coronary Arteries.* Hoeber: New York, 1961: pp 103–6.

Related topics of interest

1.3 Conduction system

Andrew Cook, Robert H Anderson

The conduction system of the heart can be divided into two major components: the sinus node and the atrioventricular conduction axis. The latter can be subdivided into the atrioventricular node (AVN); the penetrating and branching bundles; and the peripheral conduction fibers. All but the peripheral ventricular fibers are of major significance to the surgeon.

The sinus node

The anatomic landmark for the position of the sinus node is the junction between the superior vena cava (SVC) and the roof of the RA, at the superior end of the terminal groove. Usually the node, an elliptical shaped sub-epicardial structure, lies lateral to this junction, but in 10% of patients it is horseshoe shaped, extending across the junction into the interatrial groove. Its arterial supply, via the sinus nodal artery, is also somewhat variable. In approximately 55% of patients, this originates from the RCA. In the remainder, it arises from the circumflex coronary artery. Variations in its course are even more widespread. Usually, the artery arises close to the origin of the parent artery, but in circumstances where it arises more distally, it then takes a course across the RA appendage or dome of the LA. The artery usually crosses the crest of the appendage to reach the sinus node, but can enter the terminal groove from behind the SVC, or divide to pass in front of and behind the SVC. Consequently, the entire cavo-atrial junction should be considered an area of potential risk during surgery.

Propagation of atrial impulses

There is no evidence for discrete specialized tracts of conduction tissue within the RA linking the sinus to the AVN. Instead, it is now well documented that the propagation of the impulse generated by the sinus node through the atrium takes the path of least resistance, following the direction of the fibers within the atrial musculature. In this context, the RA musculature is complex, representing a mesh-like muscular bag peppered with 'holes'. The holes are the mouths of the superior and inferior caval veins, the coronary sinus, the vestibule of the tricuspid valve and the confines of the atrial septum. The mesh-like arrangement is formed by the interdigitation of atrial myocardium, and the pectinate muscles, which are extensive on the right. The conduction impulse, therefore, courses around and in between these holes along the orientation of the muscle fibers to reach the AVN. Surgical incisions through fibrous healing can produce further barriers to conduction through the atria. Given that there are no specialized tracts, however, the impulse can usually find an alternative route. A series of carefully planned incisions constitutes the basis for arrhythmia surgery.

The atrioventricular conduction axis

The key to location and avoidance of the atrioventricular conduction tissues in the normal heart is identification of the margins of the triangle of Koch and the entire atrial component of the atrioventricular conducting tissues within this area. The sides of the triangle are delineated by the tendon of Todaro, the hinge point of the septal leaflet of the tricuspid valve, and the inferior isthmus situated between the mouth of the coronary sinus and the hinge point of the tricuspid valve (Figure 1). At its apex superiorly, the triangle of Koch is bordered by the membranous portion of the AV septum. It is through this structure that the penetrating bundle passes to reach the ventricular septum. The AVN, however, is situated slightly more inferiorly within the sloping face of atrial myocardium that forms the roof of an atrioventricular muscular sandwich. Its arterial supply is via a small arterial branch running within the fibro-fatty tissue of the atrioventricular muscular sandwich, usually originating from the right but sometimes from the circumflex coronary artery.

Penetrating and branching bundles

From the AVN, the AV bundle moves towards the central fibrous body, and penetrates through it towards the left. As it does so, it passes from the AV component of the membranous septum to its ventricular component, the division being marked by the hinge point of the tricuspid valve. As a result, the conduction tissue, which has now begun to branch into the left bundle, essentially sits on top of the crest of the muscular ventricular septum, separated from ventricular myocardium only by a narrow region of fibrous tissue. As seen from the LV outflow tract, the membranous septum, located beneath the interleaflet triangle

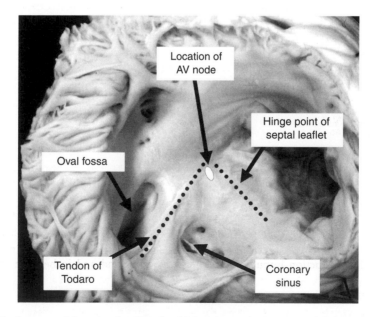

Figure 1 The features of the triangle of Koch which point to the location of the AV node. The triangle is delineated by the tendon of Todaro, the hinge point of the tricuspid valve and the coronary sinus. The node itself is located on the smooth atrial vestibule at the apex of the triangle.

between the right and non-coronary leaflets of the aortic valve, marks the site of emergence of the left bundle branch. From this point, the left bundle divides, commonly into three fascicles that run sub-endocardially down the smooth septal surface of the LV to the ventricular apex. In contrast, the right bundle branch passes as a single cord, within the ventricular myocardium from the left side, to reach the right side of the septum. Initially, it heads for a region of myocardium at the base of the medial papillary muscle of the tricuspid valve. Consequently, a line drawn from the AVN to the origin of the medial papillary muscle will delimit the course of the branching bundle. From this point, the right bundle branch runs deep within the myocardium of the body of the septomarginal trabeculation to its base, and traverses the RV cavity through the moderator band.

Further reading

1. Ho SY, Anderson RH, Sanchez-Quintana D. Atrial structure and fibres: morphologic bases of atrial conduction. *Cardiovasc Res* 2002; 54: 325–36.
2. Anderson RH, Ho SY. The morphology of the specialized atrioventricular junctional area: the evolution of understanding. *Pacing Clin Electrophysiol* 2002; 25: 957–66.
3. Anderson RH. Anatomy. In: *Paediatric Cardiology. 2nd Edn.* Anderson RH, Baker EJ, Macartney FJ et al (eds). Churchill Livingstone: London, 2002: pp 19–36.
4. Wilcox BR, Anderson RH. *Surgical Anatomy of the Heart. 2nd Edn.* Gower Medical Publishing: London, 1992.

Related topics of interest

1.4 Sequential segmental analysis

Andrew Cook, Robert H Anderson

Sequential segmental analysis represents a globally recognized method of describing congenitally malformed hearts. It enables complex cardiac malformations to be broken down into 'building blocks', which can be assessed independently and then assembled, so as to describe the connections between different components. As the name suggests, the segments of the heart and the manner in which they connect with one another are examined in sequence: beginning with the atria, then the ventricles, and finally the great arteries (Figure 1).

The morphologic method

Originally developed by Van Praagh, this system states that one component of the heart, or any variable features, should not be defined on the basis of another component that is itself variable. It follows then that each part of the heart should be analyzed with reference to the most constant component. Sequential segmental analysis of the heart begins with identifying these components within each patient.

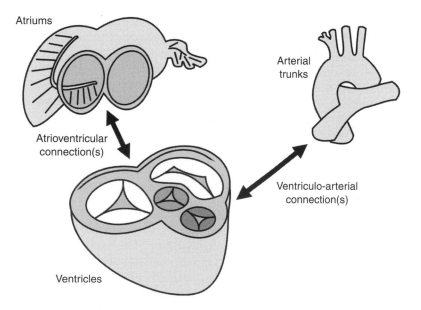

Figure 1 The building blocks of the heart are the atrial, ventricular, and arterial segments. Equally important, however, is the fashion in which the segments are, or are not, joined together. These junctions are the 'connections'.

Components

Atria

Four potential parts can be considered – the appendage, the atrial septum, the atrial vestibule, and the venous connections – with the four parts arranged around the atrial bodies. Analysis of congenitally malformed hearts demonstrated that the pectinate muscles of the appendage are the most constant feature. Currently, this feature is rarely used in clinical practice. Nonetheless, a morphologically right atrium contains pectinate muscles that extend around the tricuspid valve to the crux of the heart. Restriction of the same muscles within the appendage defines the basis of a morphologically left appendage. In this instance, the atrial wall around the remainder of the mitral valve, above its vestibule, will be smooth. Overall, this gives rise to four possible variations of atrial arrangement. In two options, the normal and the mirror-imaged arrangements, the atria are lateralized. In the others, both atria have appendages of the same morphology giving, respectively, right and left isomerism.

Ventricles

Three parts can be considered – inlet, apical trabecular and outlet portions. Both the inlet and the outlet portions are highly variable in hearts that are congenitally malformed. In contrast, the apical trabecular component is consistently found in virtually all malformations and is the best arbiter of ventricular morphology. A notable exception is seen in a truly solitary ventricle where the apical trabeculations are particularly coarse, and there is absence of the ventricular septum. In biventricular hearts, the morphologically right ventricle is defined by its coarse apical trabeculations, while the morphologically left ventricle has a much finer, criss-crossing, trabecular pattern at its apex.

Arteries

There is no independent feature to differentiate between the trunks although the branching patterns usually help. Four variants exist: an aorta, a pulmonary trunk, a common arterial trunk, or a solitary arterial trunk. The aorta not only gives rise to the coronary arteries as its first branch but also branches more distally into the arteries supplying the head and neck. The pulmonary trunk branches proximally into right and left pulmonary arteries. A common trunk supplies directly coronary, pulmonary and brachiocephalic branches, while a solitary arterial trunk is defined when the intrapericardial pulmonary arteries are absent. In this latter situation, it is not possible to determine whether the trunk present had been destined to be an aorta or a common trunk.

Connections

Once these features have been determined individually, they are joined together as 'building blocks' to assess the connections between components. Most hearts possess two separate connections across each of the atrioventricular and ventriculo-arterial junctions. If connection between two segments is as expected in the normal heart, the arrangement is designated concordant. Discordant connections occur between chambers or arterial trunks of opposite morphologic type.

Atrioventricular connections

As far as the atrioventricular connections are concerned, this presents no problems in patients with lateralized atria. For patients with isomeric appendages, the situation is less clear cut: for instance with isomeric right appendages and biventricular connections, one atrium will be connected to a morphologically right ventricle while the other morphologically right atrium will be connected to the morphologically left ventricle. Thus, one side is concordant while the other is discordant. The overall connections therefore are ambiguous, and the biventricular atrioventricular connections are described in this fashion. When considering the atrioventricular junctions, separate analysis is made for the morphology of the atrioventricular valves. Occasionally the atria are connected to a single ventricle. The possibilities are for double inlet connection, or for absence of right-sided or left-sided connection. With double inlet, both atria can be connected to a morphologically right, left, or indeterminate ventricle. When the connections are to the right or left ventricle, the complimentary ventricle is rudimentary and incomplete. When one connection is absent, the remaining atrium can also connect to a morphologically right, left, or rarely an indeterminate ventricle. In the extremely rare form termed 'double outlet atrium', one atrioventricular connection is absent whilst the single atrium is joined to both ventricular chambers.

Ventriculo-arterial connections

Similar combinations apply to the ventriculo-arterial connections, which can be concordant, discordant, double outlet, or single outlet. Double outlet can be from either the morphologically right or left ventricle, or from a solitary and indeterminate ventricle. Single outlet should be qualified by referring to the type of arterial trunk exiting the heart, and whether or not a second atretic vessel is present. As such, the single outlet can be via a single vessel, as in common or solitary arterial trunk, or can also be found in association with pulmonary or aortic atresia.

Shared connections

In some instances, either an atrioventricular or ventriculo-arterial junction is shared between two ventricles, the valvar orifice overriding the crest of the ventricular septum. In such instances, the overriding orifice is judged to arise from the ventricle supporting its greater part – the '50% rule'. This enables differentiation between discordant/concordant ventriculo-arterial connections from double outlet ventricle. When assessing ventriculo-arterial junctions, infundibular morphology and arterial relationships should be noted and described separately. These features do not alter the nature of the ventriculo-arterial connections.

Associated lesions

Once the basic connections between cardiac segments have been determined, it is necessary to document independently all the associated lesions. In the system of sequential segmental analysis there can be any number of these additional variables, including the position of the heart within the thorax, the direction of the cardiac apex, and the arrangement of the thoraco-abdominal organs. In this way, it is possible to provide a simple account of the structure of any congenitally malformed heart, even if the specific combination of connections and malformations is unique.

Further reading

1. Anderson, RH, Ho SY. Continuing Medical Education: Sequential segmental analysis – description and categorization for the millennium. *Cardiol Young* 1997; 7: 98–116.
2. Anderson RH. Terminology. In: *Paediatric Cardiology. 2nd Edn.* Anderson RH, Baker EJ, Macartney FJ et al (eds). Churchill Livingstone: London, 2002: pp 19–36.

Related topics of interest

2 Cardiac surgical physiology

2.1 Excitation-contraction coupling

Paul Roberts

A basic knowledge of cardiac electrophysiology at cellular level is essential for understanding abnormalities of cardiac conduction and contraction.

Basic electrophysiology

Repetitive and ordered cardiac contraction relies on a very precise sequence of events. It is the formation of an action potential that excites the individual cell. The sarcolemma of cardiac cells has a high-resistance, insulated phospholipid bilayer. Spaced throughout this layer are proteins that act as ion channels. Passage of ions through these channels alters the intracellular voltage potential, generating gradients with the extracellular environment.

Ion channels

Ion channels are complex proteins that span the phospholipid bilayer of the cell membrane. They contain pores through which certain charged particles may be allowed to pass. These pores are highly specific to a particular ion and have the ability to 'gate' ionic flux. Specific channels exist for potassium, sodium and calcium ions. As these channels are voltage sensitive, it is the voltage gradient across the membrane that determines whether or not an ion channel is open.

Cardiac cells at rest maintain an intracellular charge that is different to the extracellular environment. The gradient from inside to outside is known as the resting potential. In general, sodium and calcium concentrations are much higher outside the cell with potassium being much higher inside. The high intracellular concentration of potassium is maintained by the Na^+/K^+ ATP-dependent pump, which exchanges sodium ions for potassium ions. Thus, sodium ions move out of the cells in exchange for influx of potassium ions. At rest, cardiac myocytes have open potassium channels whilst others are closed. This leads to the movement of potassium ions out of the cells, leaving negatively charged ions behind. A point is reached where the potential gradient drawing potassium ions out of the cells is matched by the attractive force of the negative ions left behind. This steady state determines the resting potential, which is approximately $-90\,mV$ in ventricular muscle cells. At this stage the sodium and calcium ion channels are gated closed. Therefore, potassium ionic channels steer the cell towards $-90\,mV$, whereas sodium and calcium channels force the level towards positive. The balance and interaction of these channels produces the action potential.

The action potential

1. Cardiac muscle cells

Depolarization of an adjacent cell opens sodium channels. The influx of sodium causes the gradient to become less negative, which in turn causes more sodium ion channels to open, resulting in an even greater influx of sodium ions. This ultimately reduces the membrane potential to become transiently positive. This is responsible for phase 0 of the action potential. A transiently activated potassium channel then allows the passage of potassium ions out of the cells, returning the membrane potential to approximately zero (phase 1). Phase 2 occurs as a result of a balance of outward potassium ions with inward calcium ions. Calcium channels are slower than both potassium and sodium channels, resulting in the relatively long phase 2. Calcium ions that enter the cell during this 'plateau' phase of the action potential are responsible for the intiation of myocyte contraction. The closure of calcium channels results in the influx of potassium exceeding the exit of calcium, heralding the start of phase 3. Potassium progressively enters the cells with other ionic channels being shut. This period of repolarization returns the resting potential to −90 mV and prepares the cells for the next stimulus for depolarization. The resting period is phase 4 (Figure 1a).

2. Specialized cardiac cells

The cells of the cardiac conduction system, e.g. Purkinje fibers, behave in a similar way to cardiac muscle cells outlined above. They are slightly different, however, in that the resting potential is more negative and the upstroke of phase 0 more rapid.

Pacemaker cells (sinoatrial and atrioventricular nodes) in contrast, behave differently. They do not require initiation of the action potential, by adjacent cells, but are able to spontaneously depolarize in a rhythmic manner. This property is known as automaticity. Atrial and ventricular cells do not usually demonstrate automatic properties. However, in certain circumstances they will. An example of this is a slow (35 beats/min) ventricular escape rhythm seen in patients in complete heart block. The morphology of the pacemaker cell

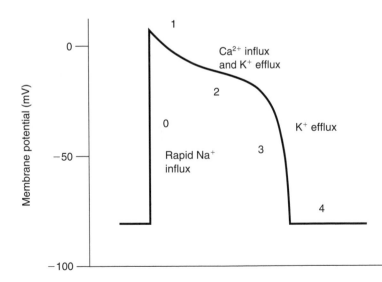

Figure 1a Myocyte action potential.

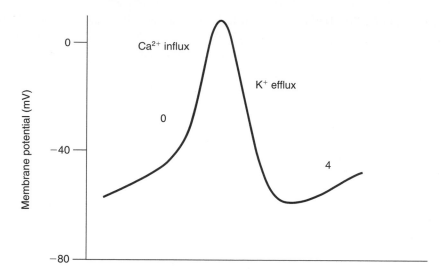

Figure 1b Pacemaker cell action potential.

action potential is also different (Figure 1b). Phase 4 of the action potential is not flat, as in cardiac muscle cells. Instead, it progressively increases due to gradual spontaneous depolarization. This is a result of a sodium channel that is different to the rapid sodium ionic transfer seen during phase 0 in cardiac muscle cells. This channel opens during repolarization, resulting in the gradual influx of sodium ions until the threshold is reached at which depolarization occurs. Phase 0 is less rapid as the rapid sodium channels are deactivated, resulting in the upstroke of the action potential being dependent on calcium influx, through relatively slow ionic channels.

Refractoriness

The action potential seen in cardiac cells is longer than that in skeletal muscle. This means that it takes longer before the cell is capable of being re-stimulated, i.e. it is refractory to further activation. This serves as a protective mechanism to prevent further rapid activation. In turn, this allows the necessary time for atrial/ventricular filling and emptying. The absolute refractory period refers to the time when the cell is completely unexcitable. This lasts from phase 0 to the beginning of phase 3. Ventricular cells have longer refractory periods than atrial, resulting in the potential for atrial cells to be excited quicker than ventricular. An example of this is atrial flutter when the atrial muscle cells are being activated at approximately 300 beats per minute.

Cardiac depolarization

Initiation of electrical impulses usually starts in the sinoatrial node. Electrical impulses are transmitted from cell to adjacent cell through gap-junctions that offer minimal resistance. The impulse is propagated through the atria to the atrioventricular node. Fibrous tissue surrounds the atrioventricular junctions, which means that the only connection of atria and ventricles is through the atrioventricular node (AVN). The AVN has small-diameter fibers of the slow pacemaker variety, which means that the impulse is protectively slowed at this juncture. The AVN therefore, controls the rate of ventricular contraction, optimizing atrial transit.

Excitation-contraction coupling

The interaction of the electrical excitation and mechanical muscular contraction is termed excitation-contraction coupling. Calcium ions are the key messenger in this process as they are integral to the electrical excitation process (action potential) and a direct activator of myofilaments. Specific proteins are responsible for mechanical contraction. Actin and myosin are involved in the contraction under the regulation of tropomyosin and troponin.

Myosin is arranged in thick filaments with globular heads and thin tails. They contain myosin ATPase, which is essential for contraction. In contrast, actin is arranged in thin helical filaments intertwined with the thick myosin filaments through myosin cross-bridges. Tropomyosin prevents contraction by lying in the grooves between the actin filaments. Troponin (I, T and C) is responsible for binding calcium ions, inhibiting ATPase activity and linking actin and tropomyosin.

During phase 2 of the action potential, calcium enters the cells. The activation of troponin by the calcium alters tropomyosin, enabling actin and myosin to interact and produce mechanical contraction. The myosin globular heads bind to the actin filaments, interdigitating thick and thin filaments to pass one another. This process is ATP-dependent and therefore utilizes energy. Ultimately, the myosin head releases actin, allowing the muscle to relax and the process to start again.

It is the concentration of calcium ions within the cytosol that determines the force of contraction. Therefore, mechanisms reducing calcium ions will reduce contractile force, i.e. become negatively inotropic. Hence, beta-adrenergic stimulation encourages calcium flux, thus increasing the force of contraction.

Clinical implications of excitation-contraction coupling

1. Antiarrhythmic drugs

All of the antiarrhythmic drugs exert their effects through actions on ionic channels. An understanding of these drugs makes the choice of appropriate antiarrhythmic easier. The Vaughan-Williams classification is based upon the pharmacological action of each group of drugs (Table 1).

2. Ion channel defects

Inherited defective ion channels are responsible for a large number of conditions: long QT syndrome, Brugada syndrome, cystic fibrosis, Liddle's syndrome (hereditary hypertension) and many myopathies such as Becker's, malignant hyperthermia, etc. Gene therapy ultimately may have a dramatic impact on the management of such conditions.

Table 1 Vaughan-Williams classification of antiarrhythmic drugs.

Class		Group name	Mechanism of action	Examples
1	A	Sodium channel blockers	Prolong action potential (by blocking several types of sodium channels)	Disopyramide, procainamide, quinidine
	B		Shorten action potential	Lidocaine (lignocaine), mexiletine
	C		Prolong action potential (by blocking outward-rectifying potassium channels)	Flecainide, propafenone, moracizine
2		Beta blockers	Indirect blockage of calcium channel opening	Atenolol, propranolol, esmolol
3		Potassium channel blockers	Prolong action potential and delay repolarization	Amiodarone, sotalol
4		Calcium antagonists	Direct blockage of calcium ion channels slows pacemaker cells, i.e. sinoatrial and atrioventricular nodes	Verapamil, diltiazem, nifedipine

Further reading

1. Ackerman MJ, Clapham DE. Ion channels – basic science and clinical disease. *N Engl J Med* 1997; **336:** 1575–86.
2. Bers DM. Cardiac excitation-contraction coupling. *Nature* 2002; **415:** 198–205.
3. Marban E. Cardiac channelopathies. *Nature* 2002; **415:** 213–18.

Related topic of interest

2.2   Cardiac conduction and arrhythmia

2.2 Cardiac conduction and arrhythmia

John Morgan

The conduction system

Heart rate and coordination of atrioventricular contraction are determined by an electrical control system comprising:

- sinus node
- atrial conduction channels
- atrioventricular node (AVN)
- His–Purkinje system.

Disease in any of these or in atrial or ventricular myocardium can cause abnormality of heart rate or incoordination of cardiac contraction.

Detailed description of the anatomy of the conduction tissues is given in Chapter 1.3. The AVN exhibits characteristic decremental conduction features: the greater the frequency of depolarization the slower the conduction through AV nodal tissues. Repolarization of atria and ventricles is organized such that those areas depolarizing first, repolarize last, an arrangement to protect against reactivation of myocardium by myocardial depolarization at adjacent sites.

Arrhythmias

- Tachycardia: (>100 bpm).
- Bradycardia: (<60 bpm).
- Irregularity of rhythm.

Symptoms

- Palpitation: often due to an abnormality of rhythm, an exaggerated awareness of sinus rhythm or an increase in stroke volume.
- Dizziness, presyncope or syncope can occur with systemic arterial hypotension, causing hypoperfusion of the brain.
- Nonspecific symptoms, including malaise, lethargy and dyspnea, may occur with persistent bradycardia. Angina may occur in tachycardia.

Cardiac rhythm investigations

Surface electrocardiogram (EKG)

The EKG deflections are arbitrarily termed P wave (atrial mass depolarization), QRS (ventricular mass depolarization), T wave (ventricular mass repolarization) and U wave (genesis disputed). The precise features of the normal QRS deflection are determined by the recording lead's orientation. Each EKG recording lead has positive and negative poles. Standard leads I, II and III are bipolar and orientated in the coronal plane; AVR, AVL and AVF ('A' for augmented, as instrumental augmentation is necessary because of the low potential at the extremities) are unipolar leads orientated in the coronal plane; and leads V1 to V6 are unipolar leads orientated in the horizontal plane.

Signal-averaged EKG
This employs computer analysis of EKG recording to identify late potential electrical activity related to myocardial depolarization in regions of myocardial abnormality which may be the substrate for re-entry ventricular arrhythmia.

Ambulatory EKG monitoring
These devices (Holter monitors) are portable mini-EKG recorders. They continuously record two EKG leads via electrodes attached to the anterior chest wall over a 24-hour period, during which the patient continues usual activities whilst keeping a diary of any symptoms so that any of these can be correlated with the EKG at the time.

Patient-activated recorders
Patient-activated devices will record a single EKG lead which can be analyzed later or transmitted by telephone to a central recording station. Their particular value is the assessment of patients whose symptoms are infrequent, but the EKG recordings are often of poor quality.

Implantable recording devices
Small subcutaneous recording devices can be implanted as a minor procedure. EKG is stored in the device prior to patient activation so that events which give rise to immediate loss of consciousness can be recorded after the event. This feature and long device life facilitate capture of infrequent events.

Tilt table testing and carotid sinus massage
Patients lie on a couch which can be tilted to 60° head up. Continuous monitoring of blood pressure, heart rate and EKG is performed. Tilting usually continues for 45 min, or is stopped if bradycardia (cardioinhibition) or hypotension (vasodepression) occurs. Sublingual nitrates or intravenous isoprenaline may be used to further stress vagotonic reflexes.

Patients with carotid sinus hypersensitivity syndrome may also have vagal cardioinhibition on inadvertent stimulation of the carotid sinus. Carotid sinus massage under controlled conditions and after assessment of carotid artery disease may unmask this.

Exercise stress testing
Exercise stress testing will demonstrate inability of the sinus node to mount a tachycardic response to physiological demand (chronotropic incompetence).

Electrophysiology study
Catheters mounted with recording electrodes are introduced through the femoral/subclavian vein under local anesthetic. These are passed to the heart using standard cardiac catheterization techniques and positioned in the atria, at the AVN and in the RV. Electrical activity

from the endomyocardium apposed to the electrodes is filtered, amplified, and recorded in unipolar or bipolar configurations as electrograms. The timing of electrical activity recorded from the endocardial surface (electrograms) at these sites and the response of electrical activity to cardiac pacing and extrastimulation (addition of premature paced beats during steady rate pacing) allows assessment of sinus and AV nodal activity and the integrity of the conduction system. Extra-stimulation techniques are also used to assess inducibility of tachycardias.

Bradycardia

Cardiac causes of bradycardia include:

Sinus node disease

This may be due to degenerative disease of the sinus node (SN), more common with increasing age, or from ischemic heart disease, viral infection and autoimmune disease. The SN may depolarize slowly or there may be a delay in electrical activity leaving the SN ('exit block').

Vasovagal syndrome

Autonomic tone is a determinant of both cardiac rate and vasomotor tone. A sudden increase in vagal tone can cause a fall in arterial pressure whether bradycardia (due to cardioinhibition) or vasodilation (due to depression of vasomotor tone) is the principal cause.

Carotid sinus syndrome is a similar entity. Hypersensitivity of the carotid sinus to mechanical pressure is the cause of a surge in vagal tone, in turn causing cardioinhibition, vasodepression and profound systemic arterial hypotension. Sinus bradycardia may be a normal finding in individuals with a high level of physical fitness and increased vagal tone.

AVN and conduction disease

AVN disease secondary to the following causes heart block:

- ischemic heart disease
- autoimmune disease
- sarcoidosis
- infection (aortic root abscess)
- prosthetic valve repair/replacement.

First degree heart block

PR interval >200 ms. In isolation it requires no treatment but may be the only manifestation of intermittent complete heart block.

Second degree heart block

- *Type 1* Cyclical elongation of successive PR intervals with eventual failure of AV conduction (P wave not succeeded by a QRS complex). It requires no treatment per se but may be the only manifestation of intermittent complete heart block.
- *Type 2* Intermittent but regular failure of AV nodal conduction, with the ventricular rate being a fixed lower ratio of the atrial rate. Prophylactic pacemaker implantation is indicated regardless of symptomatic status as progression to complete heart block is common.

Complete heart block (Third degree heart block)
Failure of AV nodal conduction with complete AV dissociation. Pacing is mandatory.

Treatments for bradycardia

Pacemaker implantation is the mainstay of therapy when a precipitating cause cannot be corrected. Pacemaker functionality is highly complex. Devices comprise single and dual chamber types, are rate responsive and may have tachycardia prevention properties as well as antitachycardia pacing algorithms.

Tachycardia

Sinus tachycardia

This may be a physiological response to exercise or stress but abnormal automaticity, either of the sinus node or an ectopic focus in either atrium or ventricle, or a re-entry excitation mechanism may cause non-physiological tachycardia.

Automatic tachycardias are due to abnormal pacemaker properties in either diseased specialized pacemaker tissue or ordinary cardiac tissue which develops pacemaker properties as a consequence of disease. For a re-entry circuit to occur an anatomical barrier to electrical conduction and a zone of slowed conduction must exist, so that the refractory period (time to recovery of excitability after depolarization) is shorter than the total conduction time around the re-entry circuit. Re-entry circuits may be the tachycardia mechanism for either supraventricular or ventricular tachycardias.

Tachycardias may be supraventricular or ventricular. Supraventricular tachycardia either originates or involves a re-entry circuit above the AV rings. Ventricular arrhythmias originate in ventricular myocardium and maintenance of the tachycardia does not involve conducting tissue in the AV rings.

Treatments for tachycardia

These include correcting the underlying cause, antiarrhythmic drug therapy, device therapy (antitachycardia pacemaker, implantable defibrillator) and curative ablative therapy (either surgical or using catheter fulguration techniques).

Further reading

1. Gray HH, Dawkins KD, Morgan JM, Simpson IA (eds). *Lecture Notes in Cardiology*. Blackwell Scientific Publications: London, 2002.

Related topics of interest

2.3 Cardiovascular homeostasis

Richard Thomas, Gareth Charlton

Cardiovascular homeostasis aims to optimize performance of the heart and vasculature in order to provide an appropriate blood flow to all tissues. It also redistributes cardiac output (CO) to those tissues or organs according to metabolic needs.

Cardiovascular homeostasis occurs at three levels

Central nervous system
Stretch receptors (baroreceptors) located in both high- and low- pressure circuits provide information on pulse rate and filling pressures. Afferent input from these (and other sources) are integrated within the vasomotor reflex centers located in the brainstem. The 'pressor' zone is an area of continuous sympathetic discharge and is closely related to both the more medial located 'depressor' zone and the vagal nuclei. Efferent transmission to heart and blood vessels is via sympathetic trunks/ganglia and the vagi.

Hormones
Hormones regulate mechanisms that are important for regulation of red cell mass, adaptation to physiological stress ('fight or flight' reaction) and acute and chronic blood pressure control. Hypothalamic response causes the adrenal medulla to release catecholamines (adrenaline (epinephrine), noradrenaline (norepinephrine)). Increased cardiac excitability and vasoconstriction lead to increased cardiac output, blood pressure and redistribution of blood from splanchnic to muscular beds. Accompanying metabolic responses include gluconeogenesis, glycolysis, lipolysis and release of ATP.

Local mechanisms
These include intrinsic cardiac reflexes and vascular autoregulation.

Cardiac homeostasis

$$\text{Cardiac output (CO)} = \text{stroke volume (SV)} \times \text{heart rate (HR)}$$

Stroke volume
Stroke volume is determined by ventricular filling (preload), contractility and afterload. Regulation of SV is mainly by intrinsic cardiac regulatory mechanisms that automatically relate preload, contractility and afterload to maintain CO.

Preload refers to ventricular end-diastolic volume and represents initial fiber length. Greater preload increases initial fiber length and stroke volume rises automatically. This is described by the Frank–Starling law: the force of myocardial contraction is proportional to initial fiber length.

Myocardial contractility has a major influence on SV. It is increased by sympathetic nervous activity, circulating catecholamines, and positively inotropic drugs. The Bowditch effect describes a force–frequency relationship whereby increased heart rate automatically increases contractility. Contractility is decreased by hypoxia, acidosis, hypercapnia, parasympathetic activity and a wide variety of drugs.

Afterload is the tension generated in the left ventricular muscle during systole and is a function of the total peripheral resistance (TPR). The Anrep effect describes the automatic adaptation to increased afterload; an initial reduction in SV leads to greater left ventricular end-diastolic volume in the following cardiac cycle and hence SV is restored.

Heart rate

Despite intrinsic rhythmicity of cardiac tissue, intrinsic ability to adapt heart rate/cardiac excitability to changing metabolic requirements in the absence of autonomic influence is limited. Efferent cardiac nerves are branches of the vagus (cholinergic) and sympathetic nerves (mainly beta-1-receptors) acting in opposing yet balanced fashion to modify cardiac activity. Relative dominance of sympathetic outflow increases heart rate (chronotropism), speed of impulse conduction (dromotropism), contractility (inotropism) and excitability by lowering threshold potential (bathmotropism). The Bainbridge reflex, however, does occur in denervated hearts and describes increased cardiac activity in response to a sudden rise in venous return.

Global vascular homeostasis

$$CO = \text{mean arterial pressure (MAP)/total peripheral resistance (TPR)}$$

Arterial blood pressure

Acute regulation of MAP is regulated by baroreceptors. Afferent activity is increased by acute elevation of MAP and passes centrally to the depressor zone from receptors located in the aorta (vagus nerve) and carotid sinus (glossopharyngeal nerve). Stimulation of the depressor zone simultaneously inhibits basal sympathetic discharge of the pressor zone and increases vagal activity. Resulting depression of cardiac excitation and vasodilatation reduce MAP. Acute falls in blood pressure stimulate the pressor zone and inhibit vagal activity by identical pathways but with opposite effects.

Total peripheral resistance

$R = 8 \times l \times \eta \times \pi^{-1} \times r^{-4}$ (Poiseuille's law: R = flow resistance; l = length; r = radius; η = viscosity). Hence a reduction in radius of only 16% will double the resistance. The arterioles are the principal resistance vessels. Viscosity is directly related to flow and depends for the most part on the hematocrit. Outside extremes of severe anemia or polycythemia; however, the effect of viscosity upon TPR is limited.

Regional vascular homeostasis

Regional vascular homeostasis ensures that CO is distributed regionally to match the demands of particular organs. This depends upon regulation of vessel diameter and autoregulation.

Vessel diameter

Arteriolar diameter is the primary determinant of vasomotor tone and organ blood flow. Neural control influences vasomotor tone via sympathetic nerves: postganglionic transmission via α_1 receptors causes vasoconstriction and β_2 receptors causes vasodilatation. Differential organ blood flow depends upon the number and type of receptors which are vessel and organ specific. Alterations in the size of capacitance vessels are controlled by similar mechanisms.

Autoregulation

This process allows tissues to regulate local blood flow independent of global perfusion to match local metabolic demands. A variety of mechanisms are important and, to an extent, organ specific. Coronary and cerebral blood flow are almost exclusively under local metabolic control. Accumulation of metabolites (H^+ ions, CO_2, adenosine diphosphate and adenosine monophosphate) and osmotically active substances (K^+) result in increased blood flow. The myogenic mechanism describes reflex vasoconstriction when vessel walls are stretched by elevations of MAP and is important in renal and cerebral autoregulation. Pulmonary vasculature is unique in demonstrating a hypoxic vasoconstrictor response, thus improving ventilation/perfusion mismatch. Locally produced vasodilators (nitric oxide (NO), kallikrein, bradykinin, prostacyclin and histamine) and vasoconstrictors (prostaglandin $PGF_{2\alpha}$, angiotensin II and endothelins) have complex actions on vasomotor tone and endothelial function.

It is likely that NO is the final common pathway for regulating vasomotor tone both in health (constitutive NO) and disease (inducible NO). Produced from L-arginine (endothelium) by the action of nitric oxide synthase it acts via increasing intracellular guanine monophosphate (GMP) and relaxes vascular smooth muscle.

Plasma volume homeostasis

Acute changes

Acute falls in blood pressure or plasma volume are detected by the juxtaglomerular apparatus (JGA) and renin release. Renin acts upon circulating angiotensinogen (from the liver) to release the decapeptide angiotensin I. This is cleaved to produce active octapeptide angiotensin II by the action of converting enzyme (from lung and kidney). Angiotensin II has the following actions: elevation of blood pressure by arteriolar vasoconstriction, stimulation of the thirst mechanism (hypothalamic), release of aldosterone (adrenal cortex), redistribution of intrinsic renal blood flow leading to reduced glomerular filtration rate (GFR) and increased salt retention. The mineralocorticoid aldosterone increases sodium reabsorption in the distal tubule, thus enhancing the sodium- and water-saving effects of a reduced GFR. The overall effect is to restore plasma volume or blood pressure by increased uptake and retention of salt (and hence water). Both aldosterone and angiotensin II feedback negatively on renin release. The action of angiotensin is terminated by breakdown in the liver and kidney.

Chronic changes

Chronic blood pressure and plasma volume regulation are achieved primarily by renal homeostatic mechanisms and are intimately related to salt and water balance.

Further reading

1. Despopoulos A, Silbernagl S. *Color Atlas of Physiology. 3rd Edn.* Thieme: New York, 1986.
2. Ganong WG. *Review of Medical Physiology. 20th Edn.* Appleton and Lange: London, 2001.
3. Whittle BJ. Nitric oxide in physiology and pathology. *Histochem J* 1995; **27**: 727–37.
4. Yentis SM, Hirsch NP, Smith GB. *Anaesthesia A to Z.* Butterworth-Heinemann: Oxford, 1995.

Related topic of interest

2.4   Cardiovascular homeostatis in pathological states

2.4 Cardiovascular homeostasis in pathological states

Richard Thomas, Gareth Charlton

Myopathic heart

Regardless of etiology, an end-stage myopathic heart demonstrates global dilatation with all chambers affected.

Regulation
Normal. Increased sympathetic tone to compensate for reduced cardiac output (CO).

Cardiac homeostasis
Low CO is associated with small, fixed stroke volume (SV). SV depends upon adequate pre-loading. Flattened Frank–Starling curve (upper range of SV is insensitive to further increases in preload). Reduction in SV is compensated by tachycardia to maintain CO.

Inadequate preload, depression of contractility and increasing afterload may lead to sudden decompensation.

Global vascular homeostasis
Left ventricular failure leads to low mean arterial pressure (MAP). Sympathetic activation causes vasoconstriction and increases total peripheral resistance (TPR). This increased after-load further depresses CO in a vicious cycle.

Regional vascular homeostasis
A low CO with increased vasomotor tone results in preferential blood flow to cardiac, muscular and cerebral beds at the expense of renal and splanchnic perfusion.

Plasma volume homeostasis
The renin–angiotensin–aldosterone system is highly active with vasoconstriction and salt and water retention.

Therapeutic strategies
- Maintain preload.
- Maintain contractility without increasing afterload (if MAP adequate consider ino-dilators).
- Aim for low-normal MAP (permitting renal and splanchnic perfusion).
- Avoid unbalanced α-adrenoceptor drug therapy (noradrenaline).
- Maintain moderate tachycardia.

Pressure-loaded heart

A chronic afterload, such as aortic or subaortic stenosis, leads to concentric LV hypertrophy. Increased LV dimensions are due to increased LV wall thickness. This adaptation preserves systolic function [ratio of end-systolic pressure (ESP) to end-systolic volume (ESV)] by maintaining contractility. However, this is achieved at the expense of diastolic function [ratio of end-diastolic pressure (EDP) to end-diastolic volume (EDV)]. This eventually results in progressive LV dilatation and heart failure. Pressure-loaded hearts have a precarious oxygen supply/demand ratio and hence predispose patients with critical aortic stenosis to sudden death.

Regulation
Normal. Sympathetic activation correlates with heart failure.

Cardiac homeostasis
Diastolic dysfunction precedes systolic dysfunction and is initially manifested as increased LVEDP with a preserved Frank–Starling curve. Normal ventricular contraction operates along a higher part of the Frank–Starling curve. However, beyond a threshold, LV dilation commences with flattening of the Frank–Starling curve.

In an afterloaded heart the SV is small and relatively fixed. Atrial transport assumes greater importance during LV filling (<40% of LVEDV) in hypertrophied hearts with diastolic dysfunction. Therefore loss of sinus rhythm can lead to rapid decompensation. Increased heart rate shortens diastole disproportionately more than systole. A low-normal (50–70 bpm) resting heart rate will therefore optimize diastolic function.

Global vascular homeostasis
MAP is usually normal. The arterial pulse pressure narrows as the stenosis progresses.

Regional vascular homeostasis
Pressure-loaded hearts have an unfavorable oxygen supply/demand ratio. Demand is increased, both by the increased work of the heart and the larger mass of ventricular muscle required to maintain contractility. Myocardial perfusion is reduced by the high EDP, decreasing coronary perfusion pressure and thus predisposing to subendocardial ischemia.

Plasma volume homeostasis
LV failure causes similar adaptations as previously described.

Therapeutic strategies
- Maintain/augment preload.
- Preserve sinus rhythm.
- Avoid tachycardia: aim for heart rates of 50–70 bpm.
- Maintain contractility.
- Maintain/augment MAP/TPR.

Volume-loaded heart

The homeostatic response depends upon whether volume loading is acute or chronic. For example, sudden mitral regurgitation (MR) triggers increased sympathetic activity as previously described.

Compensated chronic MR is usually asymptomatic. MR leads to both systolic and diastolic volume overload and eccentric LV hypertrophy with malalignment of myofibrils. LVEDP remains normal with steadily increasing LVEDV.

Once the regurgitant fraction exceeds 60% of SV, irreversible LV damage occurs. When LVEDP exceeds 20 mmHg, pulmonary venous hypertension follows, rendering the patient dyspneic. Unless surgically corrected, progressive congestive cardiac failure ensues.

Regulation
Normal. Increased sympathetic outflow occurs late.

Cardiac homeostasis
The Frank–Starling mechanism remains intact until myocardial damage occurs and the normal relationship between LVEDV and SV is lost. Tachycardia is beneficial in reducing diastolic time and the regurgitant fraction. Higher systemic diastolic pressure and lower LVEDP are seen with heart rates around 90 bpm.

Global vascular homeostasis
In aortic regurgitation (AR), TPR is characteristically low and pulse pressure is wide. This promotes forward flow for a greater proportion of the SV. Late-stage disease associated with heart failure triggers sympathetic activation as previously described, which may further accelerate decline.

Regional vascular homeostasis
In contrast to pressure-loading, chronic volume-loading places less demand on oxygen supply. In chronic AR, coronary perfusion may be compromised by a combination of low systemic diastolic pressure and increased LV wall tension.

Therapeutic strategies
- Augment preload.
- Maintain increased heart rate (90 bpm).
- Maintain contractility.
- Reduce afterload.

The transplanted heart

Regulation
Although evidence exists for partial reinnervation, the transplanted heart is effectively without efferent output from the CNS.

Cardiac homeostasis
CO is low-normal to normal due to intact intrinsic control mechanisms and preserved contractility. The relationships between CO, preload and afterload are identical to the innervated

heart in the non-stressed state. Responses to circulating catecholamine hormones are normal.

Resting heart rate is increased (typically 100 bpm) as a consequence of vagal denervation. Vagal reflexes such as the oculo-cardiac reflex are abolished.

Increasing CO initially derives from increased stroke volume (via increased preload) as heart rate will only increase once catecholamine levels rise.

Global vascular homeostasis

Baroreceptor reflexes (carotid sinus massage, etc.) are lost as a consequence of denervation from the autonomic nervous system. Drugs (atropine, glycopyrrolate, etc.) acting on the autonomic nervous system will similarly be ineffective. Mild to moderate systemic hypertension is usual in patients treated with cyclosporin for immunosuppression.

Regional vascular homeostasis

Metabolic regulation of coronary blood flow is preserved.

Plasma volume homeostasis

This may be altered at a renal level by the nephrotoxic actions of cyclosporin A, or by the sodium retention associated with steroid usage.

Therapeutic strategies

- Maintain preload.
- Maintain adequate heart rate with chronotropic agent or pacing.
- Maintain contractility.

Further reading

1. Hensley FA Jr, Martin DE. *A Practical Approach to Cardiac Anesthesia.* Little Brown & Co: Boston, 1995.

Related topic of interest

2.3   Cardiovascular homeostasis

2.5 Myocardial metabolism and oxygen flux

Crispin Weideman, Michael Herbertson

Myocardial metabolism

Energy sources

Utilization of the major myocardial fuels, namely non-esterified fatty acids (FFA), glucose and lactate, is a complex dynamic process. The breakdown of substrates to acetyl-CoA is followed by oxidation in the Krebs cycle to generate ATP. Less important substrates include amino acids (leucine and alanine) and ketone bodies.

Utilization of fuels

Myocardial fuel utilization depends upon substrate availability and physiological and pathophysiological conditions. Triggers for changes in substrate uptake and metabolism are partly linked to changes in both cytosolic adenosine diphosphate (ADP) levels and the ratio of coenzyme nicotinamide adenine dinucleotide (NAD) to its reduced form NADH.

Nutritional status
In the fasted state, FFA are the major substrate. High levels of citrate and ATP formed from FFA oxidation inhibit glycolysis. Glucose taken up by cells in these circumstances is converted to glycogen. In the non-fasted state insulin levels are higher, glucose utilization is increased, whilst FFA metabolism is reduced.

Exercise
During exercise lactate levels rise acutely (increased skeletal muscle production). Higher serum lactate inhibits glucose oxidation and FFA uptake. However, during prolonged exercise FFA metabolism increases and becomes the main energy source.

Ischemia
During mild ischemia oxidative metabolism of glucose increases and less FFA are utilized. Being a more efficient ATP generator, glycolysis may reduce oxygen consumption. However, in severe ischemia lactic acidosis inhibits glycolysis and the Krebs cycle through the key enzymes. This leads to energy shortage which impairs both systolic and diastolic function.

Sepsis
In severe sepsis there is a switch from FFA to lactate and glucose as a myocardial fuel.

ATP metabolism

ATP links substrate metabolism to electromechanical work. ATP cannot be stored in significant amounts within the myocardium, and production is tightly linked to acute energy requirements. The maintenance of aerobic metabolism is favored by the very low partial pressure of oxygen at which the mitochondrial cytochrome oxidase system functions $(6.5 \times 10^{-3}\,\text{kPa})$. The crucial role of oxygen in the oxidation of NADH to NAD^+ is linked to ADP phosphorylation.

ATP production

ATP is formed by the phosphorylation of ADP predominantly and aerobically in the mitochondria with small amounts produced by anaerobic glycolysis within the cytoplasm. Two molecules of ATP are formed for every molecule of glucose metabolized to pyruvate. The aerobic pathway produces approximately 10 molecules of ATP per acetyl-CoA metabolized, the actual amount varying according to demand. Variation in the ATP yield per atom of oxygen utilized is less than 10%.

ATP utilization

ATP supplies energy for myocardial contraction and homeostasis in the following proportion:

- mechanical work: 60–70%
- membranes active transport systems: 10–25%
- action potential generation and propagation: 5–10%.

Myocardial oxygen flux

Myocardial oxygen delivery

$$(mDO_2) \, (ml \, O_2 \, min^{-1}) = coronary \, blood \, flow \, (CBF) \, (dl \, 100 \, g^{-1} \, min^{-1}) \times arterial \, oxygen \, content \, (CaO_2) \, (ml \, O_2 \, dl^{-1} \, blood)$$

At rest, in the adult human this is approximately 50 ml O_2 min^{-1}.

$$CaO_2 = [1.39 \times haemoglobin \, (Hb) \, concentration \, (g \, dl^{-1}) \times fractional \, Hb\text{-}O_2 \, saturation + dissolved \, O_2 \, concentration \, (g \, dl^{-1}]$$

The figure 1.39 is the volume of oxygen (ml) that combines with each gram of Hb at 100% Hb-O_2 saturation. The contribution of dissolved oxygen is usually very small. CaO_2 approximates to 21 ml dl^{-1} with Hb concentration of 15 g dl^{-1} at normal oxygen saturation.

$$CBF = coronary \, perfusion \, pressure \, (CPP) \, (mmHg) \, / \, coronary \, vascular \, resistance \, (CVR) \, (dynes \, cm^{-5} \, s^{-1})$$

This is 50–100 ml $100 \, g^{-1}$ min^{-1} at rest, and can increase five-fold during exercise. CBF will be reduced by a decrease in CPP or an increase in CVR. Furthermore, CBF occurs mainly in diastole through the left ventricular wall with a more even distribution of flow throughout the cardiac cycle in the right ventricular myocardium. An increase in heart rate will shorten diastole and reduce left ventricular perfusion.

CPP = aortic root pressure – intramyocardial pressure

In normal coronary vasculature autoregulation maintains adequate CBF within a range of aortic root pressures. In the left ventricle with predominantly diastolic myocardial blood flow the end-diastolic pressure (LVEDP) becomes important. Left ventricular hypertrophy, myocardial dysfunction and ventricular distention will increase LVEDP and therefore reduce sub-endocardial perfusion.

CVR

CVR is determined by the pre-capillary resistance vessels. Small changes in the radii of these vessels alter resistance dramatically. Vasomotor control of CVR occurs through three main mechanisms:

(a) Metabolic control. Myocardial release of adenosine, triggered by myocardial work, hypoxia and ischemia, is the most important. Adenosine vasodilates by increasing cyclic adenosine monophosphate (cAMP) levels. Other metabolic dilators include protons, potassium, atrial natriuretic peptide and prostaglandins.

(b) Endothelial control. In an intact endothelium, nitric oxide ranks amongst the most potent vasodilators. With a damaged endothelium, thromboxane and endothelin produce intense vasoconstriction.

(c) Neurogenic control. Direct autonomic regulation of coronary vasculature is less important than in many other organs. Sympathetic α-receptors cause vasoconstriction through their postsynaptic effects although presynaptic α-receptors on noradrenergic nerve terminals reduce noradrenaline release with a modulating effect. Sympathetic β-receptor stimulation increases cAMP production, resulting in vasodilatation. Parasympathetic cholinergic fibers cause vasodilatation when the endothelium is intact and vasoconstriction if it is damaged.

Myocardial oxygen consumption (mVO$_2$)

The myocardium is almost entirely dependent on aerobic metabolism and has no capacity for oxygen debt. Furthermore, little oxygen is stored intramyocardially either dissolved or bound to myoglobin. With the resting myocardial oxygen extraction ratio being 75%, increased mVO$_2$ can be met only by increased CBF since resting CaO$_2$ is submaximal. Therefore the rich myocardial capillary network is essential to maintaining mDO$_2$. This system can enhance oxygen delivery during increased demand by recruiting normally unopened capillaries and preserve the linear relationship between mVO$_2$ and CBF.

Further reading

1. Opie LH. Fuels: aerobic and anaerobic metabolism. In: *The Heart*. Opie LH (ed.). Lippincott, Williams & Wilkins: Philadelphia, 1998: pp. 267–94.
2. Opie LH. Fuels: oxygen supply and coronary flow. In: *The Heart*. Opie LH (ed.). Lippincott, Williams & Wilkins: Philadelphia, 1998: pp. 295–342.
3. Priebe HJ. Coronary physiology. In: *Cardiovascular Physiolology*. Priebe HJ, Skarvan K (eds). BMJ Publishers: London, 2000: pp. 119–70.

Related topics of interest

3 Cardiovascular pharmacology

Keith D Dawkins

Angina

Many patients who come to coronary artery bypass grafting (CABG) are on multiple (nitrate, β-blocker, calcium antagonist, potassium channel-opener) therapy. Once surgical revascularization has been completed these drugs can be discontinued unless otherwise indicated (hypertension or recent acute myocardial infarction (AMI)), in which case the β-blocker should be continued. Post-CABG angina should be treated medically and cardiological opinion sought.

Hypertension

The cardiovascular and cerebrovascular complications associated with hypertension (>140/90 mmHg) increase with rises in both systolic and diastolic pressures. In the presence of coronary heart disease (CHD) hypertension should be treated aggressively. Low-dose thiazides (e.g. bendroflumethazide) should be combined with a β-blocker or an ACE inhibitor (ACEI) if there is evidence of LV dysfunction. Angiotensin II blockers (e.g. losartan, valsartan) are useful when side effects (e.g. cough) from ACEI become troublesome.

Heart failure

Left heart failure (pulmonary edema) is treated with a combination of loop diuretics and an ACEI. It is important that the dose of ACEI is titrated up to the maximum tolerated. Recent data confirmed the survival benefit with the addition of spironolactone (RALES trial), together with low-dose β-blocker (e.g. bisoprolol, carvedilol, metoprolol – CIBIS I and II, the US Multicenter Carvedilol Study, MERIT-HF). Combination drug therapy (loop diuretic, spironolactone, ACEI and β-blocker) is now known to be more effective than high-dose loop diuretic formally used.

Arrhythmias

Atrial fibrillation
Atrial fibrillation (AF) is the most common arrhythmia, accounting for approximately one-third of arrhythmia admissions. Its prevalence in the population is 0.4% increasing to 6% in patients >80 years. AF occurs in 20–50% of postoperative cardiac patients, peaking at 2–5 days. Risk factors include advancing age, LA dilatation, pre-operative AF, pneumonia and

electrolyte disturbance (hypokalemia). Sinus rhythm can be restored in 90% of patients within 6 weeks postoperatively. Because of the benign nature, many patients are offered rate control alone, using β-blocker, calcium antagonist or digoxin after correcting hypokalemia. Atrial stabilizing agents (e.g. amiodarone) may also be effective. Evidence suggests that pretreatment with β-blocker may significantly reduce the incidence of postoperative AF. Systemic anticoagulation (warfarin) is required in persistent AF because of thromboembolic risk (see below).

Ventricular arrhythmias

Ventricular ectopy is common after cardiac surgery and usually responds to correction of hypokalemia/hypomagnesemia. Sustained ventricular arrhythmias may reflect ongoing myocardial ischemia (including graft malfunction) or poor ventricular function (fibrotic arrhythmogenic foci). In these patients the emphasis has recently switched from drug to device therapy (e.g. AICD). 'Blind' treatment with antiarrhythmic agents is not recommended because of pro-arrhythmic potential.

Lipid-lowering therapy

Statins are the most effective lipid-lowering drugs for total and LDL-cholesterol reduction. Statins competitively inhibit hepatic HMG CoA reductase involved in cholesterol synthesis. Statins produce important reductions in cardiovascular events (including total mortality) in patients aged up to 75 years with CHD with a total serum cholesterol >5 mmol/liter. Statins should also be considered for all patients following CABG or percutaneous coronary intervention (PCI). Recent evidence suggests a role for statins in stabilizing arterial plaque and other beneficial effects even with normal cholesterol levels.

Statins are effective in primary prevention when lipid levels should be aggregated with other coronary risk factors, including hypertension, diabetes, smoking, age, weight and gender. When the risk of CHD exceeds 30% at 10 years, statins should be prescribed in addition to dietary measures and the correction of other risk factors. All four statins (atorvastatin, fluvastatin, pravastatin and simvastatin) are effective with minor differences in secondary effects. Side effects include myalgia, rarely myopathy and myositis, liver dysfunction (rarely hepatitis) and gastrointestinal disturbance.

In statin-intolerant patients, fibrates (e.g. bezafibrate, fenofibrate) may be used. Although less potent, they also reduce triglyceride and raise LDL-cholesterol, which may be beneficial in combined hyperlipidemias.

Antiplatelet agents and anticoagulation

Aspirin

Low-dose aspirin is an effective antiplatelet agent for secondary prevention of cardiovascular diseases. Indications include AMI, stable and unstable angina, PCI, CABG, ischemic stroke, transient ischemic attack and following carotid endarterectomy. Doses are in the range of 75–150 mg daily, except for suspected AMI and acute ischemic stroke when a dose of 300 mg is given initially. Aspirin is indicated for primary prevention of vascular events when the estimated 10-year CHD risk ≥15%.

Aspirin should be avoided in renal failure (GFR <10 ml/min) or severe hepatic dysfunction. Aspirin interacts with ACEI, β-blockers and diuretics, reducing the effectiveness or these agents, whereas the action of oral hypoglycemics may be enhanced, leading to hypoglycemia. Adverse reactions include bronchospasm and gastrointestinal hemorrhage. Aspirin is contraindicated in children <12 years, with breast feeding, and in the presence of active peptic ulceration; it should be used with caution in patients with a history of bronchial asthma, in pregnancy and in the patient with uncontrolled hypertension.

Clopidogrel

Clopidogrel directly inhibits binding of adenosine diphosphate (ADP) to its receptor and subsequent ADP-mediated activation of the glycoprotein IIb/IIIa complex. It is a powerful antiplatelet agent, particularly when used in combination with aspirin. clopidogrel acts by irreversibly modifying the platelet ADP receptor; hence platelets exposed to clopidogrel are ineffective for the remainder of their lifetime. Dose-dependent platelet inhibition occurs within 2 hours of consumption, with a steady state 40–60% platelet inhibition between 3 and 7 days. Platelet aggregation and bleeding time return to baseline values 5 days after discontinuation.

The clinical evidence for clopidogrel efficacy was derived from the randomized CAPRIE trial (clopidogrel versus aspirin) which demonstrated a reduction in ischemic stroke, myocardial infarction and other vascular deaths. Aspirin and clopidogrel are used together for routine treatment of troponin-positive acute coronary syndromes (CURE trial) and in PCI (CURE-PCI and STARS trials). Hemorrhagic risk is similar to aspirin, with increased postoperative bleeding. Therefore, clopidogrel should be discontinued 7 days prior to elective CABG. In patients with unstable angina and those undergoing PCI, a daily dose of 75 mg is given after a loading dose of 300 mg. Typically, a course of 6 months is given in unstable angina and 1–3 months after PCI (depending on stent type). Clopidogrel has replaced ticlopidine, another thienopyridine, which was associated with bone marrow suppression in 0.8% of patients.

Fibrinolytics

Fibrinolytic (or thrombolytic) drugs reduce mortality in ST-elevation AMI and also have a role in the treatment of acute massive pulmonary embolism, in acute peripheral arterial insufficiency and in selected ischemic strokes. Fibrinolytic agents convert plasminogen to plasmin which degrades fibrin containing thrombi. Selective agents (e.g. r-tPA, tenecteplase) are used with increasing frequency compared with streptokinase. Side effects mainly relate to bleeding complications, including cerebral hemorrhage.

Heparin

The heparins are a group of mucopolysaccharides (glycosaminoglycans) that act at multiple sites in the coagulation system principally by:

- combining with anti-thrombin III (heparin cofactor)
- inactivating activated Factor X
- inhibiting the conversion of prothrombin to thrombin
- secondary actions include the prevention of fibrin formation from fibrinogen.

Heparin does not have fibrinolytic activity. Unfractionated heparin is administered by intravenous or deep subcutaneous injection. Peak plasma levels occur 2–4 hours after subcutaneous administration. Because of the short half-life and the variable protein binding, unfractionated heparin is usually administered by continuous infusion (24 000–36 000 units/24 hours) monitored according to the activated partial thromboplastin time (aPTT) or the thrombin time (TT), after an initial bolus dose (5000–10 000 units). When initiating anti-coagulation, warfarin and heparin should be administered concomitantly such that heparin is continued for 2 further days after the International Normalized Ratio (INR) is within the therapeutic range. Heparin is used for the treatment of deep vein thrombosis (DVT), pulmonary embolism, acute coronary syndromes, acute arterial insufficiency, during CPB and for thromboembolic prophylaxis postoperatively.

Low molecular weight heparins (e.g. dalteparin, enoxaparin) are increasingly favored as they have superior pharmacokinetics, can be administered by once daily subcutaneous injection and do not require monitoring.

Side effects include hemorrhage, thrombocytopenia, hypersensitivity reactions and osteoporosis. Heparin can be reversed by the intravenous administration of protamine sulfate.

Glycoprotein (GP) IIb/IIIa inhibitors

These are powerful antiplatelet agents used for the treatment of acute coronary syndromes and PCI (reduced mortality and periprocedural AMI). Abciximab (ReoPro) is the Fab fragment of the chimeric human-murine monoclonal antibody 7E3 which binds to the GP IIb/IIIa receptor on human platelets, inhibiting platelet aggregation. Two other 'small molecule' IIb/IIIa inhibitors are used in the treatment of unstable (troponin +ve) acute coronary syndromes; tirofiban (Aggrastat) and eptifibatide (Integrilin). Side effects include hemorrhage (reversed with platelet transfusions) and occasional hypersensitivity reactions.

Warfarin

Warfarin, a coumarin derivative, produces an anticoagulant effect by interfering with vitamin K metabolism. Vitamin K is a cofactor in the carboxylation of numerous proteins, including the coagulation factors II, VII, IX and X. It is rapidly absorbed from the gut, has high bioavailability and reaches maximal blood concentrations in healthy volunteers 90 min after oral administration; warfarin has a half-life of 36–42 hours.

Indications for warfarin include secondary thromboembolic prophylaxis (mechanical heart valve implants, DVT and AF), thrombophilia, the antiphospholipid syndrome. Other cardiac indications include severe LV dysfunction, treatment of mural thrombus and prior to electrical cardioversion.

The adequacy of anticoagulation is monitored using the INR which relates the prothrombin time (PT) of the patient to a normal reference PT. The intensity of anticoagulation ('therapeutic range') is dependent on the indication. The target INR for most conditions is 2.5 (range 2.0–3.0), but the various guidelines do not agree on the target level for prosthetic heart valves. It is clear that the first-generation valves (ball and cage) are more thrombogenic than contemporary bi-leaflet valves. Furthermore, valves in the aortic position are less thrombogenic than those in the mitral position. INR ranges for contemporary valves in the aortic position of 2.5–3.0 and in the mitral position of 3.0–3.5 are acceptable. Long-term anticoagulation is not required for bioprostheses in the absence of AF, although some surgeons favor postoperative anticoagulation for a period of 1–3 months followed by low-dose aspirin.

Individual warfarin doses vary from 1 to 15 mg per day and there are numerous drug interactions, including antibiotics, anticonvulsants, nonsteroidal anti-inflammatory drugs (NSAIDs), fibrates and amiodarone. Most of these drugs enhance the anticoagulant effect.

There is controversy surrounding the need for a loading dose. Historically, a loading dose of 10 mg on the first two days (less in the elderly) was followed by an INR estimation on the third day, whereas the recent American Heart Association/American College of Cardiology (AHA/ACC) statement on warfarin therapy (2003) advocates a starting dose of 5 mg. There is a clear relationship between a low INR (<2.5) and thromboembolism, and a high INR (>5) and hemorrhage. In some series, one-third of patients are outside the 'therapeutic range' at any time. Bleeding in a patient on warfarin may require treatment with intravenous vitamin K_1, fresh frozen plasma or prothrombin complex concentrate (Factors II, VII, IX and X).

Further reading

1. ACC/AHA/ESC guidelines for the management of patients with atrial fibrillation. *Eur Heart J* 2001; **22**: 1852–1923. (http://www.escardio.org/scinfo/Guidelines/atrialfibrillation.pdf).
2. *British National Formulary (44)*. British Medical Association and Royal Pharmaceutical Society of Great Britain: London, 2002. (http://www.bnf.org).
3. *Guidelines on Oral Anticoagulation. 3rd edn. Br J Haematol* 1998; **101**: 374–87. (http://www.bcshguidelines.com/pdf/bjh715.pdf).
4. Hirsh J, Fuster V, Ansell J, Halperin JL. *American Heart Association/American College of Cardiology Foundation Guide to Warfarin Therapy. Circ* 2003; **107**: 1692–711. (http://circ.ahajournals.org/cgi/reprint/107/12/1692.pdf).
5. National Institute for Clinical Excellence (NICE). (http://www.nice.org.uk).

Related topics of interest

14   Postoperative complications
16.7 Percutaneous coronary intervention

4 Pre-operative assessment of cardiac surgical patients

Augustine TM Tang, Sunil K Ohri

Evaluation of patients referred for cardiac surgery aims to answer the following questions:

- Is surgery appropriate for the condition?
- Is the patient fit to undergo the planned operation?
- Is there any co-morbidity that may affect operative management?
- Is the patient agreeable to surgery given the benefit-to-risk ratio?

Whilst it is not possible to discuss every possible case scenario, the following important aspects are highlighted.

History

Angina and dyspnea feature commonly and must be assessed both in their severity and trend. Overall quality of life remains a major determinant of need for surgical intervention. Symptoms of heart failure, palpitations and syncope alert clinicians to possible sequelae of underlying cardiac disease. Other atherosclerotic complications manifestating as cerebrovascular events and lower limb ischemia should be screened for. Documentation of risk factors for coronary artery disease (smoking, hypertension, diabetes, hypercholesterolemia and family history) and valvular heart disease (rheumatic fever, bacteremic events) is important. Smokers should be persuaded to stop at least 6 weeks prior to surgery to reduce respiratory complications. Identification of important co-morbidities from past medical history is vital to the decisions on whether to operate and on the optimal surgical approach. A bleeding diathesis or hemorrhagic risk (e.g. peptic ulceration) may preclude systemic anticoagulation and hence the institution of cardiopulmonary bypass or implantation of mechanical prosthesis. A knowledge of regular medications, cardiotropic or otherwise, and any specific allergy is helpful to perioperative management. It is common to withdraw aspirin preoperatively for 7 days to minimize postoperative bleeding. Similarly warfarin may be omitted 3 days before surgery, and heparin commenced if necessary in hospital. Otherwise most regular medications including all anti-anginal, anti-hypertensive, diuretic and anti-arrhythmic drugs should be continued until surgery to avoid perioperative compromise. Symptoms of concurrent infection (viral or bacterial) alert the clinician to increased risks of postoperative respiratory, wound and prosthesis-related complications. An understanding of the social circumstances would facilitate more efficient discharge planning.

Clinical examination

In addition to searching for signs of general well-being (anemia, jaundice, cyanosis, etc.), intercurrent sepsis and nutritional status, it is important to detect arrhythmia, cardiac murmur, signs of heart failure and the state of peripheral perfusion. Carotid bruit with a recent history (6 months) of cerebrovascular events requires further investigation. The presence of abdominal aortic aneurysm and peripheral vascular disease should be assessed thoroughly. This is particularly important if saphenous vein harvesting or intraaortic balloon placement is needed. Subclavian artery stenosis manifesting as differential brachial blood pressure measurements precludes the use of an ipsilateral pedicled internal mammary artery graft. Availability and quality of other suitable conduits (saphenous vein, radial artery, etc.) for coronary grafting must be ascertained. Signs of repiratory compromise may render the patient unsuitable for 'fast-tracking' and thus warrant further investigations. Full dental assessment is necessary prior to any valvular procedure.

Investigations

- Routine – full blood count, blood biochemistry, coagulation profile, blood group typing and antibody screen, cross-matching, 12-lead EKG, chest radiographs (posteroanterior and lateral).
- Pulmonary function test and arterial blood gases – chronic smoking, obstructive or restrictive lung disease.
- Carotid artery Doppler study and angiography – carotid bruit with recent history of cerebrovascular event.
- Limb Doppler study and angiography – peripheral vascular disease.
- Abdominal ultrasound – abdominal aortic aneurysm, unexplained renal impairment, hepatic dysfunction, organomegaly.
- CT scan/MRI – mediastinal mass, pulmonary nodule, diseases of aortic root, ascending aorta, arch and thoracic aorta.
- Cardiac catheterization and angiography – coronary artery disease, left ventricular function, aortic and mitral valvular dysfunction, right heart and pulmonary artery pressures. An angiogram within 12 months of operation ought to be available and should otherwise be repeated pre-operatively except for those patients with triple vessel disease.
- Echocardiography – valvular heart disease and ventricular function.
- Radionuclide scanning – regional myocardial perfusion and reversible ischemia before revascularization for heart failure.

Consultation

The effectiveness, benefits and risks of the proposed cardiac procedure should be carefully discussed with the patient. Any additional perioperative risks associated with pre-existing co-morbidities must be highlighted. The choice of conduits for coronary artery grafting should be explained and the potential donor sites identified. In those undergoing valve replacement, the pros and cons of biological versus mechanical prostheses need addressing. Particular emphasis should be made on the implications of lifelong systemic anticoagulation in appropriate cases.

Further reading

1. Bojar RM. General preoperative considerations and preparation of the patient for surgery. Part I; 37–47 In: *Manual of Perioperative Care in Cardiac and Thoracic Surgery. 2nd Edn.* Bojar RM (ed.). Blackwell Science: Massachusetts, 1994.
2. Ferraris VA, Ferraris SP, Lough FC, Berry WR. Preoperative aspirin ingestion increases operative blood loss after coronary artery bypass grafting. *Ann Thorac Surg* 1988; **45:** 71–4.
3. Warner MA, Offord KP, Warner ME et al. Role of preoperative cessation of smoking and other factors in postoperative pulmonary complications: a blinded prospective study of coronary artery bypass patients. *Mayo Clin Proc* 1989; **64:** 609–16.

Related topics of interest

5 Cardiac imaging

David Delany

The ideal image of the heart would be a transparent, beating, three-dimensional model. There should be a clear display of anatomical connections, myocardial and valvular function and coronary artery perfusion. Pulmonary blood flow should be displayed and pulmonary vascular resistance (PVR) measurable. The status of the aorta and arch vessels should be visible and vascular compliance measurable. All this information can be obtained but only at the cost of progressively more expensive and invasive imaging technology. Therefore a cardiac surgeon has to be well versed in the efficient application of the imaging process.

The chest x ray (CXR)

Posteroanterior (PA) and lateral views should be taken. It makes no sense to assess a complex spheroidal structure in one plane only. Standard x ray department films allow measurement and sequential comparison whereas portable examinations are unreliable. The ratio of the transverse measurement of the heart to that of the thorax should be <50%, and an absolute measurement in excess of 16 cm reliably indicates cardiomegaly. Marked enlargement of the individual chambers must be present to be appreciated on the CXR. Volume overload pathologies are much more easily appreciated than those involving pressure overload. It should always be remembered that the cardiac image is only a silhouette and both pericardial effusion and juxta-cardiac mediastinal masses can simulate cardiac pathology.

Pulmonary vascularity
The assessment of pulmonary vascularity is the most useful information available from the CXR. Pulmonary venous hypertension (PVH) indicates elevated LA pressure and in the absence of mitral valve disease reflects the compliance of LV myocardium. In PVH both arteries and veins in the upper lobes are increased in size compared to the lower lobes (upper lobe diversion). Further progression resulting in interstitial edema manifests as Kerley A and B lines.

An overall increase in pulmonary vascularity is indicative of a longstanding left to right shunt or a high cardiac output (CO) state. It should be noted that acute insults to the left heart such as a ruptured papillary muscle or an acquired ventricular septal defect (VSD) present as pulmonary edema often with a very normal heart size and no suggestion of shunt vascularity.

Chronically diminished pulmonary vascularity is seen in congenital heart disease in which there is obstruction to right heart outflow such as in tetralogy of Fallot. In adults focal oligemia is sometimes seen in massive pulmonary embolism.

More complex cardiac imaging

Ultrasound, nuclear medicine, MRI, CT and cardiac catheterization with angiography are the imaging methods listed in order of increasing invasiveness. The spectrum of use of transthoracic echocardiography (TTE) and transesophageal echocardiography (TEE) is described elsewhere; because of portability and low cost it is usually the first modality used.

1. Nuclear cardiology

Historically multi-gated blood pool imaging has been used in the assessment of ventricular function. Of more importance is the contribution that nuclear medicine can make to the assessment of myocardial ischemia. MIBG myocardial imaging can be carried out in both resting and exercise states, thus providing an assessment of reversibility of myocardial ischemia. Recently, positron emission tomography (PET) has been added as an imaging strategy. In this technique a short-lived radioisotope of fluorinated glucose (FDG) yields an image of myocardial metabolism and it is claimed that this is particularly useful for detecting the hibernating myocardium. FDG is preferentially taken up by hibernating myocardium, thus appearing as hot spots (hibernating myocardium switches the predominant fuel from lipid to glucose). The problem with all nuclear-derived cardiac imaging is that the resolution suffers because of the time taken for acquisition.

2. Magnetic resonance imaging (MRI)

Many practitioners of cardiac imaging feel that MRI has the ability to fulfill all of the requirements that were listed at the beginning of this section. There is an added benefit in that potentially damaging ionizing radiation is not required. The speed of imaging has been dramatically increased in the last few years so that now breath hold sequences are available. When combined with EKG gating this provides accurate anatomical and functional cine imaging that can be applied in any plane through the heart and rendered into 3-D reconstruction. With this technique it is possible to measure ventricular mass, contractility and CO. The great vessels are well seen and by measuring flow within them it is possible to quantify shunts and valve dysfunction. Claims are made that it is possible to image the coronary arteries but this has not gained widespread clinical acceptance. It is possible to use gadolinium as a contrast agent for an accurate assessment of myocardial perfusion. Although the environment in the bore of a magnet is cumbersome, stress myocardial imaging is possible. This technique may not be tolerated by patients with claustrophobia, pacemakers or implanted defibrillators.

3. Computer tomography (CT) cardiac imaging

Over the last 15 years MRI and CT have been leapfrogging each other for pride of place as the prime non-invasive cardiac imaging modality. Just as with MRI, CT scanning times have reduced so that now with the ability to scan the heart in less than half a second and with EKG gating it is possible to obtain much higher resolution. CT also adds other dimensions to imaging. It is possible to accurately identify calcification in the heart and pericardium. This has been used to quantify the amount of calcium associated with atherosclerosis and thus devise a calcium score index which, when age adjusted, has been claimed to be a useful predictor of coronary artery disease. Conventional spiral CT has become the diagnostic tool of choice in pulmonary thromboembolism. It is also as reliable as MRI in the diagnosis of aortic pathology such as aneurysm and dissection. It is anticipated that the development of multi-slice helical scan acquisition will enable routine adoption of non-invasive coronary artery imaging.

4. Cardiac catheterization and angiography

This well-established modality is the most expensive and invasive of all the cardiac imaging strategies. It usually requires hospitalization and for pediatric patients a general anesthetic. In the investigation of complex congenital heart disease the other technologies provide useful anatomical imaging; however, only right and left heart catheterization will yield the full picture. Pressure and oxygen saturations are measured in all accessed cardiac chambers and the great vessels. Appropriate contrast injections are made and with digital cine imaging in two planes it is possible to define the cardiac chambers and the subsequent flow of contrast around the pulmonary and systemic circuits. It is possible to obtain accurate measurements of chambers and vessels and thus derive cardiac performance, blood flow and any potential shunts.

With the high prevalence of ischemic heart disease, the most commonly performed procedure is left heart catheterization and coronary arteriography. Injections are made in the left ventricle, and often in the ascending aorta, providing full assessment of both mitral and aortic valves and LV function. Subsequently, both coronary arteries are selectively injected to provide high resolution imaging of coronary artery stenoses in multiple planes.

5. Interventional cardiology

With cardiac catheterization providing access to the heart and its vessels increasingly sophisticated devices have allowed a plethora of interventions. In congenital heart disease it is possible to open up occlusions to dilated valves and vessels and to provide stenting. It is also possible to occlude undesirable vascular channels. In the field of acquired heart disease the most common intervention is coronary artery angioplasty, frequently with stenting, but it is also possible to occlude acquired defects and provide endoluminal covered stenting in the aorta.

Further reading

1. Ohnesorge BM. *Multi-slice CT in Cardiac Imaging*. Springer-Verlag: New York, 2002.
2. Bogaert J. *Magnetic Resonance of the Heart and Great Vessels: Clinical Applications*. Springer-Verlag: New York, 2000.
3. Miller SW. *Cardiac Radiology*. Mosby: New York, 1996.
4. Manning WJ, Pennell DJ. *Cardiovascular Magnetic Resonance*. Churchill Livingstone: London, 2002.

Related topics of interest

6 Echocardiography

Iain A Simpson

Introduction

Echocardiography has changed the face of diagnostic cardiology over the last 20 years, and although aspects of cardiac ultrasound imaging have become increasingly sophisticated, the basic information provided by echocardiography is relevant to everyone involved in the diagnosis and treatment of heart disease in the modern era. Cardiac surgeons have long been familiar with diagnostic cardiac catheterization and coronary angiography, yet echocardiography has until recently remained in the realms of cardiologists. With the advent of intraoperative echocardiography and particularly transesophageal echocardiography (TEE), an understanding of cardiac ultrasound is now an important aspect of cardiac surgical training.

Cardiac ultrasound modalities

Established modalities:

- M-mode echocardiography
- Two-dimensional echocardiography
- Spectral Doppler ultrasound
- Colour Doppler flow mapping
- Transesophageal echocardiography.

Evolving modalities:

- Contrast echocardiography
- Stress echocardiography
- Tissue Doppler imaging
- Three-dimensional echocardiography.

Clinical applications

Pre-operative assessment

- Valve disease
- LV function: regional and global
- Aortic pathology.

Intraoperative assessment

- Mitral/aortic reconstructive surgery
- Complex congenital heart disease
- Epiaortic assessment of atherosclerotic plaques
- Regional myocardial ischemia.

Postoperative assessment

- Hypotensive patient.

Valve disease

Generally transthoracic echocardiography (TTE) combined with Doppler ultrasound and TEE can provide accurate assessment of the severity of valve pathology. Precise quantification of the severity of valve stenosis is usually possible, whereas in valve regurgitation accurate estimation is more difficult and is based on a variety of echocardiographic and Doppler ultrasound parameters.

Aortic stenosis

Echocardiography can provide structural information on the aortic valve including leaflet mobility and calcification. It can also demonstrate the presence and severity of associated LV hypertrophy and/or LV systolic impairment.

Doppler ultrasound is more useful in quantifying the severity of stenosis, the maximum velocity of the stenotic jet measured by continuous wave Doppler predicting the aortic valve gradient. A simplified Bernoulli formula computes the valve gradient where the predicted pressure drop $= 4V^2$ (V = maximum velocity across the valve). In patients with severe LV impairment this approach underestimates the transvalvular gradient and hence aortic stenosis. Be wary of missing severe aortic stenosis in a patient with an apparently low gradient. In this situation using Doppler ultrasound to calculate the functional aortic valve area is more representative. Overestimating the severity of aortic stenosis can occur in patients with associated severe aortic regurgitation. This is less of a problem clinically as the the severity of the aortic regurgitation per se will almost certainly merit valve replacement.

One should always be cautious in a patient with clinical signs of significant stenosis and EKG/echocardiographic signs of LV hypertrophy yet Doppler ultrasound has predicted a low gradient even in the presence of good LV function. This may represent technical problems and an underestimation, or the patient may not have severe aortic stenosis and the hypertrophy is caused by hypertension or hypertrophic obstructive cardiomyopathy (HOCM). If there is a discrepancy between the clinical and echocardiographic findings further imaging and cardiac catheterization may be advisable. As HOCM can cause LV outflow tract obstruction and mimic aortic stenosis, one must be wary of operating on a patient with an apparently high aortic valve gradient who may turn out to have HOCM and a normal aortic valve.

Mitral stenosis

Echocardiographic assessment of mitral stenosis is usually quite straightforward and provides an accurate estimate of severity, and identification of valve thickening, restriction and calcification as well as LA dilatation. Doppler ultrasound provides an accurate estimate of the true functional severity of mitral stenosis using an estimate of the rate of mitral diastolic velocity reduction (mitral pressure half-time). This enables fairly accurate estimation of mitral valve area (cm²): MVA = 220/mitral pressure half-time.

TEE is extremely valuable in clarifying the severity of stenosis, presence of LA thrombus and suitability of the valve for balloon mitral valvuloplasty.

Valve regurgitation

Accurate assessment of the severity of valve regurgitation (semiquantitative) is more difficult, although valuable information on the morphology of regurgitation and the effects on cardiac function can usually be obtained. This is true for both mitral and aortic valve regurgitation.

- Valve morphology
  - 2-D and TEE

- Functional assessment
  - Chamber dilatation and impact on ventricular function

- Quantitative assessment
  - Spectral Doppler and color flow mapping.

Quantitative assessment includes the width and spatial distribution of the color jets of regurgitation in combination with the zone of flow convergence on the LV side of the mitral valve and the aortic side of the aortic valve. In addition, the intensity of the spectral Doppler signal and the effects on forward flow are taken into account.

Aortic pathology

TEE is essential for the assessment of aortic pathology and falls into the following areas:

- aortic endocarditis
- Marfan syndrome
- aortic dissection
- aortic intramural hematoma
- aortic atheroma
- aneurysm/rupture of the sinus of Valsalva.

Of these, aortic dissection and intramural hematoma are probably the most important. TEE can provide a rapid, clear and accurate diagnosis of aortic dissection allowing immediate surgical intervention. This is particularly useful when the dissection involves the ascending aorta (Stanford Type A). The technique is complimentary to other imaging modalities, particularly MRI, each having advantages and disadvantages (Table 1).

Table 1 Transesophageal echocardiography versus magnetic resonance imaging.

	Advantages	Disadvantages
TEE	Rapid diagnosis Performed in ICU Real-time imaging	First part of arch not seen No imaging of abdominal aorta
MRI	Good imaging of arch Abdominal aorta and organ perfusion	More time consuming Requires patient transfer Time-averaged images

Valvular reconstruction

TEE is now an essential part of the assessment of patients undergoing mitral reconstructive surgery. It can provide key information to assess the suitability of the valve for surgical repair, determine the relative contribution of the individual leaflets and their segments to the regurgitation and assess the presence of chordal rupture and commissural involvement. In addition, it can guide the type of repair and assess the end result for valve competence and the presence of systolic anterior motion. It also plays a similar role in the expanding field of aortic valve conservation surgery.

Assessing the postoperative hypotensive patient

In a hypotensive, ventilated patient in the ICU following surgical intervention, TEE provides rapid information on the underlying cause:

* LV dysfunction
* underfilling requiring volume expansion
* pericardial tamponade requiring surgical drainage
* valve dehiscence or impaired leaflet motion.

Further reading

1. Izzat MB, Sanderson JE, St. John Sutton MG. *Echocardiography in Adult Cardiac Surgery.* Isis Medical Media: Oxford, 1999.
2. Gray HH, Dawkins KD, Morgan JM, Simpson IA (eds). *Lecture Notes in Cardiology.* Blackwell Scientific Publications: London, 2002.

Related topics of interest

7 Anesthesia for cardiac surgery

David A Hett

Almost all patients presenting for cardiac surgery have pre-existing hemodynamic abnormalities, and the aim of cardiac anesthesia is to induce and maintain anesthesia without causing myocardial or other organ injury. This requires extensive monitoring and close cooperation between the anesthetist, perfusionist and surgeon.

Pre-operative management

The pre-operative visit allows the anesthetist to discuss with the patient premedication; induction, including siting of lines for invasive monitoring; and the possibility of elective postoperative mechanical ventilation. Clinical assessment includes evaluation of non-cardiac medical problems. The cardiological aspects of the patient should have been fully evaluated and relevant investigations including chest x ray, EKG, echocardiography and angiography should be available for inspection. Results of recent blood tests should also be ready for the pre-operative visit. A full drug history should be obtained and clear instructions given to continue therapy up to the time of operation. Traditionally 'heavy' premedication was used including long-acting benzodiazepines in combination with opioids to minimize angina in ischemic heart disease. With improved medical control this is not necessary and short-acting benzodiazepine alone is sufficient and less likely to precipitate pre-operative hypoxia.

Induction and maintenance of anesthesia

A variety of drugs can be used safely to induce anesthesia in the cardiac patient. It is essential to understand the underlying cardiovascular pathophysiology and how it interacts with the anesthetic agents.

Monitoring

Electrocardiogram (limb and V5 chest leads), oxygen saturation, end-tidal carbon dioxide, invasive and non-invasive blood pressure should be routinely monitored before induction. Post-induction central venous access is usually gained via the internal jugular approach. The routine use of pulmonary artery catheters is popular in the USA. However, in the UK they are reserved for high-risk cases (especially those with poor left ventricular function) since no benefit has been demonstrated in low-risk patients. Transesophageal echocardiography is likely to become more commonplace in the future but is especially useful in surgery for valve repair and congenital defects. It is also helpful in weaning from cardiopulmonary bypass in difficult cases.

Induction

The aim is to achieve sleep without upsetting the myocardial oxygen supply/demand ratio. The most common approach is to use a moderate dose of opioid such as fentanyl 10 μg/kg or remifentanil 1 μg/kg before administering a small dose of thiopental, propofol or midazolam by slow intravenous injection. This technique maintains hemodynamic stability and avoids myocardial depression. A non-depolarizing muscle relaxant is then used to facilitate endotracheal intubation: pancuronium through its vagolytic and sympathomimetic actions may result in tachycardia and hypertension which is undesirable in ischemic heart disease. Although these could be prevented by anti-anginal drugs such as beta blockers; vecuronium may be preferable since it lacks such cardiotropic side effects.

Maintenance

The aim is to maintain anesthesia without exacerbating myocardial ischaemia. This means avoidance of tachycardia or hypertension. Whilst anesthetic agents alone may preserve the oxygen supply/demand ratio it may be necessary to use other vasoactive drugs to achieve total hemodynamic control. Adequate depth of anesthesia is commonly reached using moderate doses of opioid such as fentanyl 10–30 μg/kg supplemented by an inhalational agent such as isoflurane. Despite the 'coronary steal' phenomenon, isoflurane does not sensitize the myocardium to catecholamines and maintains cardiac output better than some counterparts.

Management of cardiopulmonary bypass (CPB)

Anticoagulation

Contact between blood and the CPB circuit results in massive activation of the clotting cascade, and heparin is therefore used to prevent coagulation during CPB. A bolus of 300 IU/kg is given centrally before CPB, and an activated clotting time (ACT) should be measured after 1 minute to assess its effectiveness. A target of 480s or 3 × baseline value is sufficient to prevent clotting whilst on CPB.

Anesthesia during CPB

Anesthesia during CPB can be maintained by administering inhalational agents into the oxygenator. Alternatively, a propofol infusion, which due to its short duration of action, lack of accumulation and venodilator effect, is ideal for this purpose.

Myocardial protection

Aortic cross-clamping renders the heart ischemic and without myocardial protection this will cause irreversible damage and a low output state postoperatively. Myocardial protection can be achieved by hypothermia, cardioplegia (crystalloid or blood) or inducing ventricular fibrillation. Each technique has its own advantages and limitations.

Temperature

Hypothermia reduces the oxygen requirement of tissues which become ischemic during CPB. Blood and surface cooling can reduce the core temperature and the subsequent reduction in oxygen requirements allows for lower flow rates on full CPB.

Weaning from CPB

Preparation for weaning from CPB includes normothermia (nasopharyngeal temperature at 37°C), management of dysrhythmias by DC cardioversion and pacing, correction of acid–base and electrolyte imbalance and the reinstitution of ventilation. Weaning is then guided by the ventricular function, which can be optimized by adequate filling, stable sinus rhythm, and the use of inotropes and vasoactive agents until separation from CPB is complete. Mechanical circulatory support (e.g. intraaortic balloon pump) may be required if these measures fail.

Reversal of heparin

Protamine sulfate is given at a dose of 1–2 mg/100 units heparin used before CPB with an aim to revert to baseline ACT. Being highly negatively charged, it binds to the positively charged heparin and prevents any further binding to antithrombin III.

Postoperative management

The patient is transferred to the Intensive Care or High Dependency Unit for a period of postoperative ventilation. Full monitoring is continued in this period and attention is paid to fluid balance, postoperative bleeding, temperature, hemodynamic stability and electrolyte and acid–base disturbance. Weaning from the ventilator may occur after 2–4 hours or whenever the patient is rewarmed, bleeding becomes minimal, and the hemodynamics stable. Adequate analgesia is then established, electrolyte and acid–base imbalances are corrected, sedation is stopped, and when the patient is awake and obeying commands with adequate ventilation, extubation can occur.

Further reading

1. Gothard J, Kelleher A. *Essentials of Cardiac and Thoracic Anaesthesia*. Butterworth Heinemann: Oxford, 1999.
2. Tuman KJ, McCarthy RJ, Spiess BD et al. Does choice of anaesthetic agent significantly affect outcome after coronary artery surgery? *Anesthesiology* 1989; **70**: 189–98.
3. Hensley FA, Martin DE. *A Practical Approach to Cardiac Anaesthesia*. Little, Brown & Company: Boston, 1995.

8 Cardiopulmonary bypass

8.1 The extracorporeal circuit

Terry Gourlay, A Fisher, Kenneth M Taylor

History

Although the perfusion technology has evolved, the principles of the cardiopulmonary bypass (CPB) machine have remained consistent since the earliest clinical application by Gibbon in 1953. The aims are to provide:

- adequate gas exchange whilst the heart and lungs are out of the circulation
- adequate systemic blood flow
- means of controlling body temperature to any desirable level
- facilities for salvage and safe re-transfusion of blood from the surgical field.

Technological advances have resulted in the development of membrane oxygenators, which are far superior in their ability to oxygenate blood than earlier disk and bubble oxygenators. The materials used both for the construction of oxygenators, CPB tubing as well as the cannulae required for the institution of bypass have continued to evolve to improve the delivery of flow to the patient and limit the systemic inflammatory response to CPB. The indications for CPB has also expanded over the years to include removal of intracranial masses where profound hypothermia/low flow/circulatory arrest is used, thoracic tumor/major airway resection, pulmonary embolectomy, pulmonary transplantation, venovenous bypass for liver resections, caval reconstructions for renal tumors, resuscitation of hypothermic accident victims and the development of long-term support for the injured pulmonary bed in the form of extracorporeal life support (ECLS).

Structure of the CPB circuit

The tubing set is made of inert medical grade plastic (e.g. PVC) varying in diameter to provide adequate systemic flow on CPB. The latter is determined by patient size (BSA), temperature and nature of CPB (partial versus complete). Average adult size is $\frac{1}{2}$ inch for venous and $\frac{3}{8}$ inch for arterial tubing. Systemic heparinization is mandatory to prevent coagulation activated by the extracorporeal circuit. Adequacy of anticoagulation is monitored by activated clotting time (ACT $\geq 2.5 \times$ baseline). Heparin bonded circuits aim to dampen systemic inflammation triggered by CPB and may also reduce systemic heparin requirement.

The arterial pump and the blood oxygenator perform the primary functions of CPB. Modern membrane oxygenators incorporate heat exchangers for the control of body temperature. Heat exchange failure is very uncommon but may result in the leak of water into blood; initially this will result in unexplained increase in the reservoir volume followed by acidosis due to hemolysis and subsequent hemoglobinuria. There are two types of membrane oxygenators used for short-term support: flat sheet polypropylene and hollow-fiber micro-porous, polypropylene membranes. The micropores permit efficient exchange of O_2 and CO_2, but over many hours of use the efficiency declines due to the leakage of serum through the micropores reducing the rate of gas transfer. A falling venous saturation and a reduced arterial PaO_2 in the face of a rising FiO_2 may indicate oxygenator failure.

Two types of pumps are currently employed:

- roller pumps
- centrifugal (kinetic) pumps.

Roller pumps are occlusive and may be used to deliver pulsatile flow, which has been associated with better tissue perfusion during CPB. Currently, centrifugal pumps deliver non-pulsatile laminar perfusion but have the potential benefits of reduced blood trauma and protection against air embolism. Furthermore, because of their non-occlusive nature, the afterload governs the flow rate and it is therefore safe to clamp the line delivering flow to the patient without pressure overloading the system. There is a risk that flow may be reversed if the pressure developed by the centrifugal pump falls below that of the patient; a minimum revolution rate is therefore recommended (800 rpm) to avoid sucking blood back through the arterial cannula.

Ancillary functions of the CPB are:

- Blood salvage – blood from the surgical field is suctioned back to the CPB machine using additional roller pump(s) where it is filtered (20 µm) to remove particulate debris before entering the main blood reservoir.
- Delivery of blood cardioplegia – blood is taken from a dedicated port on the outlet side of the oxygenator. A roller pump delivers a mixture of blood and cardioplegia. The proportion of cardioplegia and blood is governed by the differential diameter of the tubes passing through the roller pump-head. Using this in conjunction with a heat exchanger enables blood cardioplegia to be delivered at any given temperature.

Monitoring during CPB:

- Patient parameters: EKG, arterial pressure, CVP, pulse oximetry (SaO_2), end-tidal CO_2, core temperature.
- Pump parameters: arterial line oxygen saturation, venous line oxygen saturation, gas flow and oxygen concentration, temperature of water in heat exchanger, temperature of pump blood, blood flow rate, arterial line pressure, cardioplegia line pressure.

Safety devices:

- Power failure alarm and automatic backup.
- Bubble detector, alarm and automatic pump cut-out.
- Temperature sensor and alarm.
- Venous reservoir level sensor, alarm and automatic pump cut-out.

CPB circuit management

Important parameters, which can be modulated during CPB, include PaO_2, $PaCO_2$, blood pressure, temperature and the hematocrit (Hct). The relationship between these parameters and oxygen delivery is described by the equation:

$$\text{Oxygen delivery} = 10 \times \text{pump flow} \times [1.34 \times Hb \times SaO_2] + 0.003 \times PaO_2$$

Where pump flow is in l/min, saturation is a decimal figure, Hb is g/100 ml and PaO_2 is mm Hg.

Hemodilution encountered in CPB is due to the priming of the pump-oxygenator with asanguinous fluid. Although reducing oxygen delivery, moderate hemodilution is well tolerated due to improvements in tissue perfusion by lowering plasma viscosity. In adults, Hct of 20 is often acceptable during CPB. In children, higher Hct may be desirable to limit water retention and to this end pump priming with blood may be employed with or without modified ultrafiltration.

The level of hemodilution may be predicted by the formula:

CPB Hct = patient's blood volume $\times$ pre-CPB Hct / (patient's blood volume + prime volume)

Similarly, oxygen delivery may be modified by alteration in the pump flow. At 37°C a cardiac index of 2.4 l/min/m² is normally maintained, which is reduced with hypothermia. An index of 2.4 l/min/m² is sufficient to maintain anesthetised cardiac patients although resting CI is >3.0 l/min/m².

Core temperature is controlled by the heat exchanger. Blood is channelled through the heat exchanger prior to patient delivery where its temperature is modified by water flowing on the opposite side of the heat exchange surface. The Hct, blood and water flow rates may influence the efficiency of the heat exchange surface. Although the heat exchanger may be very efficient the core temperature of the patient may rise or fall depending on independent factors governing the blood/tissue interface: e.g. re-warming of peripheries may be accelerated by the use of vasodilators in the re-warming phase.

Filtration during CPB

Arterial line screen filters (40 μm) reduce the embolic load to the brain and other organs. Arterial line filters are not employed in ECLS circuits because of the risk of filter occlusion from accumulation of embolic material with prolonged ECLS (days to weeks) using reduced heparinization (ACT 200–300 s). Leukocyte-depleting filters (polyester depth filters) may replace conventional arterial line filters in the future. A growing body of clinical evidence reports clinical benefits of removing activated neutrophils from blood during CPB as well as delivering neutrophil-depleted blood cardioplegia. Ultrafiltration and modified ultrafiltration may have the benefits of hemoconcentration during CPB, particularly in pediatric patients when a higher Hct is required to maintain oxygen delivery and attenuating tissue injury by removing cytokines (interleukins IL-6 and IL-8).

Further reading

1. Gravlee, Davis, Kurusz, Utley (eds). *Cardiopulmonary Bypass Principles and Practice. 2nd Edn.* Lippincott Williams: Philadelphia, 2000.
2. Mora CT. *Cardiopulmonary Bypass: Principles and Techniques of Extracorporeal Circulation.* Springer-Verlag: New York, 1995.
3. Taylor KM (ed) *Cardiopulmonary Bypass-Principles and Management.* Chapman and Hall Medical: London, 1986.
4. Casteneda AR, Jonas RA, Mayer JE, Hanley FL. *Cardiac Surgery of the Neonate and Infant.* WB Saunders: Philadelphia, 1994.
5. Society of Perfusionists of Great Britain and Ireland. *Recommendations for Standards of Monitoring and Alarms During Cardiopulmonary Bypass.* London, 2001. (www.sopgbi.org)

Related topics of interest

8.2 End-organ injury

George Asimakopoulos, Kenneth M Taylor

Introduction

Inflammation is the initial, non-specific attempt of vascularized tissue to eliminate injurious agents. Inflammatory mechanisms may become exaggerated and damage the host. If control is lost of local inflammation or when there is a systemic inflammatory response, mediators are released into the circulation, which may affect injury to tissues remote from the initial injury. This phenomenon occurs when patients undergo cardiopulmonary bypass (CPB) and is one manifestation of the systemic inflammatory response syndrome (SIRS). This has been defined by the following criteria:

- temperature >38°C
- heart rate >90/min
- respiratory rate >20/min

Or,

- pCO_2 <32 mmHg
- leukocyte count >12 000/mm^3

Or,

- leukocyte count <4000/mm^3

Or,

- immature leucocytes forms >10% of neutrophils.

SIRS is initiated by:

(1) contact activation of blood
(2) leukocyte and endothelial activation following ischemia-reperfusion
(3) leukocyte and endothelial activation caused by endotoxin, probably from the splanchnic bed
(4) operative trauma.

Post-perfusion syndrome, including accumulation of interstitial fluid, organ dysfunction and occasionally organ failure are recognized complications of CPB.

Molecular and cellular components of the systemic inflammatory response

Several molecular cascades play a role in inflammation:

Factor XII

Surface activation of Factor XII (Hageman factor) is pivotal in the development of the inflammatory response and the intrinsic coagulation pathway. This process directly activates complement factor 5 (C5) and neutrophils.

Complement

Complement is a system of proteins that are activated in the early phase of the inflammatory response. Complement consists of 9 proteins (C1–C9) and their split products, e.g. C3a and C3b. Complement may become activated by antibody/antigen complexes (classical pathway), or the 'alternative pathway' by the contact of C3 with foreign surfaces. Activated complement products promote vasodilation, increased vascular permeability, leukocyte activation, leukocyte mobilization, chemotaxis and adhesion and phagocytosis of organisms by neutrophils and macrophages. Both pathways are activated during CPB.

Cytokines/chemokines

Cytokines such as the interleukins (ILs) are small molecular weight proteins secreted by leukocytes and other cells in response to external stimuli. Interleukins act as important messengers of the inflammatory response. The pro-inflammatory cytokines tumor necrosis factor α (TNFα) and IL-1 are secreted by activated monocytes and in turn activate neutrophils, macrophages and endothelial cells. Activated monocytes and endothelial cells produce IL-6; plasma levels reach a peak 4 hours after CPB. IL-8 is a chemokine, which is a chemoattractant for leukocytes. The IL-8 found in plasma post-CPB originates from endothelial cells. IL-10 has anti-inflammatory actions since it inhibits the generation of pro-inflammatory cytokines. Production of IL-10 increases significantly within 24 hours post-CPB.

Adhesion molecules

Specific adhesion molecules mediate the interaction between leukocytes and endothelial cells. At times of endothelial dysfunction, e.g. following myocardial reperfusion injury, up-regulation of adhesion molecules enhances neutrophil-mediated tissue damage. Adhesion molecules that regulate leukocyte–endothelial cell interaction can be divided into three main groups: the selectins, the integrins and the immunoglobulin superfamily. The leukocyte integrin CD11b/CD18, in particular, participates in the firm adhesion of leukocytes to endothelium and is up-regulated significantly during CPB.

Neutrophils

Activation of neutrophils and their mobilization towards injured tissues are critical steps in inflammation. Although neutrophils are an important defense against invading organisms, when activated via SIRS they may cause tissue damage by releasing proteolytic enzymes and oxidative products. Tissue injury is dependent upon the ability of neutrophils to adhere to endothelium. Therefore, neutrophil-mediated tissue injury is associated with an up-regulation of integrins (CD11b/CD18). Blocking of these integrins in animal models has reduced post-CPB lung dysfunction.

Monocytes

CPB causes significant activation of monocytes. Activated monocytes release pro-inflammatory cytokines, which may cause further activation of neutrophils and endothelial cells.

Endothelial cells

The endothelium becomes activated after exposure to certain cytokines. Although endothelial permeability increases post-CPB, the mechanisms involved remain unidentified. Activated endothelium expresses cell adhesion molecules, and plasma levels of endothelial-derived factors such as von Willebrand increase post-CPB.

Organ dysfunction

Whilst ischemia of atherosclerotic origin may be the primary cause of organ dysfunction, SIRS is regarded as a major contributor. CPB-associated dysfunction of the brain, heart, lungs, kidneys and gut has been widely reported.

Brain

Cerebral dysfunction following CPB is well recognized and ranges in severity from frank stroke (2% incidence) to more subtle changes in cognitive function (20–40%). Cerebral damage may be caused by:

- substantial fall in cerebral blood flow
- macroembolism, e.g. atherosclerotic debris from the ascending aorta
- microembolism – both gaseous and particulate
- SIRS.

Myocardium

Currently there is no ideal method of myocardial preservation, and evidence of injury is evident with all currently adopted techniques. The role of CPB-related ischemia-reperfusion injury and its impact upon myocardial dysfunction remains debatable. Myocardial injury as measured by the release of troponin I or T and CK-MB is reduced following off-pump coronary artery bypass grafting (OPCAB) surgery compared to CPB.

Lungs

Pulmonary dysfunction post-CPB is evidenced by increased pulmonary vascular permeability, neutrophil sequestration, water content and pulmonary vascular resistance. Clinically these changes manifest as reduced lung compliance and increased arterial-alveolar gradient. Studies to date have not shown differences in lung dysfunction when comparing OPCAB and CABG with CPB.

Kidneys

Large studies in patients undergoing CPB have found a significant increase in creatinine levels in 7–11% of patients whilst 3–4% of patients suffer acute renal failure. Pre-existing renal dysfunction, advanced age (>70 years), low output syndrome and emergency operation are independent risk factors for postoperative renal dysfunction.

Gastrointestinal tract

The gut undergoes injury, which may be mediated by hypoperfusion of the intestinal mucosa. Gut dysfunction is evident with increases in gut permeability. As a result of this injury, the splanchnic bed may become a source of inflammatory mediators such as cytokines, oxygen free radicals, leukotrienes and arachidonic acid metabolites. Importantly, the gut is a source of endotoxins, which may enter the bloodstream when gut barrier function is compromised.

Further reading

1. Paparella D, Yau TM, Young E. Cardiopulmonary bypass induced inflammation: pathophysiology and treatment. An update. *Eur J Cardiothorac Surg* 2002; **21**: 232–44.
2. Asimakopoulos G, Taylor KM. The effects of cardiopulmonary bypass on leucocyte and endothelial adhesion molecules. *Ann Thorac Surg* 1998; **66**: 2135–44.
3. Taylor KM (ed). *Cardiopulmonary Bypass – Principles and Management.* Chapman and Hall Medical: London, 1986.
4. Smith PLC, Taylor KM (eds). *Cardiac Surgery and the Brain.* Edward Arnold: London, 1993.

Related topics of interest

9 Thermoregulation in cardiac surgery

Adrian Mellor, Charles D Deakin

Accidental hypothermia is common during all surgical procedures, but cardiac surgery uses deliberate hypothermia to reduce oxygen consumption (8% per °C temperature reduction) and protect vital organs from ischemia.

Temperature regulation

Under normal circumstances temperature is under strict physiological control with core temperature maintained at 37 ±0.2 °C. Temperature sensors in the core and periphery relay afferent impulses to the hypothalamus. Efferent mechanisms consist of hypothermia-induced cutaneous vasoconstriction, shivering and hyperthermia-induced vasodilatation and sweating.

Temperature monitoring

Temperature is usually measured using either a thermistor or thermocouple, both of which respond rapidly to small changes in temperature.

Core temperature is considered to be the temperature of blood perfusing deep tissues such as the heart, liver and brain. Temperatures are not, however, uniform throughout the body and temperatures measured at different sites have different physiological significance. The commonly used sites for measurement of core temperature in clinical practice are the nasopharynx, distal esophagus, axilla, pulmonary artery, rectum and tympanic membrane. All these sites are considered to represent core temperature and there is little variation between them in a normothermic state. Axilla, rectum and bladder lag behind the rapid changes in true core temperature seen during cardiopulmonary bypass (CPB) and are therefore not suitable for use in patients undergoing rapid changes in core temperature.

Peripheral temperature varies considerably at different sites. Over the scalp and chest wall it approaches core temperature, whereas in the extremities it may be 4–5°C below core temperature. Peripheral temperature, however, is usually measured from a representative single site such as skin over the thigh.

Hypothermia during cardiac surgery

Passive cooling

General anesthesia and surgery impair thermoregulatory responses to hypothermia and cause cooling through several mechanisms:

- *Peripheral vasodilation* on induction of anesthesia redistributes heat from the warm core to cold periphery, resulting in a drop in core temperature of 0.5–1.0 °C.
- *Reduced metabolic heat production* (15–40%) particularly through decreased brain metabolism and reduced respiratory muscle activity.
- *Increased heat loss* by radiation (40%), convection (30%), evaporation (20%) and respiration (10%). Most loss occurs through peripheral vasodilation, evaporation from the body surface (particularly cleaning fluids) and evaporation from exposed body cavities.
- The *thermoregulatory threshold* that triggers shivering and vasoconstriction is reduced by approximately 3–4 °C. These heat-producing mechanisms are not activated until core temperature falls to below approximately 32 °C. The body becomes poikilothermic before the threshold.
- *Neuromuscular-blocking drugs* paralyze skeletal muscle and prevent heat production by shivering.
- *Cooling effect of cold anesthetic gases* minimized by using heat and moisture exchange filters.
- *Cooling effect of cold intravenous fluids* – 500 ml blood at 4 °C will drop core temperature by 0.3 °C.

Active cooling
Active cooling is facilitated by the use of a counter-current heat exchanger mounted in the CPB circuit. On initiating bypass, core temperature falls rapidly followed by a reduction in skin temperature. This results in rapid cooling of the heart, brain and other vital organs. Even without active cooling, the temperature drifts lower on CPB due to the lack of thermal insulation of the extracorporeal circuit.

Effects of cooling on arterial blood gases
Arterial carbon dioxide tension ($PaCO_2$) falls with hypothermia as gases are more soluble in cold blood. This leads to two alternative methods of managing the arterial blood gases on hypothermic bypass:

- *pH-stat* – $PaCO_2$ is corrected for temperature, resulting in relative hypercarbia. This causes cerebral vasodilatation, which may be beneficial to bring about rapid cerebral cooling for cases involving deep hypothermic circulatory arrest.
- *Alpha-stat* – this method does not correct for temperature and may be beneficial in terms of reducing cerebral blood flow and hence embolic events in adults.

Rewarming during cardiopulmonary bypass

Active rewarming via the integral heat exchanger preferentially heats the core organs because peripheral blood flow is reduced by vasoconstriction. Temperature differential between pumpblood and body is restricted to approximately 10 °C to minimize risk of gas embolism (particularly during cooling). Blood should not be superheated within the exchanger (>39 °C) to avert denaturing proteins. Rewarming is usually considered adequate when core temperature reaches 37.0 °C and peripheral temperature reaches 34.5 °C. It is vital to avoid overheating of the brain (indicated by nasopharyngeal temperature >37 °C). However, on separation from CPB, peripheral rewarming is usually incomplete. As a result of post-bypass vasodilation, heat is rapidly transferred from a warm core to cooler periphery, resulting in an 'afterdrop' in core temperature. The degree of postoperative hypothermia correlates poorly both with core temperature on separation from CPB and core–peripheral temperature gradient but is related to the degree of peripheral rewarming before separation from CPB. As water mattresses are of limited effectiveness, the magnitude of postoperative hypothermia can be reduced by improving the degree of peripheral rewarming on bypass using:

(1) Pulsatile flow on cardiopulmonary bypass.
(2) Prolonged heat exchanger rewarming.
(3) Forced air rewarming (e.g. Bair Hugger).
(4) Pharmacological vasodilation of the periphery (e.g. sodium nitroprusside or GTN).

Physiological effects of postoperative hypothermia

On admission to intensive care, most patients are cold (centrally and peripherally) and vaso-constricted. The elevated systemic vascular resistance (SVR) may result in hypertension, increased afterload, and give a false impression of cardiovascular stability. The net effect of the combination of the effects listed below is to produce a metabolic acidosis. Postoperative rewarming leads to vasodilatation and unmasks relative hypovolemia, resulting in hypotension.

Any patient with a core temperature below 36.0°C is hypothermic. Even core temperatures just 1.0–1.5°C below normal are associated with adverse outcomes:

Metabolic
- Prolonged action of anesthetic drugs.
- Left shift of the oxygen dissociation curve, impairing oxygen delivery.
- Increased postoperative stress response (resulting in hyperglycemia).

Cardiac
- Increased blood viscosity increasing cardiac work.
- Increased left ventricular afterload.
- Increased arrhythmic potential (VF when <30°C).
- Increased inotrope requirements.

Respiratory
- Prolonged ventilation requirements.

Hematological
- Impaired coagulation (clotting cascade is enzyme dependent; platelet function is impaired by hypothermia).
- Thrombocytopenia.
- Leuckopenia.

Postoperative rewarming

Prevention of heat loss is as important as active rewarming in minimizing postoperative hypothermia. A single drape reduces heat loss from convection and conduction by 30%.

Warming intravenous fluids is also important. The administration of one unit (500 ml) of blood at 4°C requires 50% of basal metabolic heat to rewarm it to 37°C over one hour.

Active heating can be achieved by:

- heated humidified respiratory gas
- circulating water mattresses
- fluid warmers
- forced-air warming.

Forced-air rewarming is the only effective method of rewarming patients postoperatively. Additional infusion of a vasodilator (e.g. GTN) dilates surface vessels and increases the rate of heat uptake.

Further reading

1. Phillips R, Skov P. Rewarming and cardiac surgery: a review. *Heart Lung* 1988; 17: 511–20.
2. Sessler DI. Perioperative thermoregulation and heat balance. *Ann NY Acad Sci* 1997; **813**: 757–77.
3. Deakin CD, Petley GW, Clewlow F. Measurement of rewarming from hypothermic cardiopulmonary bypass. A review. *Cardiovasc Engineering* 1998; **3**: 36–42.
4. Sessler DI. Perioperative heat balance. *Anesthesiology* 2000; **92**: 578–96.

Related topics of interest

10 Hypothermic circulatory arrest

Irving Shen, Ross M Ungerleider

Deep hypothermia with circulatory arrest (DHCA) remains an essential adjunct in aortic and pediatric cardiac surgery. In profound hypothermia, the core temperature is gradually lowered to 18–20°C using cardiopulmonary bypass (CPB). Perfusion is discontinued, the patient's blood volume is drained into the pump reservoir, and cannulae can be removed, facilitating surgery in a bloodless field.

Indications

(1) Any cardiopulmonary procedure or repair of complex congenital cardiac defects that requires an asanguineous field (e.g. repair of tiny pulmonary arteries in patients with excessive systemic to pulmonary collateral flow).
(2) Repair of the distal ascending aorta or the aortic arch.
(3) Atherosclerotic disease or heavy calcification of the aorta that would make clamping of the aorta hazardous.
(4) Control and repair of massive hemorrhage as a result of cardiac or aortic laceration in redosternotomy.

Methods

In the past, hypothermia was achieved using surface cooling by submerging the patient in an ice water bath after induction of general anesthesia. Currently, core cooling is achieved on CPB using established techniques.

The heart may fibrillate during cooling (<32°C). Left ventricular distention can occur in some instances (e.g. in patients with severe aortic valve insufficiency or in patients with excessive systemic to pulmonary collateral blood flow). This can be prevented by venting the left ventricle and/or the pulmonary artery. Alternatively, the aorta can be cross-clamped and the heart arrested with cardioplegic solution once the ventricle fibrillates.

Hematocrit management
As blood viscosity increases with systemic cooling, blood flow through the microcirculation may become impaired. Hemodilution is frequently employed during hypothermic CPB to provide adequate oxygen delivery and prevent sludging in the capillary beds. A hematocrit of approximately 20% is targeted for hypothermic CPB down to 18–20°C. Recent data in children, however, suggests that the problem of blood viscosity is more theoretical than real and that a higher hematocrit (approximately 30%) may be better during the cooling phase before DHCA.

Rate and duration of cooling

The brain is the most sensitive organ least tolerant to ischemia during DHCA. Rapid cooling must be avoided as this will lead to wide temperature gradients between the brain and surrounding tissues. Non-uniform cooling will lead to cerebral rewarming during the circulatory arrest period, which can result in neurological injury. It is important to cool for at least 20–25 minutes prior to induction of DHCA to ensure adequate suppression of cerebral metabolic activity.

Neuro protection and monitoring

There is no direct way to monitor cerebral metabolism clinically, and therefore indirect measures must be employed to determine the degree of cerebral protection during DHCA. Since cerebral metabolism is a direct function of brain temperature, nasopharyngeal temperature is used clinically as an indirect measurement of cerebral cooling. In fact, monitoring temperature at various sites in the body, including esophageal, blood, rectal, bladder, and nasopharyngeal, can ensure uniform cooling throughout the body.

Other ways to monitor cerebral metabolism during cooling include measuring internal jugular venous saturation (saturation >95% signifies minimal cerebral oxygen extraction) and monitoring electroencephalographic (EEG) activities. Using silent EEG activity as an end-point for cooling is not always reliable because EEG activity does not always become silent at a consistent body temperature.

Various strategies can be used to minimize the deleterious effect of DHCA. Packing the patient's head with ice during the period of cooling and DHCA has the theoretical advantages of more rapid and uniform cooling and prevention of rewarming during the arrest period. This appears to be more effective in neonates and infants than in adults, presumably due to the larger surface area to volume ratio of their head. Drugs added to the pump prime or given to the patient just prior to DHCA have not been consistently shown to be efficacious. Intravenous methylprednisolone (10 mg/kg) given at least 8 hours prior to DHCA appears to decrease both the systemic inflammatory response and the deleterious effect of DHCA on cerebral metabolic recovery.

The acid–base management strategies used during cooling have a significant effect on cerebral blood flow and metabolism. Carbon dioxide (CO_2) solubility in blood increases at low temperature and this leads to alkalemia during cooling. The more commonly employed alpha-stat acid–base management allows blood to remain alkalemic during cooling. In pH-stat acid–base management, CO_2 is added to the bypass circuit in order to normalize the blood pH. CO_2 is a potent cerebral vasodilator, and using pH-stat acid–base management during cooling can significantly increase blood flow to the brain, leading to more rapid and homogenous cooling. However, excess CO_2 can cause tissue acidosis at the time of DHCA and may be the reason for significant impairment in cerebral metabolic recovery after DHCA using pH-stat cooling alone. There is now evidence that when pH-stat acid–base management during cooling is changed to alpha-stat for a few minutes prior to the onset of DHCA, the acidotic effects of pH-stat with respect to cerebral metabolic recovery is avoided.

Safe DHCA time

The possibility of brain injury appears to increase with the duration of circulatory arrest period. Therefore, the period of DHCA should be limited to an absolute minimum required to achieve surgical objectives. Usually 30–40 minutes of uninterrupted DHCA is considered safe at a nasopharyngeal temperature of 18–20°C. Continuous low–flow cardiopulmonary bypass or DHCA interrupted by intermittent periods of low-flow reperfusion (50 ml/kg/minute for 1–2 minutes) may provide better end–organ protection than a prolonged period of uninterrupted DHCA. In adults, using continuous retrograde cerebral perfusion during DHCA can extend the length of 'safe' arrest period with decreased postoperative neurologic complications.

Reperfusion and rewarming

When CPB is re-established after DHCA, a period of cold reperfusion for approximately 10 minutes before active rewarming results in increased cerebral blood flow. Too aggressive rewarming or warming the body core temperature to above 36°C can increase the risk of neurologic injury and must be avoided.

Complications

All the major organ systems can be adversely affected by a period of DHCA. Coagulopathy and platelet dysfunction often result in excessive bleeding postoperatively. The systemic inflammatory response to CPB and DHCA often results in capillary leak, profound tissue edema and organ dysfunction.

The brain, however, is the most sensitive organ with the greatest risk for injury after circulatory arrest. Neurologic injury may be global or related to blood flow watershed areas as a result of diffuse cerebral ischemia. Seizures are usually temporary, do not require long-term therapy and are caused by air embolism. Choreoathetosis, although rare, can occur after DHCA. This most commonly occurs 2–6 days after surgery and the symptom severity usually improves with time. In some severe cases, choreoathetoid movements or hypotonia can be permanent. The exact pathophysiology of choreoathetosis is unclear but it is most likely due to ischemic injury to the basal ganglia. With the advent of pH-stat cooling and limiting the duration of DHCA by employing intermittent or continuous low–flow perfusion, many of the clinically recognizable complications are decreasing.

Further reading

1. Greeley WJ, Kern FH, Meliones JN, Ungerleider RM. Effect of deep hypothermia and circulatory arrest on cerebral blood flow and metabolism. *Ann Thorac Surg* 1993; **56**: 1464–6.
2. Jaggers J, Shearer IR et al. Cardiopulmonary bypass in infants and children. In: *Cardiopulmonary Bypass: Principles and Practice. 2nd Edn.* Gravlee GP, Davis RF, Kurusz M, Utley JR (eds). Lippincott, Williams & Wilkins: Philadelphia, 2000: pp 633–61.
3. Phoon CK. Deep hypothermic circulatory arrest during cardiac surgery: effects on cerebral blood flow and cerebral oxygenation in children. *Am Heart J* 1993; **125**: 1739–48.

Related topics of interest

11 Myocardial preservation

11.1 Cardioplegia

Sir Bruce E Keogh

Myocardial preservation encompasses strategies employed during cardiac surgery to produce a motionless bloodless operating field, enabling precise surgical repair without compromising myocardial function. The most effective strategies commence pre-operatively, continue throughout surgery and extend into the postoperative period. These strategies aim to optimize myocardial oxygen supply/demand balance and minimize ischemia.

Pre-operative phase

Baseline medical management should optimize myocardial oxygen supply/demand pre-operatively. Ideal strategy varies with cardiac pathophysiology:

- stable coronary disease: maintain 'status quo' with anti-anginal medication until surgery
- unstable coronary disease: intravenous nitrates to improve coronary perfusion and heparin to reduce thromboembolic risks ± intra-aortic ballon pump (IABP) when medical therapy fails.

A balance must be struck between myocardial work and coronary perfusion pressure. Loss of coronary perfusion pressure from excessive coronary/systemic vasodilation may be harmful.

Operative phase

Ideally, the surgeon needs a quiet bloodless operative field achievable by various means. Whichever method is chosen the principle of minimizing myocardial ischemia remains unchanged. The early work of Melrose confirmed hyperkalemic cardioplegia as a safe and reversible method of diastolic cardiac arrest. The delivery medium has been shifting from crystalloid to blood because of the latter's superiority in:

- providing oxygen and nutrients
- buffering
- minimizing intracellular edema
- distributing cardioplegia evenly
- scavenging oxygen free radicals (superoxide dismutase, catalase, glutathione, plasma proteins, urate, vitamins C and E).

Further pioneering work of Buckberg found that myocardial oxygen consumption is reduced by 90% with electromechanical arrest. This observation combined with evidence that profound hypothermia may aggravate the depletion of energy reserves and delay metabolic and functional recovery resulted in a reappraisal of warm blood cardioplegia. Increasing recognition that all cardioplegic techniques are dependent on adequacy of distribution and frequency of replenishment, particularly when warm blood cardioplegia is used, focused attention on improving distribution and minimizing ischemic time. To some extent both issues were addressed by the advent of retrograde coronary sinus delivery in the early 1990s. This cardioplegic technique was designed to improve delivery beyond arterial stenoses. Furthermore, the potential for continuous retrograde infusion of warm blood cardioplegia addressed concerns that normothermia would substantially shorten the lethal ischemic time between doses. However, subsequent evidence supported intermittent delivery of warm/tepid cardioplegia at intervals of 10–20 min.

Myocardial protection for off-pump coronary artery bypass grafting (OPCAB) surgery is assuming increasing importance with its rising popularity. The heart sustains short periods of regional ischemia well when target coronary arteries are occluded. However, many surgeons routinely insert intracoronary shunts to limit ischemia whilst others induce ischemic-preconditioning prior to protracted coronary occlusion during anastomosis. Hemodynamic monitoring (CI, SVO_2) plays a key role in optimizing myocardial performance and protection during OPCAB surgery.

Although most surgeons generally prefer one or two methods of myocardial protection it is important to appreciate the pros and cons of other techniques:

Myocardial protection with cardiopulmonary bypass
1. Continuous coronary perfusion with ordinary, normokalemic blood
Blood is delivered continuously to the myocardium on either a beating or fibrillating heart under mild hypothermia. The aorta is cross-clamped and coronaries are perfused through an aortic root cannula or through direct coronary cannulation. This technique may be used for aortic valve surgery with poor LV function or for repeat mitral surgery through the right chest without aortic cross-clamping.

Potential pitfalls:

- Risk of selectively perfusing the left anterior descending coronary artery (LAD) or circumflex artery with direct coronary cannulation, particularly if the left-main is short.
- When used, fibrillation should be induced electrically but maintained by hypothermia. Electrical fibrillation reduces sub-endocardial perfusion compared with spontaneous fibrillation – this is particularly hazardous in ventricular hypertrophy.
- In the presence of coronary disease, decompression may alter collateral flow to ischemic areas.
- Excessive flow (>300 ml/min) may induce cellular damage and with longer procedures myocardial edema will reduce compliance.

This technique is well tolerated with good results in short procedures.

2. Moderately hypothermic intermittent global ischemia
Commonly known as intermittent aortic cross-clamping, it is a popular technique for uncomplicated CABG and to facilitate minor modifications of a distal anastomosis without further cardioplegia. The heart is electrically fibrillated prior to aortic cross-clamping. This induces global ischemia with fibrillation, followed by anoxic arrest and electrical silence on the EKG. The mechanism of protection/tolerance is associated with myocardial preconditioning.

Key points for this approach are:

- Cardiac decompression is important prior to aortic cross-clamping to prevent myocardial distention and myofibrillar disruption.
- Mild hypothermia (32–34°C) increases permissible global ischemia to approximately 15 min and dampens the amplitude of fibrillation.

It is inexpensive, simple and compares favorably with cold blood/crystalloid cardioplegia. Aortic trauma and thromboembolism are potential concerns, particularly in arteriopaths.

3. Profoundly hypothermic global ischemia
This technique relies on cardiac arrest during profound hypothermia and is generally reserved for major aortic/arch procedures.

4. Cardioplegic arrest
Cardioplegic solutions induce diastolic arrest by altering the resting potential ($-90\,mV$) and ionic gradients in the myocyte. The trans-membrane potential changes rapidly with ionic flux, principally Na^+, K^+, Ca^{++} and Cl^-.

There are two main cardioplegic methods:

(1) The most popular strategy is to prevent repolarization by increasing the $[K^+]$ in the extracellular fluid ('extracellular' solutions).
(2) The less common approach is to block depolarization by lowering the extracellular $[Na^+]$ ('intracellular' solutions).

The cardioplegic solution may be delivered in crystalloid or blood, antegradely into the coronary arteries and/or retrogradely via the coronary sinus. The crystalloid form is always cold (4–10°C), but blood cardioplegia can be hypothermic or normothermic. Despite its simplicity, crystalloid solution is being superseded by blood cardioplegia.

Unresolved controversy in cardioplegia centers around both the temperature and route of administration. The key to understanding cardioplegic techniques lies in an appreciation of the relative contributions of electromechanical activity and temperature to oxygen consumption and energy demands of the myocardium. Cold temperature left-shifts the oxygen dissociation curve substantially so that at 20°C only 50% of the hemoglobin-bound oxygen is released. At 10°C this becomes <40%. This is offset by reduced myocardial oxygen requirement and the increased blood solubility of oxygen. Around 5–20°C a fully O_2-saturated solution can support adequate oxygenation without hemoglobin. Furthermore, hypothermia causes enzyme dysfunction, membrane instability, intracellular calcium sequestration, inefficient energy utilization, reduced oxygen uptake and disturbed osmotic homeostasis. Since electromechanical arrest and not hypothermia is the major determinant of oxygen consumption, Lichtenstein proposed continuous warm blood cardioplegia to ensure aerobic arrest and eliminate reperfusion injury. He demonstrated clinical superiority over continuous cold blood cardioplegia. In practice, however, visualization is impaired by continuous administration, and intermittent warm blood cardioplegia is preferred by many.

An oxygen debt accumulates during global ischemia with reduced intracellular high-energy phosphates. A burst of warm cardioplegia ('hot shot') given immediately before aortic unclamping provides substrate resuscitation and myocardial recovery. Removing the clamp restores antegrade coronary perfusion. Further myocardial energy regeneration occurs during this period before electromechanical work resumes with cardioplegia washout.

Retrograde administration through the coronary sinus and venous system at

100–250 ml/min pressurizing to 30–50 mmHg delivers cardioplegia across capillaries into the Thebesian veins and coronary arteries (inherent 25–30% 'wastage'). Distribution is generally good but less predictable than antegrade with inconsistent RV protection. It is particularly useful for coronary re-operations and in valve procedures when surgery can continue during cardioplegia delivery.

Reperfusion phase

Restoration of coronary perfusion triggers a complex cascade of ischemia-reperfusion injury (IRI) leading to disruption of endothelial and myocyte integrity. Reperfusion of ischemic tissue generates oxygen free radicals (OFR) by intra-mitochondrial reduction of oxygen. Neutrophils in the reperfusate are activated and generate more OFR. The highly reactive OFRs oxidize sulfydryl bonds (S–H bond scission) and polyunsaturated lipids essential to cell membrane integrity. The resultant sarcolemmal damage triggers calcium influx, overload and insensitivity with subsequent contractile impairment. Simultaneously, there is depletion of NADPH and increased sodium/calcium exchange. Similarly, endothelial injury and dysfunction occurs with increased microvascular permeability. Intracellular and interstitial edema compresses adjacent capillaries, reducing perfusion and exacerbating ischemic injury – no reflow phenomenon. The clinical spectrum of IRI ranges from reversible myocardial stunning lasting minutes/days to the dramatic and fatal condition of stone heart. Strategies to minimize IRI include:

- avoiding ischemia
- low-pressure reperfusion
- hypocalcemic reperfusion
- adding OFR scavengers to the reperfusate
- neutrophil depletion.

IRI plays a prominent role in revascularization following recent acute occlusion and myocardial infarction. In the latter situation, the timing of surgery becomes an important consideration and enters the arena of myocardial protection.

Postoperative phase

Avoid excessive functional demands on the heart:

- afterload reduction
- heart rate control
- maximize oxygen delivery
- minimize oxygen consumption.

Further reading

1. Buckberg G. Oxygenation cardioplegia: blood is a many splendoured thing. *Ann Thorac Surg* 1990; **50:** 175–7.
2. Buckberg GD. Myocardial temperature management during aortic clamping for cardiac surgery. *J Thorac Cardiovasc Surg* 1991; **102:** 895–903.
3. Barner HB. Blood cardioplegia: a review and comparison with crystalloid cardioplegia. *Ann Thorac Surg* 1991; **52:** 1354–67.
4. Intermittent aortic cross-clamping and cold crystalloid cardioplegia for low risk coronary patients. *Ann Thorac Surg* 1996; **61:** 834–9.

Related topics of interests

11.2 Non-cardioplegic techniques

Kyriakos Anastasiadis, Ravi Pillai

Background

Optimum myocardial protection for CABG remains controversial. Cardioplegia in its various forms is now the most common method used. Alternatives such as ventricular fibrillation and systemic hypothermia with or without aortic cross-clamping are still in use and produce acceptable results. The reintroduction of OPCAB has further popularized non-cardioplegic techniques.

Low cardiac output, significant inotropic requirement and the need for IABP or other mechanical assist device are indicators of impaired myocardial function probably from inadequate myocardial protection. Sixty-five percent of post-CABG mortality can be directly attributed to cardiac failure. Myocardial injury may occur during reperfusion with production of oxygen free radicals (OFR). Different cardioplegic reperfusion techniques can limit OFR injury but do not prevent the fall in high-energy phosphates. This is particularly important in high-risk patients who may not tolerate perioperative ischemia-reperfusion injury.

There is a sigmoidal relationship between myocardial ischemia and damage. The rate of recovery is dependent on the extent of damage and not on the duration of ischemia. Systemic hypothermia enhances myocardial protection by reducing metabolism. The importance of temperature in the development of regional necrosis after myocardial ischemia in the beating heart is becoming apparent. Recent studies have shown that the proportion of the ischemic risk zone that becomes necrotic is directly correlated with temperature. Thus, mild hypothermia (approximately 32°C) is a useful adjunct to the cross-clamp fibrillation technique. Below this temperature, it becomes more difficult to cardiovert to sinus rhythm between distal anastomoses. Sequential construction of the grafts permits proximal anastomoses to be undertaken with the heart beating.

Recent prospective randomized trials have shown the efficacy of the cross-clamp fibrillation technique (CCF) in myocardial revascularization. This produced similar or better results than cardioplegia in terms of postoperative cardiac enzyme release and LV diastolic dysfunction. With cardioplegic protection significant correlation between the duration of aortic clamping and cardiac enzyme release was found.

Thus the beneficial effects of cardioplegic arrest are countered by a reduced total aortic clamping in CCF. Cardioplegia delivery even when guided by measurement of myocardial temperature does not eliminate tissue acidosis.

There is concern over increased perioperative cerebral microemboli and postoperative neuropsychological disturbances with CCF (with multiple aortic clamping) although the evidence is inconclusive.

Cross-clamp fibrillation

Using CPB, with the heart empty (±venting) ventricular fibrillation is induced by DC current and the aorta is cross-clamped. Good systemic venous drainage and the avoidance of ventricular distention prevents subsequent subendocardial ischemia. Each graft is constructed sequentially, with the distal anastomosis performed with the heart fibrillating. This is followed by the proximal anastomosis, if the conduit is a free graft, whilst the heart is reperfused and beating (DC cardioversion may be required after removal of the aortic cross-clamp). This sequence allows the evaluation of blood flow in each graft along with EKG assessment to detect regional ischemia. The ability to easily distinguish between coronary arteries and veins can be potentially of great benefit. This is particularly important with intramyocardial arteries. Non-coronary collateral flow which interferes with cardioplegic arrest may be beneficial in CCF by improving oxygen delivery during the ischemic period.

Ischemic preconditioning

The 'protective' effect in CCF may be due to 'ischemic preconditioning'. First described by Murray in 1986 it was regarded as the most powerful form of endogenous protection against ischemia-reperfusion injury in most differentiated tissues including the heart. Repeated brief insults of sublethal ischemia followed by reperfusion protects the myocardium during a subsequent prolonged episode of ischemia by preserving the myocardial ATP content and resulting in improved recovery of contractile function after reperfusion. The mechanism may involve adenosine receptors. Experimentally, the phenomenon of distant organ protection has been demonstrated (e.g. preconditioning the kidney may protect the heart). Two windows of protection has been observed: the first is immediately following ischemia and lasts approximately 12 hours and the second operates between 24 and 36 hours after the initial insult. Preconditioning is most likely to benefit patients when it is used to protect against ischemia induced by coronary artery occlusion during surgery. Sequential construction of distal and proximal anastomoses allows increasing areas of myocardium to be reperfused during the procedure. Data suggest that preconditioning or cardioplegia afford similar and substantial protection (first window) of post-ischemic contractile and vascular function, while combination of the two affords no significant additional protection.

Off-pump CABG (OPCAB)

Hemodynamic stability during cardiac manipulation for complex, multivessel OPCAB is critical for optimal myocardial protection. There is concern over myocardial injury caused by transient occlusion and stabilization of the coronary arteries in a beating, working heart. Although intraluminal shunts are used to avoid ischemia during graft anastomosis, blood flow through the shunts can be affected by upstream pressure and inherent resistance, resulting in reduced flow during hypotension or severe proximal stenosis. For these reasons different patterns of active (with a pump) or passive (from the aorta) coronary perfusion are suggested to provide adequate oxygen supply, improving regional ischemia. Devices that offload and support the RV have also been employed, adding to hemodynamic stability when revascularizing the posterior wall of the heart. Ischemic preconditioning has also been used in OPCAB for regional protection.

OPCAB has been associated with reduced metabolic derangement and myocardial damage upon reperfusion. Myocardial protection during OPCAB is multifactorial. Careful, individualized choice of graft sequence and maintenance of stable systemic hemodynamics are of central importance. Recently refined techniques for non-traumatic rotation of the heart and visualization of coronary anastomoses allow precise and controlled grafting of all coronary territories in the majority of cases. Improved anesthesia has facilitated the performance of OPCAB and enhanced outcomes. Studies demonstrated less enzyme release in OPCAB compared to conventional CABG with CPB and cardioplegia. OPCAB may also offer superior protection of other organs although this has not been consistently demonstrated.

The increasing number of elderly arteriopaths needing CABG that cannot be safely performed with aortic manipulation makes OPCAB with 'no touch aorta' technique (pedicled arterial and Y grafts) an attractive approach.

Further reading

1. Murray CE, Jennings RB, Reimer KA. Preconditioning with ischemia: delay of lethal cell injury in ischemic myocardium. *Circulation* 1986; **74**: 1124–36.
2. Casthely PA, Shah C, Mekhjian H et al. Left ventricular diastolic function after coronary artery bypass grafting: a correlative study with three different myocardial protection techniques. *J Thorac Cardiovasc Surg* 1997; **114**: 254–60.
3. Pillai R, Wright JEC. Ventricular fibrillation with intermittent aortic cross clamping in coronary heart surgery. In: *Surgery for Ischaemic Heart Disease*. Pillai R, Wright J (eds). Oxford University Press: New York, 1999: pp 149–54.
4. Buckberg GD. Overview: procedure versus protection: an impossible separation. *Semin Thorac Cardiovasc Surg* 2001; **13**: 29–32.

Related topics of interest

12 Blood conservation

12.1 Pharmacological approach

David Royston

The rationale of any pharmacological intervention in cardiac surgical patients is to avoid the need for transfusion of blood or hemostatic products.

At-risk patient groups

Epidemiological studies in over 14 000 patients have found that prolonged bypass time (>100 min but especially >150 min), increased age, creatinine greater than 200 μmol and procedures other than primary myocardial revascularization alone are risk factors for postoperative bleeding. Recent ingestion of platelet active agents, especially aspirin, has not been shown as a consistent risk factor for excessive bleeding in these recent series.

Prophylactic therapy

The majority of at-risk cardiac surgical patients will receive prophylactic therapy. The available agents for this are either the lysine analog antifibrinolytics (tranexamic acid or epsilon-aminocaproic acid) or the serine protease inhibitor aprotinin.

Lysine analogs
Availability, uses and suggested dose
Epsilon-aminocaproic acid is not available for human use in the UK and many European countries but is used routinely in North America. Tranexamic acid is licensed for prophylactic use in surgical patients with localized fibrinolysis such as those with hemophilia having dental extractions and patients having prostatectomy or conisation of the cervix. Recommended dose for these indications is 0.5–1.0 g three times a day. Total dose should not exceed 50 mg kg^{-1} day^{-1}. There is no specific license for the use of tranexamic acid in patients having cardiac surgery and it is contraindicated in patients with a history of thrombotic disease. Studies in cardiac surgical patients have used total doses between 0.5 and 20 mg.

Efficacy
Drains loss
Meta-analysis showed that drain loss is reduced by about 20–40%. When pooled together an analysis of tranexamic acid dose versus chest tube drainage does not demonstrate a dose–response effect. Reduction in drain losses was not further enhanced by increasing dosage above 1.5 g.

Red cell transfusions

Reduction in transfusion is less consistent. Meta-analysis of data related to epsilon-aminocaproic acid showed no benefit to reduce transfusions. For tranexamic acid there was an overall effect but this was not consistent. There was no evidence of any benefit in patients who may have received aspirin prior to surgery and an inconsistent effect in patients having higher risk surgeries such as reoperations (odds ratio 0.8; CI 0.45–2.3).

Hemostatic product transfusions

There is limited data to show any reduction in the transfusion of hemostatic products in patients receiving tranexamic acid. The largest study reported thus far shows no significant benefit of either lysine analog in reducing the need for hemostatic products after primary myocardial revascularization.

Resternotomy for bleeding

The meta-analysis by Laupacis also showed that the incidence of resternotomy for bleeding was not influenced by the prior administration of tranexamic acid. A second analysis amalgamating data for tranexamic acid and epsilon-aminocaproic acid did show a significant reduction in resternotomy rate.

Safety

There are no formal studies of the safety of lysine analogs in heart surgery. Concerns have been raised about the effects of lysine analogs on renal function. There are no prospective randomized studies that support this concern. There are multiple anecdotal and small series reports of thrombosis and death in patients who have received prophylactic lysine analogs. These reports include drug administration for menorrhagia (thrombotic complications affecting cerebral, renal and retinal vessels), sub-arachnoid hemorrhage and also with complex cardiac surgery. Use of lysine analogs when there is fibrinolysis associated with disseminated intravascular coagulation (DIC) is known to be associated with adverse outcome.

Aprotinin

Availability, uses and suggested dose

Aprotinin is registered for prophylactic use to prevent bleeding and the need for blood transfusions associated with heart surgery. The dose regimen licensed within the UK is administration of a loading dose of 280 mg (2×10^6 KIU: 200 ml of the commercially available solution) followed by an infusion of 70 mg (500 000 KIU) h^{-1}. A further bolus of 280 mg (2×10^6 KIU: 200 ml of solution) is added to the prime volume of the perfusion system to combat the effects of hemodilution. A low-dose regimen (1×10^6 KIU loading and 1×10^6 KIU in pump-prime), without continuous infusion is used in lower risk patients in some centers. There is no evidence to support the use of aprotinin therapy in pediatric practice. There is little evidence for efficacy to reduce use of blood and products in patients having aortic surgery utilizing hypothermic circulatory arrest. The meta-analysis by Levi and colleagues showed a two-fold reduction in mortality in patients given high-dose aprotinin. The reason for this is unknown.

Efficacy

Drains loss and red cell transfusion

Large-dose aprotinin therapy has been shown to be extremely effective, and safe, in preventing blood loss and the need for blood and blood products in patients having open-heart surgery. The current literature contains over 40 reports of randomized placebo-controlled studies which have shown that high-dose aprotinin therapy reduced drain losses (range 35–81%), the total amount of transfusions (range 35–97%) and the proportion of patients transfused (range 40–88%). There is a consistent benefit to reduce transfusions of red cells. This effect appears to be dose-related and is observed in patients undergoing reoperations and in those patients taking antiplatelet agents, as well as in patients considered at lower risk for bleeding and those requiring transfusions.

Hemostatic product transfusions
There is a consistent reduction in the need for platelets, fresh frozen plasma and cryoprecipitate in patients given prophylactic aprotinin therapy. Use of the high-dose regimen is reported to produce a five-fold reduction in need for hemostatic products in higher risk patients. As with drains loss and red cell transfusions there is a dose–response effect on hemostatic product use.

Resternotomy for bleeding
A significant reduction in resternotomy rate is reported in all meta-analysis published thus far.

Safety
There have been multiple studies related to safety aspects of aprotinin therapy. In particular any effects on graft patency and thrombotic risk, renal dysfunction and hypersensitivity reactions have been the focus of most studies.

Thrombotic risk
There are multiple anecdotal reports of thrombosis associated with aprotinin in heart surgery. In other forms of surgery and when there is fibrinolysis secondary to DIC, aprotinin (in conjunction with heparin) is reported to improve outcome and prevent further thrombotic risk. This may be especially relevant in patients having surgery with hypothermic circulatory arrest.

Graft patency, assessed by computed tomography, was unaffected by aprotinin therapy. The largest ($n=870$) multicenter study of graft patency using angiography showed that the apparently higher incidence of saphenous vein graft failure was not significant once other known risk factors for this complication had been fully considered (e.g. distal run off).

Renal function
There is no evidence, from controlled studies, to show a deleterious effect of aprotinin on clearance of water, electrolytes or creatinine. In placebo-controlled studies plasma creatinine was not significantly affected by the use of high-dose aprotinin except in patients after insertion of ventricular assist device. Patients with established renal dysfunction show no deleterious effects of the use of high-dose aprotinin. However, there is evidence to show that the plasma half-life of aprotinin is extended in patients with renal dysfunction. The total dose of aprotinin should be reduced in this situation

Hypersensitivity reactions
The largest series reported thus far was of 248 patients who were known to have received aprotinin previously. Nine of these patients had a hypersensitivity response on re-exposure.

The majority of these were transient flushing and occasionally bronchospasm, but two patients experienced severe cardiovascular effects requiring administration of adrenaline (epinephrine) and noradrenaline (norepinephrine). Hypersensitivity reactions were most common in patients re-exposed within 6 months of the first exposure, primarily the pediatric population. In patients re-exposed more than 6 months after the first exposure the incidence was <1%, which is the same as that reported on first exposure.

Rescue therapy

In patients who are actively bleeding postoperatively there is no evidence for efficacy of the lysine analogs and this therapy has been associated with an increased incidence of myocardial infarction. Placebo-controlled studies have shown that aprotinin will reduce bleeding (but no need for transfusion) when given postoperatively. Entry criteria for this study was loss of >400 ml in 3 hours.

In patients with a post-bypass platelet function abnormality there is evidence that the use of desmopressin (DDAVP) may be beneficial to reduce bleeding. The dose of DDAVP is 0.3 $\mu g \, kg^{-1}$ given in 50 mL of saline and infused over a 20 min period. Significant hypotension occurs in about 40% of patients given this dose.

Further reading

1. Alderman EL, Levy JH, Rich JB et al. Analyses of coronary graft patency after aprotinin use: results from the International Multicenter Aprotinin Graft Patency Experience (IMAGE) trial. *J Thorac Cardiovasc Surg* 1998; **116**: 716–30.
2. Hardy JF, Belisle S, Dupont C et al. Prophylactic tranexamic acid and epsilon-aminocaproic acid for primary myocardial revascularization. *Ann Thorac Surg* 1998; **65**: 371–6.
3. Laupacis A, Fergusson D. Drugs to minimize perioperative blood loss in cardiac surgery: meta-analyses using perioperative blood transfusion as the outcome. The International Study of Perioperative Transfusion (ISPOT) Investigators. *Anesth Analg* 1997; **85**: 1258–67.
4. Royston D. Aprotinin versus lysine analogues: the debate continues. *Ann Thorac Surg* 1998; **65**: S9–S19.
5. Levi M, Cromheecke ME, de Jonge E et al. Pharmacological strategies to decrease excessive blood loss in cardiac surgery: a meta-analysis of clinically relevant endpoints. *Lancet* 1999; **354**: 1940–7.

Related topics of interest

12.2 Non-pharmacological approach

Malcolm Dalrymple-Hay

Introduction

Although transfusion rates vary significantly among institutions, the percentage of patients receiving homologous blood transfusion associated with cardiac surgery is between 60 and 75%. Continuous attempts should be made to reduce this.

Why avoid transfusion?

There are a number of adverse effects associated with the use of banked blood:

(1) Transmission of blood-borne pathogens from homologous donors. (Estimated risk HIV: 1 in 550 000; hepatitis C: 1 in 3300.) The possibility of transmitting spongiform encephalopathies, notably new variant Creutzfeldt–Jakob disease (CJD) via blood transfusions has led to leukodepleted products. The risk of transmission is unknown.

(2) Transfusion reactions; hemolytic, allergic and febrile.

(3) Cost: in some countries blood donors are unpaid; however, the collection, processing, testing, inventory and administration of each unit of blood adds incrementally to the cost of the procedure.

(4) The use of homologous transfusion has been associated with an increased risk of bacterial infection following CABG and a decrease in immune function, which may increase the severity of an infection.

No blood conservation policy is complete without consideration of both pharmacological and non-pharmacological methods. It should always be remembered that meticulous surgical hemostasis is the cornerstone of any blood conservation program. This may be supplemented by judicious blood pressure control and use of positive airway pressure in the early postoperative period. The transfusion trigger (level of hemoglobin) depends on the physiological state of the patient: 9.5 g/dl is generally regarded as a suitable figure for higher-risk patients (elderly, poor lung function, recent myocardial infarction). Lower-risk patients may tolerate a lower hemoglobin level down to 7 g/dl. Appropriate use of transfusion triggers will have an important impact on blood conservation.

Non- pharmacological methods

(1) Autologous blood predonation:
    (i) weeks preoperatively
    (ii) prior to commencement of cardiopulmonary bypass (CPB).
(2) Use cell salvage intraoperatively.
(3) Autotransfusion of washed shed postoperative mediastinal fluid.

Autologous blood predonation: weeks pre-operatively

Autologous blood predonation in this scenario is rarely used in a cardiac setting for a number of reasons: there are a number of generally accepted contraindications, many of which apply to the population undergoing cardiac surgery (see Table 1).

Table 1 Autologous blood predonation: contraindications.

Absolute	Non cardiac	Anemia, hemoglobinopathies
		Hypovolemia, dehydration, malnutrition
		Active bacterial infection (e.g. dental, urinary, cutaneous)
		Significant carotid artery disease, recent transient ischemic attacks
	Cardiac	Unstable angina pectoris
		Significant left main coronary artery stenosis
		Aortic valve disease – stenosis (gradient >70 mmHg, area <0.5 cm^2)
		– insufficiency (syncopal attacks)
		Uncontrolled congestive cardiac failure
Relative		Uncontrolled hypertension
		Body mass <30 kg
		Limited venous access
		Iron deficit
		Intercurrent illness

The 35-day shelf life of packed red cells is also a major constraint as operating schedules must be strictly adhered to, in order to avoid expensive wastage of predonated units.

There is little data available as to the efficacy of this form of predonation in cardiac surgery.

Autologous blood predonation: prior to commencement of cardiopulmonary bypass

Autologous blood can be protected from the damaging effects of CPB by removing one to two units shortly before instituting CPB. This has variably been shown to preserve red cell mass and reduce transfusion requirements. Similar contraindications exist as for predonation but given the ability to commence CPB rapidly these are more flexible.

Alternatively, plasmapheresis can be performed immediately prior to surgery. This has the advantage of removing platelets and clotting factors without reducing red cell mass. The sequestered platelets and clotting factors are spared the detrimental effects of CPB and infused following separation from CPB. There is controversy as to reduction in transfusion requirement and blood loss postoperatively.

Intraoperative use of cell salvage

During the procedure all shed blood not returned to the CPB circuit via the cardiotomy suckers can be scavenged using a cell saver system. Cell savers are able to scavenge all fluid including non-heparinized and heparinized blood.

The fluid is washed, filtered and centrifuged to produce concentrated red cells, the hematocrit and hemoglobin of which are approximately 60 and 20 g/dl, respectively.

No other blood constituents are saved by this method; the washing process has been shown to eliminate platelets, plasma proteins including clotting factors and fibrinogen degradation products.

The use of intraoperative cell salvage has again been variably shown to reduce transfusion requirement postoperatively but a recent meta-analysis concluded in its favor.

A continuous autotransfusion circuit is needed for intraoperative cell salvage for Jehovah's Witnesses patients who would otherwise refuse blood transfusion. The use of recombinant erythropoietin pre-operatively in these high-risk patients to increase the hemoglobin level provides an added margin of safety.

Autotransfusion of washed shed postoperative mediastinal fluid

Shed mediastinal blood is collected via pleural and pericardial drains postoperatively. In some centers this has been reinfused straight back into the patient. Utilizing a cell salvage system this shed fluid can be processed in the cell saver if and when a patient requires a transfusion postoperatively. The washing process removes the abundant fibrinogen degradation products found within this fluid which would otherwise inhibit fibrin polymerization and create a coagulopathy. Clinical trials found no increase in sternal infection and coagulopathy after reinfusion of washed fluid. The oxygen-carrying capacity of these red cells is unknown but it has been demonstrated that red blood cells of shed mediastinal blood have a normal membrane stability (osmotic fragility) compared with circulating red blood cells after CABG, or stored red blood cells.

A minimum volume (approximately 500 ml) of postoperative drainage, however, is required to produce a meaningful volume after washing. Autotransfusion of washed mediastinal fluid has been shown to decrease transfusion requirement.

Further reading

1. Helm RE, Klemperer JD, Rosengart TK et al. Intraoperative autologous blood donation preserves red cell mass but does not decrease postoperative bleeding. *Ann Thorac Surg* 1996; **62**: 1431–41.
2. Scott WJ, Pett SB, Follis F et al. Blood conservation practices; a survey of VA cardiac surgery programmes. *Chest* 1991; **1001**: 945–56.
3. Fergusson D, Blair A, Henry D et al. Technologies to minimize blood transfusion in cardiac and orthopedic surgery. Results of a practice variation survey in nine countries. International Study of Peri-operative Transfusion (ISPOT) Investigators. *Int J Technol Assess Health Care* 1999; **15**: 717–28.
4. Dalrymple-Hay MJR, Pack L, Deakin CD et al. Autotransfusion of washed shed mediastinal fluid decreases the requirement for autologous blood transfusion following cardiac surgery – a prospective randomised trial. *Eur J Cardiothorac Surg* 1999; **15**: 830–4.

Related topics of interest

13 Cardiac intensive care

Neil McGill, Ravi Gill

As many comprehensive texts exist on the subject of cardiac intensive care, this short review will focus on several important aspects of postoperative management: patient transfer, sustained hypotension, oliguria, excessive bleeding, hypothermia and extubation.

Patient transfer

Safe transfer of the patient from the operating room to the intensive care unit (ICU) can only be undertaken when the patient is stable, fully monitored and accompanied by appropriate personnel. The ICU should receive instructions on the arrival time, ventilator settings and drug infusions needed. On arrival at the ICU there should be a systematic handover that details the patient's past medical history, pre-operative evaluation and intra-operative course. This should be followed by a full clinical examination and appropriate investigations (blood tests, imaging, etc.).

Sustained hypotension

The cause can be frequently diagnosed from the history, clinical examination and the charts. The most serious causes include massive bleeding, tamponade and myocardial ischemia, all of which may require immediate re-operation. The physiological causes can be divided into the components of cardiac output (pre-load, contractility, after-load and rate) and systemic vascular resistance. Classically, pre-load is related to end-diastolic fiber length, and can be assessed by measuring end-diastolic pressure (central venous pressure for the RV, and pulmonary capillary wedge pressure or LA pressure, for the LV). The most common reason for reduced pre-load is hypovolemia, although cardiac tamponade, pneumothorax and arrhythmias can also contribute. Optimal pre-load can be estimated by monitoring the filling pressures and/or cardiac output during volume expansion. If the filling pressures increase without improvement in blood pressure/cardiac output, then pre-load is probably optimal. It is important to appreciate that the traditional Beck's triad (hypotension, jugular venous distention and muffled heart sounds) is present in <50% of postoperative cardiac tamponade. Sudden cessation of chest tube bleeding with increased filling pressures, hypotension, reduced ECG electrovoltage and pulses paradoxus may suggest the diagnosis. Confirmation includes mediastinal widening on chest x ray and pericardial fluid/RV diastolic collapse on echocardiography. Tamponade needs immediate drainage.

After-load is related to ventricular systolic wall tension. The normal heart will increase contractility when faced with an increased after-load to maintain stroke volume. This compensation may be limited in the diseased/compromised heart. For the RV it is an increase in pulmonary vascular resistance (from hypoxia, acidosis, hypercapnia) and for the LV an increase in systemic vascular resistance (acidosis, hypothermia, excessive inotropes/vasopressor, hypovolemia) that increases after-load and reduces cardiac output. Treatment is directed at the cause.

Hypotension may result from many arrhythmias. Approximately 30% of all routine coronary surgery cases may develop fast atrial fibrillation postoperatively. Tachyarrhythmias must be treated aggressively with appropriate anti-arrhythmic agents/potassium/magnesium and/or synchronized DC cardioversion. Pacing in an appropriate mode (e.g. sequential AV) for bradyarrhythmia may restore cardiac output.

Surgical trauma, chronic volume/pressure overload, inadequate myocardial preservation, untreated ischemia, hypoxemia, electrolyte and acid–base disturbances may all impair contractility and cause hypotension. Treatment should be directed at the etiology. This involves cardiac output monitoring using a pulmonary artery catheter or echocardiography. Once heart rate, pre-load and after-load are optimized, contractility can be manipulated with inotropic agents. Adrenaline (epinephrine) is a naturally occurring catecholamine with both alpha and beta (beta-1 and beta-2) adrenergic effects. The overall effects are to increase cardiac output through increases in contractility, after-load and heart rate. Although it dilates coronary arteries, oxygen demand will be increased and may outstretch supply. Dobutamine is a synthetic catecholamine with beta-1 adrenergic effects (decrease both pulmonary and systemic vascular resistances). It is less chronotropic than dopamine and may be superior for the treatment of myocardial failure. Dopamine has dopaminergic and beta-adrenergic effects at low dosages ($<5\,\mu g/kg/min$). Dopaminergic action causes vasodilatation in the splanchnic, renal, coronary and cerebral vascular beds. At doses of $5–10\,\mu g/kg/min$ beta-1 receptor effects predominate and at higher doses alpha affects emerge leading to progressive vasoconstriction. Amrinone and milrinone are phosphodiesterase inhibitors with positive inotropic and vasodilating (systemic and pulmonary) effects. They are useful for improving diastolic function post-CPB. Response to inotropic/vasoactive agents should be monitored through cardiac output and hemodynamic studies. If cardiac output remains depressed despite optimum pre-load, inotropic and after-load manipulation mechanical assistance may be considered (intra-aortic balloon pump/ventricular assist devices).

Excessive bleeding

The definition varies but may result from pre-existing or CPB-induced coagulopathies, inadequate heparin reversal and technical problems. The distinction between surgical bleeding and coagulopathy underpins the management strategy. Avoidance of unnecessary blood/blood product transfusion relies on timely and appropriate investigation. Coagulation is assessed on ICU admission to guide subsequent decisions should excessive bleeding occur. Assessment includes activated clotting time, prothrombin time, activated partial thromboplastin time, platelet count and fibrinogen assay. The mechanism of coagulopathy can be further investigated by thromboelastography, which quantifies the viscoelastic properties of the developing clot, and can be conducted quickly and inexpensively. Furthermore, it can assess many different components of clot formation. A normal thromboelastogram, however, does not always exclude coagulopathy as, for instance, the prothrombin time more sensitively predicts deficiencies in the APTT pathway.

Oliguria/anuria

Oliguria (<0.5 ml/kg/h) and anuria (excluding mechanical blockage) may reflect acute renal failure (ARF), a potentially fatal complication following cardiac surgery. Renal ischemia from low output state and pre-existing renal disease are the principal causes among a complex etiology. Chronic/acute elevations in serum creatinine pre-operatively pose major risks for postoperative ARF. Prophylactic use of dopamine, mannitol and furosemide (frusemide) have been met with variable success. Therapeutic measures include ensuring adequate MAP (>75 mmHg) and cardiac index (>2.5 l/min/m²), instituting volume replacement, dopamine and loop diuretics. Hemofiltration/dialysis is indicated in non-responders for volume overload, hyperkalemia, acidosis and uremia.

Hypothermia

Refer to Chapter 9.

Extubation

Extubation should be done by a nurse/physician capable of performing immediate re-intubation and bag and mask ventilation. Appropriate tubes, drugs, suction and ventilation facility should all be present at the bedside. Essentially, in the absence of respiratory disease, pulse oximetry in conjunction with respiratory rate is often sufficient to judge successful weaning: given that the following conditions apply, extubation will probably proceed successfully.

- $SaO_2 > 92\%$ with FiO_2 <0.4
- pressure support < 20 cmH$_2$O and PEEP <5 cmH$_2$O
- respiratory rate <20/min
- core temperature >36°C
- no residual neuromuscular blockade
- cardiovascular stability
- adequate hematocrit (>0.24 in low-risk patients).

In the presence of pulmonary disease or heart failure, correct timing of extubation becomes more critical and should always be physician-led. Early extubation should not be attempted with marginal cardiac function when even brief hypoxia could be dangerous. In patients with heart failure or fluid overload, forced diuresis is often necessary before extubation can proceed. Once cardiorespiratory stability is achieved on full ventilation the respiratory support mode is changed to allow the patient to regulate their own breathing. With sedation lightened and improved pulmonary toilet, the level of pressure support and positive end-expiratory pressure (PEEP) is gradually reduced. Inotropic support is continued until after extubation. Prognostic variables for failure to wean include:

- tidal volume <5 ml/kg
- vital capacity <10 ml/kg
- minute volume <10 l/min
- maximum inspiratory pressure < -20 cmH$_2$O
- respiratory rate/tidal volume (shallow breathing index) >100.

Trends in PO_2, PCO_2, and base excess on blood gas monitoring are more helpful than isolated measurements.

Further reading

1. Bojar RM. Post-ICU care and other complications. In: *Manual of Perioperative Care in Cardiac and Thoracic Surgery. 2nd Edn.* Bojar RM (ed). Blackwell Science: Oxford, 1994: pp 259–98.

Related topics of interest

14 Postoperative complications

Augustine TM Tang, Sunil K Ohri

A number of common events may occur after transfer of patients from intensive care to the ward. They are considered below.

Pyrexia

Differential diagnosis of postoperative pyrexia requires careful clinical assessment of the likely source of infection supplemented by microbiological examination of appropriate specimens (sputum, urine, stool, venous blood, indwelling cannulae, wound exudate). A high index of suspicion must be maintained, coupled with prompt investigations, particularly in the presence of valvular prosthesis/synthetic materials/conduits. Antibiotic treatment should be culture-directed and commenced according to clinical need. Leukocytosis (neutrophilia), tachycardia, rigors and sweats and persistent pyrexia indicate significant sepsis and need for early treatment. Prolonged (>7 days) and mutiple-agent therapy may be required in some situations (infective endocarditis, sternal osteomyelitis, mediastinal sepsis).

Arrhythmia

Tachyarrhythmia

Supraventricular tachyarrhythmia (SVT) can occur in up to 40% of postoperative cardiac patients, with atrial fibrillation and atrial flutter being the most common. Sinus tachycardia without a clear predisposition may herald SVT, prompting some surgeons to advocate treatment. Most SVTs are primary and relate to sympathetic overactivity often exacerbated by metabolic derangements (low serum potassium and/or magnesium). However, secondary causes including hypoxia, pericardial effusion and myocardial ischemia must be considered. Symptomatic patients (palpitations, sweating, hot flushes) without significant hemodynamic compromise may be treated pharmacologically (potassium supplement, amiodarone, digoxin, beta-blocker, calcium channel antagonists, etc.) and monitored. Acute hypotension may require prompt volume replacement and synchronized DC cardioversion. Atrial flutter is generally more responsive to electrical cardioversion than fibrillation.

Bradyarrhythmia

Conduction defects and heart block may give rise to symptomatic bradyarrhythmias. Precise diagnosis of the rhythm disturbance, pre-existing EKG abnormalities, extent of surgery and nature of pathology all guide prognosis and the need for permanent pacing. Ambulatory 24 hour EKG recording may be necessary for decision making in some instances. Intravenous access (central lines preferable) for chronotropic drug therapy and temporary pacing should be gained immediately. Epicardial pacing electrodes introduced at surgery may allow prompt external pacing.

Poor oxygenation

Pre-existing pulmonary disease, recent smoking, acute lung injury (from CPB, barotrauma), pleural effusion, pneumothorax, atelectasis, sputum retention, pulmonary embolism and chest infection rank among the commonest causes of inadequate oxgenation in the early postoperative period. Careful clinical evaluation combined with arterial blood gas measurement and chest x ray usually secure the diagnosis. Early ambulation with vigorous chest physiotherapy are effective preventive measures. Oxygen therapy and ventilatory support (CPAP, BIPAP, Bird respirator, endotracheal ventilation) may be used as supportive treatment while the underlying cause is addressed, e.g. active bronchial toilet (nasopharyngeal suction, mini-tracheostomy and bronchoscopy), antimicrobial therapy or intercostal chest drainage.

Poor urine output

Oliguria often results from a combination of pre-renal and renal causes. Diagnosis relies on reviewing risk factors (age >70, diabetes, hypertension, pre-existing renal impairment or kidney disease, prolonged CPB, low output state), evaluation of fluid balance and volemic state, hemodynamic parameters, peripheral perfusion and biochemical markers of renal function (serum creatinine and blood urea). Hypovolemia is treated by appropriate volume repletion guided by changes in CVP. A low CO state requires careful assessment and appropriate therapy (manipulation of preload, afterload and inotropic action) often combined with invasive monitoring. Diuresis can be induced with loop diuretics, mannitol, aminophylline and metolazone. Dopamine used at a low dose (2.5–4.0 µ/kg/min) often improves urine output by its combined actions on the heart and kidney. Frequent monitoring of serum biochemistry, volume and acid–base status reveal the effectiveness of treatment and predict the need for renal replacement therapy. Nephrotoxic agents (ACE inhibitor, NSAID, selected antibiotics, etc.) should be withheld if not considered essential.

Wound complications

Simple erythema of wound margins may indicate inflammatory reaction to sutures and not infection. Purulent discharge is the hallmark of wound infection. Subcutaneous abscesses must be drained, usually by opening part or all of the wound. Local measures (wound dressings) usually suffice for superficial infections of the conduit harvest site. Microbiological culture of exudate/wound swab may guide antimicrobial treatment in cases of sternotomy wound infection, progressive or deep infection of donor wounds and systemic sepsis. Deep sternal wound infection is often accompanied by copious discharge, sternal instability and chest pain. Diagnosis of mediastinitis and infective sternal dehiscence prompts immediate sternal debridement followed by appropriate repair (rewiring or plastic reconstruction) often combined with mediastinal irrigation (diluted antiseptic/antibiotic solution). Negative pressure therapy with a purpose-designed vacuum dressing system has emerged as a useful tool in bridging to reconstruction particularly for unstable/critically ill patients and those after failure of primary reconstruction. Non-infective sternal dehiscence sparing the manubrium may respond to external chest splinting and observation alone. More extensive or progressive sternal instability requires wound exploration and re-wiring.

Anticoagulation control

Systemic anticoagulation is often indicated following cardiac surgery (prosthetic valvular replacement, atrial fibrillation, dilated cardiac chamber, intracardiac thrombus, coronary endarterectomy) for variable duration. Full anticoagulation within the target range (INR 2.0–4.5 with mitral prosthesis towards the upper range) can be achieved with oral agents (coumarins including warfarin and nicoumalone) but instant effect requires intravenous heparin (monitor APTR: range 2.0–2.5). Warfarin interacts with many drugs commonly used in postoperative cardiac patients (e.g. amiodarone, aspirin, simvastatin and certain antibiotics), resulting in altered anticoagulant effect. Coupled with a delayed onset of action (2–3 days), frequent coagulation monitoring is necessary during hospitalization.

Drugs (diuretics, antiplatelet, ACEI, analgesic, anti-lipid)

A number of pharmacological agents are frequently indicated in the postoperative cardiac surgical patient:

- Diuretics – used temporarily to correct volume overload from pump-prime and fluid retention during the early postoperative phase; may be continued after discharge in chronic heart failure.
- Antiplatelet agents – aspirin, glycoprotein IIb/IIIa receptor antagonists used to mitigate progression of occlusive disease in native coronary vessels and grafts.
- Lipid-lowering drugs – agents used to reduce cholesterol and triglyceride levels have been shown to offer effective secondary prevention against the effects of coronary atherosclerosis.
- Angiotensin inhibitors – ACE inhibitors or angiotensin II antagonists are indicated in patients with impaired ventricular function or chronic hypertension. Monitoring of renal function and serum biochemistry is important. Beta-adrenergic antagonists (carvedilol) may be useful for moderate systolic heart failure.
- Analgesia – mild to moderate pain from surgical trauma is usually controlled effectively by oral analgesics such as acetaminophen, codeine-based products and/or NSAIDs.
- Antiarrhythmic agents – the commonly used drugs (digoxin, amiodarone, beta-blockers, calcium channel antagonists) have many unwanted effects so that their use should be monitored and stopped appropriately. Elective cardioversion following a mandatory period of systemic anticoagulation and transesophageal echocardiography (TEE) to exclude intracardiac thrombus may be necessary in failure of pharmacological cardioversion after 6 weeks of full treatment.

Further reading

1. Bojar RM. Post-ICU care and other complications. In: *Manual of Perioperative Care in Cardiac and Thoracic Surgery. 2nd Edn.* Bojar RM (ed). Blackwell Science: Oxford, 1994: pp 259–98.
2. Lee JH, Geha AS. Postoperative care of the cardiovascular surgical patient. In: *Glenn's Thoracic and Cardiovascular Surgery. 6th Edn.* Vol II. Baue AE, Geha AS, Hammond GL, Laks H, Naunheim KS (eds). Appleton & Lange: Connecticut, 1996: pp 1777–92.
3. Tang ATM, Ohri S, Haw M. Novel application of vacuum assisted closure technique for the treatment of sternotomy wound infection. *Eur J Cardiothorac Surg* 2000; **17**: 482–4.

Related topics of interest

15 Risk stratification and performance monitoring

Sir Bruce E Keogh, Robin Kinsman

Introduction

The popularization of coronary surgery as a new, expensive and very invasive treatment for angina in the early 1970s spawned a careful evaluation of this new therapy. A series of ambitious, randomized studies established the indications for CABG and provided the substrate for risk stratification and prediction of early operative mortality. As a result coronary surgery, with its high volume with an easily definable outcome, is now used as a model for outcome measurement.

Whilst this allows surgeons to offer better informed consent than for many other therapies there is another aspect. The explosion in communications media including popular magazines and the Internet has meant that the public have a growing understanding of risks and benefits from surgery and therefore a greater appreciation of differences in outcomes between institutions. The patient is evolving into a consumer who expects detailed specifications of his treatment and this has brought with it an intolerance of inequalities in quality of care and a burgeoning of healthcare regulation.

The most public examples of this transformation have been the public disclosure of individual surgeon's results for coronary surgery in New York and Pennsylvania and the public inquiry into pediatric cardiac surgical deaths at the Bristol Royal Infirmary in England. On both sides of the Atlantic there is a focus on how to measure institutional and individual surgeons' performance in such a way that takes account of differing casemix and also triggers an early alarm for review in order to ensure transparent levels of patient safety and avoid the ignominy of public disclosure being the first warning sign of inferior performance. This requires individual surgeons to adopt a responsible and professional attitude to regular assessment of their own performance. So what tools are available?

The first and most basic approach is the measurement of simple mortality rates for coronary surgery. For example, in surgery conventional measures of outcome are in hospital or 30-day mortality and length of stay in hospital. This data is widely available in hospital information systems and national Department of Health databases. Data quality varies from country to country but because of the large numbers of cases it permits international comparisons of healthcare provision.

Risk stratification

The above approach has limitations for measuring institutional performance because even neighboring institutions may have different expertise and different casemix. The risk that any one patient will not survive surgery is dependent on a number of different factors, some of which can be quantified (age, gender and co-morbidities). Risk scoring systems attempt to take account of these risk factors and convert them into a numeric risk score, which represents the probability of death or some other outcome for an individual. The higher the score, the greater the predicted risk. Over the years, a variety of risk stratification systems have evolved which range from simple additive systems such as the Parsonnet/Euro scores to highly complex statistical algorithms used by large regional and national databases. These categorize patients into different risk groups which permit rational comparisons of outcomes between groups of patients, institutions and individual surgeons.

It is essential that risk stratification is specific to type of cardiac surgery (e.g. CABG versus valve replacement). Thereafter, age, urgency, LV function, gender and whether the operation is a first or a redo procedure are the most important variables. The scoring for additional co-morbidities brings relatively small incremental benefit to the predictive models. The variables influencing outcome are remarkably similar in different branches of surgery.

Conventionally, surgical results are presented as an average outcome over a given time frame. In practical terms data is analyzed over defined time periods: 1, 2 or 3 years to ensure sufficient case-load analysis. Even so, these short series represent only snapshots in time, which may be unrepresentative of overall performance. Risk-stratified surgical results have been presented as a risk-adjusted mortality ratio (or standardized mortality ratio) which is the observed mortality divided by the expected mortality: average performance yields a ratio of 1. Results are generally analyzed over a 3-year time frame to attenuate chance variability.

Tracking individual surgical performance

A surgeon can monitor performance on a day-to-day basis using the Cumulative Summation (CUSUM) plot. The standard CUSUM chart plots a cumulative number of events against time. In the context of cardiac surgery, an event might be an adverse outcome, such as postoperative death, and time might be defined by the date-order in which operations were performed. In order to standardize the time frames, the first operation would be given the operative sequence number of 1, the second operation, an operative sequence number of 2, and so on. The calculation of the standard CUSUM value is relatively simple. Each of the observed outcomes is given a numerical value: the adverse outcome a value of 1 and other outcomes a value of 0. The end result is a stepwise graph where the average mortality is reflected in the gradient of the plot. This is a useful visual tool for spotting clusters of deaths or a deterioration or improvement in performance, but it is not very sophisticated.

Adding risk stratification enhances the value of the standard CUSUM. In standard CUSUM plots a death attracts a value of 1 so the plot moves up one unit. This is not necessarily a fair reflection of performance. So, in a risk-stratified CUSUM plot a death attracts a value related to the predicted risk of surgery. A patient with a predicted mortality risk of 20% who dies will attract a value of 0.8 rather than 1. Control limits may define good or bad performance.

An alternative way of presenting the same data is the Variable Life Adjusted Display (VLAD) plot (Figure 1). As with the standard CUSUM method, the VLAD may be used to examine any event rate as long as a suitable predictor exists for that event, such as death.

This plot attempts to provide a visual representation of performance against the predicted outcome rate. It may trend up or down over time.

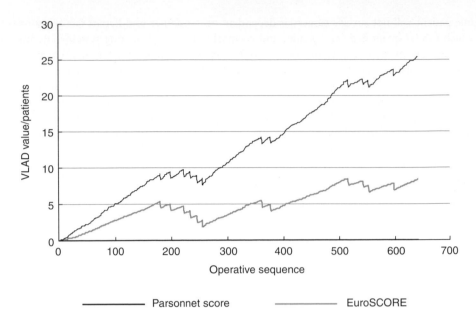

Figure 1 VLAD plots using different risk predictors for a series of 640 consecutive CABG operations at one hospital in the UK.

Effectively, when the analysis begins the VLAD plot is set to zero. If a patient survives the operation, overall VLAD-value increases in a manner that relates to the patient's mortality risk. If the patient had 60% risk of death then the value increases by 0.6, if the patient has 10% mortality risk VLAD-value increases by 0.1, and so on. However, if the patient dies following the operation then the VLAD-value decreases. For the patient with a predicted mortality risk of 10% the decrease would be 0.9, whereas for the patient with a risk of 60% the decrease would be only 0.4. The death of a high-risk patient is therefore weighted.

With each operation the VLAD-value increases or decreases according to the risk of the operation, and at various times the net value will be positive, negative or zero. An overall positive value implies that more patients have survived than one would expect according to the risk model, whereas an overall negative value implies that more patients have died than expected. A zero value is exactly what the risk model predicts. Transitions from overall positive to overall negative values and back again are commonplace and reflect the nature of normal surgical practice.

Mortality is a readily measurable end-point but a poor indicator of quality of care, cost-effectiveness or use of resources. Mortality does not differentiate the average surgeon delivering stable patients from theater from the under-performing surgeon compensated by excellent intensivists. Using death as a benchmark for a surgeon's performance, even with risk stratification, is not particularly sensitive due to the overall low mortality rate. This model may be refined by evaluating morbidity outcomes, such as insertion of an intra-aortic balloon pump postoperatively, new acute renal failure, cardiac arrest and return to theater for a new cardiac procedure, ventilation >72 hours, intensive care stay >96 hours and discharge from hospital >12 days. This approach may take us closer to measuring surgical performance and quality of care in cardiac surgery.

Further reading

1. Parsonnet V, Dean D, Bernstein AD. A method of uniform stratification of risk for evaluating the results of surgery in acquired heart disease. *Circulation* 1989; **79**: I3–I12.
2. Roques F, Nashef SA, Michel P, Gauducheau E et al. Risk factors and outcome in European cardiac surgery: analysis of the *EuroSCORE* multinational database of 19030 patients. *Eur J Cardiothorac Surg* 1999; **15**: 816–22: discussion 822–3.
3. Shroyer ALW, Grover FL, Edwards FH. 1995 coronary artery bypass risk model: the Society of Thoracic Surgeons Adult Cardiac Surgery National Database. *Ann Thorac Surg* 1998; **65**: 879–84.
4. Steiner SH, Cook RJ, Treasure T. Monitoring surgical performance using risk adjusted cumulative sum charts. *Biostatistics* 2001; 2.
5. Lovegrove J, Valencia O, Treasure T, Sherlaw-Johnson C, Gallivan S. Monitoring the results of cardiac surgery by variable life adjusted display. *Lancet* 1997; **350**: 1128–30.

PART B   ADULT CARDIAC SURGERY

16 Myocardial revascularization

16.1 Imaging in ischemic heart disease

Michael Stewart, Huon Gray

A number of techniques are available to investigate ischemic heart disease (IHD), define coronary lesions, and assess their impact on myocardial perfusion and function. Coronary angiography is currently the clinical gold standard.

Coronary angiography

1. Technique

A modified percutaneous femoral Seldinger technique is commonly used. Alternatively, a direct radial/brachial artery puncture or brachial artery cut-down is utilized. After arterial puncture a guidewire is introduced into the artery over which a sheath with indwelling dilator is advanced. Various pre-formed catheters are used to engage the coronary ostia with the Judkins or Amplatz shapes being most popular. A pigtail catheter is advanced across the aortic valve into the LV to perform contrast ventriculography. A transvalvular gradient is assessed on pull-back. On completion, the sheath is removed and hemostasis assured by either manual pressure or a collagen plug.

2. Indications

- Unstable angina.
- Inadequate medical control of stable angina.
- Angina associated with a high-risk non-invasive test.
- Post-infarct (myocardial infarction (MI)) angina.
- Ischemic cardiomyopathy.
- Pre-operative assessment in patients requiring valve surgery.
- Non-invasive test indicating high risk of future cardiac events.
- Multiple risk factors for coronary artery disease (CAD).
- Risk of CAD and occupation rendering diagnosis important.
- Survivors of cardiac arrest.

3. Purpose

To define coronary anatomy and the degree of luminal stenoses. Information is obtained on the location, length, geometry and severity of the coronary lesions and collateral circulation.

4. Limitations

- Inability to detect early intramural atherosclerosis.
- Plaque rupture and thrombosis often involve non-flow limitating lesions presenting as acute coronary syndrome and MI.
- As coronary angiography provides a 2-D picture, views from two orthogonal planes are required to assess complex 3-D coronary luminal lesions.
- Overlying side branches interfere with lesion assessment.
- The absence of normal reference segments in diffuse CAD can underestimate luminal obstruction. Intracoronary ultrasound, pressure wire assessment and stress myocardial perfusion imaging may be required to delineate the functional significance of coronary artery lesions.

5. Risks and common complications (Table 1)

Table 1 Risks and common complications.

Common complication	Risk (%)
Mortality	0.11
Myocardial infarction	0.05
Cerebrovascular accident (CVA)	0.07
Vascular complication	0.43
Contrast reaction	0.37
Local arterial complication	3.0

Risk factors for procedural complications are:

- cardiogenic shock
- within 24 hours of acute MI
- renal insufficiency
- severe cardiomyopathy
- advanced age
- severe vascular disease.

6. Contraindications

- Renal insufficiency, particularly in the presence of diabetes.
- Fever or active infection.
- Acute gastrointestinal bleeding.
- Decompensated congestive heart failure or acute pulmonary edema.
- Severe hypertension.
- Severe anemia.
- Recent stroke.
- Severe coagulopathy.
- Other life-threatening co-morbidities.

7. Standard nomenclature in coronary artery disease.

Clinical investigators in the CASS, Thrombolysis in Myocardial Infarction (TIMI) and BARI trials have standardized descriptions of the coronary artery segments and the severity of coronary artery lesions. Coronary artery location is described with reference to a standard coronary map. Stenosis severity is visually estimated or more accurately determined digitally from a ratio of the minimal luminal diameter to reference vessel diameter. A semi-quantitative measurement of lesion severity is proposed by the TIMI investigators based on contrast flow through a stenosis (Table 2).

Table 2 A semi-quantitative measurement of lesion severity proposed by TIMI investigators.

Contrast flow	TIMI grade
Prompt antegrade flow and rapid clearing	3
Slowed distal filling but full opacification of distal vessel	2
Small flow and incomplete opacification of distal vessel	1
No contrast flow	0

8. X ray projections

- Standard views include right and left oblique.
- Caudal and cranial projections; modified where necessary to achieve optimal imaging of relevant coronary anatomy.

9. Contrast agents

Nonionic contrast agents with fewer side effects are preferred but are more expensive than older ionic counterparts.

Intravascular ultrasound (IVUS)

A trans-catheter ultrasonic probe can be introduced into coronary arteries over an angioplasty wire. Direct imaging of the lumen and vessel wall enables assessment of atheroma and calcification within the vessel. Generally IVUS is undertaken during coronary angioplasty to determine the optimal intervention needed, e.g. stenting.

Intracoronary pressure wire

A fine wire with a pressure transducer allows measurement of the intracoronary pressure. By comparing pressure beyond a lesion with aortic pressure at the catheter tip one can quantify the hemodynamic significance. Flow limitation can be assessed more accurately by measuring the pressure gradient across a lesion after administering a potent coronary vasodilator, e.g. adenosine.

Myocardial perfusion imaging

By comparing two radionuclide images of myocardial perfusion at rest and under stress (exercise or pharmacologically, e.g. dobutamine/dipyridamole), the functional importance of CAD can be accurately assessed. Myocardial perfusion imaging is more sensitive and specific in identifying CAD than exercise EKG. Computerized image analysis and the development of single-photon emission computed tomography (SPECT) further improved its diagnostic accuracy. Pharmacological stress permits the assessment of patients who are unable to exercise. Late redistribution after reinjecting a perfusion agent 4 hours following a rest study may identify hibernating myocardium suitable for revascularization.

1. Perfusion agents

Thallium 201(Tl-201) is a potassium analog which is actively transported into cells via the sodium–potassium pump (Na–K ATPase). This agent is ideally suited for assessing myocardial viability as its accumulation is proportional to regional myocardial blood flow. The initial injection reflects the instantaneous myocardial blood flow. Tl-201 continuously washes in and out of myocardial cells so that its late redistribution reflects the distribution of intracellular potassium, or myocardial viability.

Technetium Tc-99m (sestamibi) is a short-lived radiotracer that mixes with the LV blood pool. It can be used as a rapid bolus injection for first-pass radionuclide angiocardiography or by labeling erythrocytes for equilibrium radionuclide angiocardiography from which ventricular function can be derived.

2. Imaging protocols

A rest–stress protocol utilizing Tc-99m evaluates LV regional and global function. Stress–rest myocardial perfusion imaging, using Tl-201 or Tc-99m, allows visualization of the LV myocardium. Tc-99m produces superior image quality and is the agent of choice for assessing myocardial ischemia. Tl-201 provides a delayed redistribution image without additional radionuclide doses for assessing myocardial viability. Cellular Na–K ATPase activity is deranged in hibernating myocardium. A delayed 4-hour image or repeat study 24 hours later can detect Tl-201 redistribution in hibernating tissue.

3. Drugs interfering with perfusion imaging

Beta-blockers, nitrates and calcium channel blockers should be withheld for ≥48 hours whilst amiodarone and digoxin for 1 week before imaging. If dipyridamole is used, caffeine should be avoided immediately prior to the test

4. Positive emission tomography (PET)

PET utilizes fluorodeoxyglucose (FDG) as radioactive tracer, which is taken up more avidly by ischemic myocardium. The sensitivity and specificity for detecting myocardial viability approaches 90%. PET produces better images than SPECT but has a very short half-life (75 s) and requires immediate scanning at peak stress, usually induced by dipyridamole.

Magnetic resonance imaging (MRI)

MRI may contribute to the assessment of proximal CAD but currently is not routinely employed in clinical practice. MRI is particularly useful for assessing LV function/mass and demonstrating cardiovascular structural abnormalities. With technological advancement, 3-D visualization of the coronary vessels as well as MR coronary angiography is impending.

Further reading

1. British Cardiac Society Guidelines and Medical Practice Committee, and Royal College of Physicians Clinical Effectiveness and Evaluation Unit. Guideline for the management of patients with acute coronary syndrome without persistent ECG ST segment elevation. *Heart* 2001; **85**: 133–42.
2. ACC/AHA/AACP-ASIM. Guidelines for the management of patients with chronic stable angina. *J Am Coll Cardiol* 1999; **33**: 2092–197.
3. Braunwald E. Heart disease. *A Textbook of Cardiovascular Medicine. 5th Edn.* WB Saunders: Philadelphia, 1997.
4. Scanlon PJ, Faxon DP, Audet AM et al. ACC/AHA guidelines for coronary angiography. A report of the American College of Cardiology/American Heart Association Task Force on Practice Guidelines (Committee on Coronary Angiography). *J Am Coll Cardiol* 1999; **33**: 1756–824.
5. Management of stable angina pectoris. Recommendations of the Task Force of the European Society of Cardiology. *Eur Heart J* 1997; **18**: 394–413.

Related topics of interest

1.2   Coronary circulation
2.5   Myocardial metabolism and oxygen flux
5   Cardiac imaging
6   Echocardiography

16.2 Conventional coronary surgery

Sunil K Ohri

Background

Since the development of coronary surgery (CABG) in the 1960s by pioneers such as Favaloro and Johnson, CABG has evolved into many diverse approaches. Conventional CABG may be considered as coronary revascularization using saphenous vein and a single thoracic artery as bypass conduits with CPB. Suitable candidates need to undergo standard investigations such as exercise testing, selective coronary angiography and, when indicated, echocardiography, nuclear imaging and PET scanning.

Indications

These have been well defined by trials in the 1970s of surgery versus medical management, and have been more recently confirmed by meta-analysis. The controversy, which has developed with the advent of angioplasty/stent technologies, surrounds the optimal revascularization approach. Currently, stenting in highly selected patients has a re-intervention rate of 15% at 1 year with increased failure reported in diabetic patients and small vessels. The early (1 year) data of drug eluting stents is promising with restenosis rates of <5% at 1 year. However the long-term efficacy and durability of the surgical approach remains to date the gold standard.

Elective CABG is indicated for patients with:

- severe angina (chronic, post-infarct, recurrent or unstable) despite medical therapy
- left main stem stenosis
- triple vessel disease involving LAD with impaired LV function.

Urgent/emergency CABG is indicated for patients with:

- myocardial infarction with unstable angina/refractory ischemia
- myocardial infarction with refractory ventricular arrhythmias
- myocardial infarction with cardiogenic shock, which may be combined with concomitant procedures such as VSD closure and valvular operations
- acute failure of PTCA and/or stenting (incidence 0.1–0.5%; mortality 10–12%).

Surgical strategy

Choice of conduit

The choice of conduit needs to be tailored to the patients' needs and co-morbid states. Complete arterial revascularization is becoming increasingly popular since the Achilles heel of conventional saphenous vein (SV) conduit is myointimal hyperplasia and late graft failure.

Half of all vein grafts are occluded at 10 years and 50% of patent grafts demonstrate significant stenoses. However, in the modern era of secondary prevention with the routine use of aspirin and statins, vein graft patency is expected to improve. The Cleveland Clinic has shown the substantial advantage of grafting the LAD using the left internal thoracic artery (LITA) compared to SV (11% mortality advantage at 10-year follow-up). LITA patency is >90% at 10 years. More recent data have supported the potential benefit of bilateral ITA grafting, but only when the second ITA is grafted to the circumflex territory. Other alternative conduits include the radial artery (5-year patency of 80%), lesser SV (3-year patency 60%), cephalic vein (5-year patency 45%), cryopreserved homograft vein (1-year patency 15%), gastroepiploic artery (1-year patency 90%), inferior epigastric artery and prosthetic grafts.

Conduit harvesting

The long SV remains the mainstay conduit for grafting non-LAD territories due to its ease of harvest and excellent handling qualities. It has been demonstrated that vein handling and distention play a critical role in venous endothelial injury, which may influence subsequent graft patency. SV should be carefully distended using heparinized autogenous blood. Using bridging incisions rather than one continuous incision or employing endoscopic vein harvesting (EVH) techniques may reduce postoperative morbidity. Two approaches are currently employed for EVH. One approach utilizes a single incision at the level of the knee to insert an endoscopic port. Through the port a dissector can be inserted to create an operating tunnel along the course of the SV. The vein is visualized with attached light source and camera on a color monitor. The operating tunnel is distended with insufflated CO_2 under pressure. The vein is dissected to the sapheno-femoral junction; all tributaries are endoscopically divided with bipolar diathermy. A stab incision at the groin is used to identify and divide the vein. Additional length may be obtained by reversing the vein dissection towards the ankle. The alternative EVH system employs similar principles except that the operating tunnel is held open by dissection and not CO_2. The incisions should not be closed until heparin is reversed with protamine to avoid hematomas; legs should be wrapped in a pressure bandage. The wound morbidity of EVH is <5%, enabling better and early ambulation together with cosmetic benefits. There is no evidence of histologic difference between venous endothelium harvested by EVH or open technique. These techniques have now been successfully employed to harvest the radial artery.

Harvesting of the ITA may be undertaken either as a skeletonized vessel or as a pedicled graft with surrounding muscle and veins. A harmonic scalpel may reduce lateral thermal injury to the LITA. The advantages of a skeletonized vessel include a longer conduit, reduced devascularization of the chest wall and less sternal wound complications; this may be particularly beneficial when bilateral ITAs are planned for diabetic patients. Traction on the sternum should be limited to avoid postoperative neuropraxias and maintain sternal integrity. The LITA should be trimmed to the minimum length required to avoid the distal one-third which has a smaller lumen and is prone to vasospasm. Vasodilators may be applied following harvesting including GTN, nitroprusside, papaverine and phenoxybenzamine. To prevent endothelial injury intraluminal delivery of drugs should be avoided. Thoracoscopic ITA harvesting is usually a prelude to a LAST/MIDCAB, OPCAB, robotic surgery or LAST approach in the awake patient.

Myocardial preservation

There are many approaches including cardioplegia (antegrade and/or retrograde, cold or warm, intermittent or continuous), cross-clamp fibrillation and hypothermia/fibrillation without cross-clamping.

Anastomotic approaches

Hand sewn

- Continuous suturing.
- Interrupted using conventional suture material or nitinol clips.

Automated

Distal anastomotic devices, such as the Ventrica® (Ventrica, Inc., california) magnetic anastomosis, are still undergoing evaluation. Two proximal anastomotic guns are now available for clinical use; both use nitinol stents to secure the vein to the proximal aorta without the need to apply an aortic clamp. The potential neurological advantages remain unproven but potential benefits may be obtained in redoaortas and arteriopaths.

Endarterectomy

This should be avoided whenever possible due to the increased risk of perioperative MI and death. The RCA is often a potential target; alternatively, the PDA may be grafted, which will also avoid subsequent risk of stenosis at the RCA crux.

Redo CABG

Percutaneous stenting of stenosed grafts should always be considered prior to redo CABG as the mortality from the latter is approximately twice that of first-time CABG. This is due to risk of damaging existing grafts on re-entry. A patent LITA graft compounds this problem. Alternative strategies should then be considered such as OPCAB surgery, thus avoiding the need to dissect out a patent LITA for grafting anterior or right-sided vessels. A left thoracotomy may be employed to graft the circumflex territory. Myocardial preservation may be more difficult in the face of diffuse coronary disease, necessitating a combined antegrade and retrograde delivery of cardioplegia and down newly constructed grafts. Old vein grafts should not be handled to avoid coronary embolism. Stenosed vein grafts should not be ligated, particularly to the LAD territory after adding an LITA graft, as LITA flow may be insufficient in the initial perioperative period.

Results

Current operative mortality for elective first-time CABG is 2–2.5% despite a rise in the mean age of patients with more co-morbidities. The attrition rate of venous conduit remains at 2–4% annually. Disease progresses at an advanced rate in the proximal portion of grafted vessels; at 5 years 40% of grafted vessels occlude proximal to patent grafts. Initially 90% of patients attain either complete relief of angina or substantial improvement with increased quality of life. Graft attrition results in recurrent angina in 20% at 5 years and 40% at 10 years.

Further reading

1. Loop FD, Lytle BW, Cosgrove DM et al. Influence of the internal mammary artery on 10 year survival and other cardiac events. *N Engl J Med* 1986; **314**: 1.
2. Dalrymple-Hay MJR, Alzetani A, Costa R, Ohri SK. Endoscopic vein harvesting with the aid of carbon dioxide insufflation. *Ann Thorac Surg* 2001; **71**: 739–41.
3. Yusuf S, Zucker D, Peduzzi P et al. Effect of coronary artery bypass graft surgery on survival: overview of 10-year results from randomized trials by the Coronary Artery Bypass Graft Surgery Trialists Collaboration. *Lancet* 1994; **344**: 563–70.

Related topics of interest

16.3 Arterial grafting techniques

Brian F Buxton, Jai Raman

The type, quality and ultimately the patency of a conduit are pivotal in determining the results of CABG. The current gold standard is the left internal thoracic artery (ITA) grafted to the left anterior descending coronary artery (LAD) which has a failure rate of <1% per year. The most commonly used arteries for CABG are the ITA and radial artery (RaA). The current focus is on the optimal use of these conduits. The gastroepiploic (GEA) and inferior epigastric (IEA) arteries play a minor role.

Grafting strategy

The type of arterial reconstruction depends upon the preference of the surgeon. Common strategies involve the use of one, or both ITA grafts supplemented by one or both RaA. The final configuration will be determined by the number and position of the target arteries, and may be influenced by other factors such as age, on- or off-pump techniques, calcification of the aorta and valve surgery. A number of anastomotic techniques are necessary for the most efficient use of arterial grafts and the ability to achieve extensive and even complete arterial grafting. These techniques are Y-grafting, sequential anastomoses and graft extension. The final decision of how and where to use these techniques is made once the heart is exposed.

Harvesting

ITA

This is usually harvested with a pedicle which contains transversus thoracis muscle fascia, extra pleural tissue, nerves and lymphatics. Skeletonization, where the arteries are removed without any surrounding tissues, or semiskeletonization, leaving the collateral veins, is becoming increasingly popular because of reduced chest-wall devascularization, denervation and sternal infection. Also, additional graft length may result from skeletonization. Where possible, both the right and left ITAs are left in-situ – that is, attached to the subclavian artery and only used as a free graft when length is inadequate. A carefully performed extra pleural technique is favored in elderly patients and those with poor lung function. A skeletonized or semiskeletonized right ITA will reach many of the left- or right-sided arterial targets without a graft extension. Passage of the in-situ ITA graft posterior to the thymus will ensure protection on sternal re-entry.

RaA

Anatomic and physiologic testing provide the basis for safe harvest of the RaA. The modified Allen test is very reliable and has been validated by a number of techniques including oximetry, Doppler ultrasound or digital diastolic artery pressure. Doppler ultrasound assessment has the advantage of providing anatomic, physiologic and pathologic data – e.g. level of the brachial bifurcation, the presence of calcium in the wall of the RaA – and confirms ulnar collateral flow when the RaA is occluded. Return of blood flow to the ischemic hand (within 10 s) with the RaA occluded validates the safety of RaA harvesting.

The RaA has a higher prevalence of intimal disease (fibrointimal hyperplasia or atherosclerosis) compared with the ITA. This is related to age, diabetes, smoking and peripheral vascular disease. Medial calcification (Mönckeberg's arteriosclerosis) occurs more frequently with age. The RaA is usually harvested with its collateral veins using an atraumatic technique with double clipping of the branches. Other techniques such as the use of harmonic scalpel and skeletonization are being investigated. The RaA is harvested from one or both sides: recognized complications include altered sensation, wound hematoma and infection. Avoidance of a leg incision allows early mobilization and may lead to a shorter hospital stay.

Alternative arterial grafts
A number of arterial grafts have been used infrequently, usually when other vessels are not available. They are the GEA, IEA, splenic, subscapular/thoracodorsal, inferior mesenteric, ulnar arteries and the descending branch of the lateral circumflex femoral artery.

Standard grafting techniques

Arterial free graft (AFG)
Arterial free grafts can be used in a similar fashion to SVGs. Proximal anastomosis to the ITA conserves the length of the arterial conduit. The early results suggest there is minimal impact on the patency of the left ITA or the AFG which takes origin from the ITA as a Y-anastomosis. The Y-graft technique is simple to perform and is applicable to OPCAB. It is performed high on the left ITA at about the level where the internal thoracic enters the pericardium. Grafts are brought through the pericardium, the left ITA–LAD anastomosis is performed first, followed by distal AFG anastomosis (commonly, the RaA).

Sequential anastomotic techniques
When the arterial conduit is grafted parallel to the coronary target a longer anastomosis (2–3 times the diameter of the native coronary artery) is constructed and this requires additional length of arterial conduit. The diamond technique is used where the conduit and the coronary artery are anastomosed at a right angle. The size of this anastomosis is kept small to prevent distortion of either native coronary artery or the graft. An advantage of this technique is that a shorter length of conduit is needed.

Graft extension techniques
The use of graft extension techniques increases the flexibility of in-situ ITA grafting, particularly on the right side. Early patency rate of graft extension techniques is similar to that using a direct left ITA to coronary artery anastomosis. Whether there is any reduction of late graft patency through use of extension techniques requires further investigation.

Combined techniques
A common combination is the ITA/RaA Y-grafting technique used in association with sequential grafting. Graft extension with a sequential anastomosis is a less popular technique.

Clinical outcome

Bilateral ITA graft has been shown to improve the clinical outcome. Lytle et al. have shown an improved survival and a decreased re-intervention rate for 2001 patients having bilateral, compared with 8123 with a single ITA graft. Weinschelbaum et al. in 1023 patients, reported an operative mortality of 2.5% for patients having radial and ITA grafts. There was a 98% graft patency in 62 patients at a mean of 25 months. They concluded that revascularization using ITA and RaA grafts is safe and complications are not higher than with SVGing. Tatoulis et al., in 6646 patients who had at least one RaA as the graft of second choice, found that the operative mortality and myocardial infarction rates were 0.8% and 1%, respectively. This observational study confirmed that the RaA was a safe and versatile graft.

Graft patency

The right or left ITA, when grafted to the LAD, has a 10-year patency of 90–95%, with a 1% annual failure rate. The patency rate for the RaA graft at 1 year is about 90% and at 5 years is approximately 87%.

Competitive flow

Should an arterial graft be used for low-grade stenosis (<60%)? Current information suggests that the failure rate of arterial grafting increases 2–3 fold when grafted for low-grade stenosis. Although there is an increased failure rate using the left ITA graft to the LAD with a low-grade stenosis, the 10-year results are superior to saphenous vein. A high tolerance for competitive flow in the ITA compared with the RaA graft has been reported. Coronary stenosis <70% predicted increased failure rate of the RaA compared with a stenosis <40% before an increased failure of the ITA.

Target artery

Grafting of the left- compared with the right-sided vessel offers superior patency.

Free graft versus in situ

Detaching the right ITA from the subclavian artery increases the failure rate by a factor of about 2. Nonetheless, the patency rate of the free right ITA is about 80% at 10 years. Detaching the left pedicled ITA graft reduces long-term patency by only 2–3%.

The size of the arterial graft and the native coronary artery

Studies found no correlation between graft patency and the diameter of either the ITA graft or the recipient artery.

Sequential anastomosis

Angiographic results for sequential anastomosis have generally been satisfactory. However, these angiogram reports have been difficult to evaluate because of the complex pressure gradients and flows in the various segments of the sequential graft. Ochi reported 21 of the 24 sequential GEA grafts remained patent. Dion et al. concluded that sequential ITA grafting optimizes arterial revascularization. The 5-year patency is excellent, identical to that of single ITA grafting and appears similar to early postoperative patency. The need for re-intervention has been extremely low (3.1%) over the whole follow-up.

Y-grafts

The early results for Y-grafts have been favorable, Maniar reported a 99% patency ($n=165$) of the left ITA beyond the 'Y' anastomosis at 1 year. Royse reported 92% patency at 1 year of the left ITA graft beyond the anastomoses ($n=198$). The early patency of the RaA graft proximal to a sequential anastomosis also appears satisfactory; however, there is concern about the fate of the RaA graft distal to a sequential anastomosis. More recently, Royse reported a 25% early graft failure after the sequential anastomosis at 12 months and Maniar et al. have reported a 50% failure rate at 1 year when the RaA is grafted to the distal RCA with a low-grade stenosis.

RaA trials

Trials comparing the patency of the RaA with the saphenous vein and with the right ITA are in progress. The Multicenter RaA Patency Study (RAPS) compares the patency of the RaA with SVGs in the second and third grafting position with the left ITA grafted to the LAD. The Radial Artery Patency and Clinical Outcome (RAPCO) Trial is a randomized study comparing the patency of the RaA with the free RITA or the SVG. About 560 patients have been enrolled in each of these trials since 1996 and results are awaited. The Complete Arterial Revascularization and Conventional Coronary Artery Surgery Study (CARACCAS) compares complete arterial revascularization with conventional coronary artery bypass grafting. The results of all three trials are awaited.

Further reading

1. Buxton BF, Ruengsakulrach P, Fuller J et al. The right internal thoracic artery graft – benefits of grafting the left coronary system and native vessels with a high grade stenosis. *Eur J Cardiothorac Surg* 2000; **18**: 255–61.
2. Dion R, Glineur D, Derouck D et al. Long-term clinical and angiographic follow-up of sequential internal thoracic artery grafting. *Eur J Cardiothorac Surg* 2000; **17**: 407–14.
3. Possati G, Gaudino M, Prati F et al. Long-term results of the radial artery used for myocardial revascularization. *Circulation* 2003; **108**: 1350.
4. Royse AG, Royse CF, Tatoulis J et al. Postoperative radial artery graft angiography for coronary artery bypass surgery. *Eur J Cardiothorac Surg* 2000; **17**: 294–304.
5. Weinschelbaum E, Macchia A, Caramutti V et al. Myocardial revascularization with radial and mammary arteries: initial and mid-term results. *Ann Thorac Surg* 2000; **70**: 1378–83.

Related topics of interest

16.4 Arterial grafting: rationale and outcome
16.2 Conventional coronary surgery

16.4 Arterial grafting: rationale and outcome

David Taggart

The clinical and prognostic benefits of coronary revascularization for certain subgroups of patients with ischemic heart disease are well accepted and each year, on a worldwide basis, approximately 700,000 patients undergo CABG. Most patients require three or more bypass grafts and this is conventionally performed using a single internal thoracic artery (ITA) and supplemental saphenous vein grafts. While CABG provides excellent short- and intermediate-term outcome the long-term results are limited by vein graft failure. The rationale for arterial revascularization is based on the biological, angiographic and clinical superiority of arterial conduits.

Vein graft failure and its consequences

Approximately 10–15% of vein grafts occlude within a month of CABG mainly due to thrombotic occlusion. Over the following years, myointimal hyperplasia results in progressive stenosis of the vein graft so that by 10 years after CABG, 50% of grafts are occluded and half of the remaining patent grafts are severely diseased. In contrast, the patency of left ITA grafts exceeds 90% at 10 years. Aspirin and statins improve vein graft patency rates over the medium term but the long-term benefits remain unproven.

The consequences of vein graft failure are increased mortality, myocardial infarction and recurrence of angina requiring re-interventions in up to one-third of patients within 10 years of CABG. Patients requiring redo surgery face a substantially increased perioperative mortality and morbidity and consume significantly more resources.

Rationale for arterial grafts

1. Biological

Arterial conduits (internal thoracic artery, radial artery (RaA) and gastroepiploic artery) are structurally distinct from coronary arteries but morphologically and physiologically resemble coronary arteries more than vein grafts. The endothelium of arterial conduits, in particular the ITA, produces more nitric oxide (NO) and prostaglandins than vein grafts. NO is a powerful vasodilator and inhibitor of thrombus formation, platelet aggregation and smooth muscle cell proliferation. Furthermore, the laminar flow in the ITA graft, in contrast to more turbulent flow in vein grafts, produces high shear stress, which further stimulates NO production.

2. Angiographic data

Ten years after CABG 90–95% of ITA conduits remain patent and disease-free, whereas 75% of vein grafts are occluded or severely diseased. This difference was initially attributed to the fact that the left ITA was invariably placed to the LAD and that inferior patency rates of vein grafts to other coronary vessels were due to inferior run off in those territories. More recent evidence has demonstrated that arterial conduits, and in particular the ITA, with few exceptions, have better patency than vein grafts, regardless of coronary targets.

Lower ITA patency rates, however, have been observed in the following situations:

- ITA placed to the RCA (due to disease progression at the crux)
- ITA used as a free graft from the aorta (due to size and wall stress discrepancy)
- ITA placed to coronary artery without a severe stenosis (<60%) (due to competitive flow)
- right ITA placed through the transverse sinus (conflicting evidence regarding patency).

The RaA is more prone to spasm than the ITA graft but appears to have better patency rates (about 90% at 5 years) than vein grafts, particularly when postoperative vasodilators (e.g. calcium channel blocker) are used. The long-term patency rate of RaA grafts is, however, not yet known.

3. Clinical results

Even in the absence of data from randomized trials the clinical and survival advantages of a single ITA graft are widely accepted. These were firmly established in 1986 when the Cleveland Clinic reported that the use of an ITA to the LAD, in contrast to vein graft, improved survival (by 11% after 10 years) and reduced the risks of recurrent angina, myocardial infarction and the need for re-interventions.

Although bilateral ITA grafts have been used for over 20 years there have been no randomized trials comparing this strategy to single ITA grafts. In a large observational study with over 8000 single and 2000 bilateral ITA patients, followed for 10 years, the Cleveland Clinic reported survival benefits for bilateral ITA patients, which was observed in all age groups and included diabetic patients and those with ventricular dysfunction. In a meta-analysis of observational studies, involving almost 16000 patients (comprising 11269 single and 4693 bilateral ITA patients matched for age, gender, LV function and diabetes) the bilateral ITA group had significantly better survival (HR for death=0.81, 95% CI: 0.70–0.94). Furthermore, the Cleveland Clinic has reported a marked reduction in redo surgery from 40% in patients with a single ITA to less than 10% in patients with bilateral ITA 10 years after CABG.

Indications for arterial revascularization

- Life expectancy greater than 5 years.
- Younger patients.
- Patients with poor venous conduits.
- Patients with known or suspected aortic disease (OPCAB using pedicled and composite arterial conduits eliminates aortic manipulation).

Contraindications to arterial revascularization

Suggestions that arterial revascularization increases perioperative mortality and morbidity, and in particular the risk of myocardial and respiratory injury, are unfounded. There is a slight increase in the risk of sternal dehiscence in diabetic patients with harvest of both ITA grafts but this can be reduced by using skeletonized harvesting technique. Contraindications to the use of both ITA include:

- obese or diabetic patients
- severe respiratory impairment
- severely impaired ventricular function (need for inotropes may promote spasm in arterial conduits in patients with a limited life expectancy in any event)
- emergency revascularization in hemodynamically unstable patients.

Further reading

1. Loop FD, Lytle BW, Cosgrove DM et al. Influence of the internal thoracic artery graft on 10-year survival and other cardiac events. *N Engl J Med* 1986; **314**: 1–6.
2. Yusuf S, Zucker D, Peduzzi P et al. Effect of coronary artery bypass graft surgery on survival: overview of 10-year results from randomized trials by the Coronary Artery Bypass Graft Surgery Trialists Collaboration. *Lancet* 1994; **344**: 563–70.
3. Lytle BW, Blackstone EH, Loop FD et al. Two internal thoracic artery grafts are better than one. *J Thorac Cardiovasc Surg* 1999; **117**: 855–72.
4. Taggart DP, D'Amico R, Altman DG. The effect of arterial revascularization on survival: a systematic study comparing bilateral and single internal thoracic arteries. *Lancet* 2001; **358**: 870–5.

Related topic of interest

16.5 Off-pump coronary artery revascularization

Gianni D Angelini, Raimondo Ascione

The demographics of the modern surgical population undergoing coronary artery bypass grafting (CABG) include increasing numbers of elderly and other high-risk patients with co-morbid disease. Coronary surgery on the beating heart has emerged to satisfy the demand of minimizing the morbidity associated with cardiopulmonary bypass (CPB), reduction of costs and resource while maintaining quality of care and patient satisfaction. Initially a mini-invasive approach was used through a left anterior small thoracotomy (LAST) to graft the left internal thoracic artery (LITA) to the left anterior descending (LAD) coronary artery. Subsequently, the off-pump coronary artery bypass surgery (OPCAB) via median sternotomy has become a more commonly used procedure due to the need for multiple coronary revascularization. Recent evidence suggests that the OPCAB procedure reduces neurological events, vascular complications, atheroemboli, coagulopathy, vasomotor changes, fever and reperfusion injury to the myocardium and lungs, which are associated, at least in part, to the use of CPB and cardioplegic arrest.

Patient selection

LAST
- Single-vessel disease of the LAD.
- The patients most likely to benefit are those in whom coexistent pathology increases the risks associated with CPB, young patients in whom progression of the disease is likely, elderly patients, and where a midline sternotomy itself carries a possible risk (redo operation).

OPCAB
- There are currently no absolute pre-operative exclusion criteria.

Anesthetic aims

Intraoperative
- Mean arterial pressure at 50–60 mmHg or above with increments of metaraminol 0.5–1.0 mg or volume as requested by hemodynamic condition.
- Heart rate at less than 70 beats per min with increments of esmolol.
- Systemic temperature between 36 and 37°C.

Postoperative
- Forced air warming to reach a stable nasopharyngeal temperature of 37°C.
- Early extubation (2–3 hours).

Surgical techniques

LAST
- Left anterior mini-thoracotomy (8–15 cm) at the 4th or 5th intercostal space to allow the best exposition of the mid-portion of the LAD.
- LITA harvesting under direct vision or via thoracoscopic harvesting.
- Anastomosis facilitated by stabilizer, blower-humidifier, and shunt.

OPCAB
- Following median sternotomy the pericardium is opened with no traction sutures to increase the freedom of heart manipulation.
- Exposition of coronary vessels: the vessels of the anterior wall (left anterior descending and diagonals) are under direct vision, whereas the vessels of the diaphragmatic wall (posterior descending artery) and lateral wall (obtuse marginal branches) need to be exposed with appropriate surgical maneuvers. The operating table is positioned at 20° Trendelenburg to increase the pre-load and assist the tilting and twisting of the heart towards the right. The table is then rotated to the right towards the surgeon. These two maneuvers produce counter-clockwise rotation of the heart and facilitate access to the circumflex system and posterior descending coronary artery. Traction on a folded cotton tape stitched to the posterior pericardium, halfway between the inferior vena cava and the left inferior pulmonary vein, facilitate the exposition of both the posterior and lateral wall.
- Stabilization of all the coronary anastomotic sites around the heart is obtained with a pressure-based reusable device, or alternatively a suction-based disposable stabiliser.
- Coronary incision is then performed and visualization may be enhanced with a blower-humidifier.
- Insertion of an intracoronary shunt, with appropriate size, is performed to avoid myocardial ischemia during the construction of the anastomosis. However, some surgeons prefer coronary occlusion with a suture or silastic sling.
- Anastomosis is performed with Prolene suture according to the chosen venous or arterial conduit and removal of the shunt just prior to tying the knots.

Results

Retrospective experiences from many centers suggest that LAST and OPCAB surgery offer a reduced mortality and morbidity, and similar angiographic results when compared with conventional surgery with CPB and cardioplegic arrest. Furthermore, prospective randomized studies, in elective patients, have shown a similar mortality and a highly reduced postoperative morbidity and cost, while maintaining quality of care, when comparing OPCAB surgery with conventional CABG.

Further reading

1. Calafiore AM, Angelini GD, Bergsland J, Salerno TA. Minimally invasive coronary artery bypass grafting. *Ann Thorac Surg* 1996; **62**: 1545–8.
2. Nataf P, Lima L, Benarim S et al. Video-assisted coronary bypass surgery: clinical results. *Eur J Cardiothorac Surg* 1997; **11**: 865–9.
3. Benetti FJ, Naselli G, Wood M, Geffner L. Direct myocardial revascularization without extra-corporeal circulation. Experience in 700 patients. *Chest* 1991; **100**: 312–16.
4. Puskas JD, Wright CE, Ronson RS et al. Off-pump multivessel coronary bypass via sternotomy is safe and effective. *Ann Thorac Surg* 1998; **66**: 1068–72
5. Ascione R, Lloyd CT, Gomes WJ et al. Beating versus arrested heart revascularization: evaluation of myocardial function in a prospective randomized study. *Eur J Cardiothorac Surg* 1999; **15**: 695–90.

Related topics of interest

16.6 Minimally invasive approaches

Douglas G West, Anthony C de Souza

Introduction

Cardiac procedures are conventionally performed through a sternotomy or thoracotomy, with CPB and cardioplegic arrest to provide a motionless and bloodless operating field. The convenience and safety of this approach is at the expense of considerable trauma to the body. Complications associated with standard incisions and CPB have prompted efforts to minimize access and eliminate or refine CPB.

Minimizing access

Coronary artery surgery

Minimal approaches must offer access to coronary targets, room for CPB or off-pump stabilization and also allow ITA harvesting.

The minimally invasive direct coronary artery bypass (MIDCAB) procedure involves a left anterior small thoracotomy (LAST) incision, permitting a left ITA (LITA) to LAD anastomosis is superior to stenting with a lower re-intervention rate. The incision (8–12 cm) can be cosmetically placed in the submammary fold, with superior reflection of the pectoral muscles, and chest entry is generally through the 5th intercostal space. ITA harvesting through this incision may be limited in length and requires considerable soft tissue and rib retraction. The latter may cause fracture and severe pain. A thoracoscope introduced through either the LAST or a separate lateral port improves LITA dissection. MIDCAB also exposes the diagonal artery but the circumflex territory is best approached through a more lateral left thoracotomy. The right ITA can be harvested for grafting the RCA through a small right minithoracotomy. Excessive postoperative pain is a drawback despite superior cosmesis.

The right gastroepiploic artery may be harvested and anastomosed to PDA or LAD through a sub-xiphoid incision which allows elevation of the rib cage. Division of the diaphragmatic insertion improves exposure but increases postoperative pain.

The partial or ministernotomy requires a shorter midline skin incision followed by a limited superior or inferior midline sternotomy. The bone incision is diverted laterally into an intercostal space. An inferior partial sternotomy ending in the left first interspace is termed the 'C' incision; a superior partial sternotomy ending in the right 4th/5th interspace constitutes the 'J' incision; a mirror image incision (ending in the left 4th/5th space) is the reverse 'J'. Conversion to full sternotomy is simple. Parasternal and transternal incisions have been described but conversion is difficult and the risk of ITA damage limited their popularity.

Valve surgery

Aortic valve surgery has been approached successfully through a 'J' or reversed 'J' sternotomy, allowing access for aortic and right atrium (RA) cannulation. Transverse sternotomy through the 2nd/3rd interspace, preserving the manubrium and sternoclavicular joints, has been abandoned because both ITAs required division. De-airing of the heart is more difficult and flooding of the operative field with CO_2 is commonly employed. The mitral valve has been approached through small right anterior thoracotomy, parasternal or 'C' sternotomy using femoral CPB, trans-septal approach and external retractors to optimize exposure. The Cleveland Clinic popularized partial sternotomy in aortic and mitral surgery. Right parasternal incisions are now rarely used because of bony instability, sacrifice of the right ITA and the difficulty of conversion to full sternotomy.

Thoracoscopic assistance

VATS techniques improve visualization in minimal access procedures, as in mitral surgery, and enhance maneuverability, e.g. ITA harvest. Single lung ventilation $\pm CO_2$ insufflation increase working space within hemithorax.

In MIDCAB totally thoracoscopic ITA harvest is now established. Thoracoscopy improves access to the proximal ITA compared to LAST alone (Table 1).

Table 1 Standard thoracoscopy access ports and instrumentation.

Access ports	Instrumentation
5th interspace mid-axillary line	30° endoscope
3rd interspace anterior-axillary line	Dissecting instrument
7th interspace anterior-axillary line	grasper/Kittner pledget

LITA is mobilized to the 5th interspace using preferably a Harmonic Scalpel® with inherently less smoke and lateral thermal spread. Pericardiotomy parallel and anterior to the phrenic nerve (approximately 2 cm lateral to thymus) usually exposes the LAD. The arteriotomy target is identified and adequate LITA length confirmed. Endoscopic view of a transthoracic needle accurately locates the LAST to directly above the LAD. This technique allows off-pump LITA-LAD anastomosis through a 5–6 cm incision. The pectoral muscles are split and not divided and rib retraction is unnecessary when using a dedicated retractor (Heart Port®). This endoscopic approach – Endo ACAB (Endoscopic Atraumatic Coronary Artery Bypass) – is believed to reduce postoperative pain compared to conventional MIDCAB.

In mitral valve surgery, thoracoscopy improves visualization for both repair and replacement through right minithoracotomy. The endoscope introduced through either the thoracotomy or a separate lateral port provides additional lighting, better exposure of the annulus and the commissures in particular.

CPB modifications

CPB is essential for minimal access valvular surgery and is occasionally used for MIDCAB. Specially designed cannulae facilitate institution of RA-to-aorta CPB through limited incisions. The Heart Port® system provides percutaneous arterial and venous cannulation for femoral CPB. A cannula is threaded through the femoral artery upstream to the ascending aorta for antegrade flow. A balloon 'endoclamp' passed retrogradely into the ascending aorta is inflated to isolate the aortic root, permitting subsequent cardioplegic arrest and venting.

Venous return is provided by a catheter advanced via the femoral vein into the inferior vena cava (IVC) and RA with potential augmentation by internal jugular cannulae draining the SVC. This endovascular technique carries the risk of balloon migration, arch vessel obstruction and aortic damage/dissection. Intraoperative TEE and improved cannulae ameliorated but failed to abolish such complications.

Various small incisions and special cannulae (Seldinger technique) exist for CPB. Flexible vascular clamps, e.g. Chitwood clamp, permit aortic cross-clamping through minimal incisions, thus avoiding the risk of a balloon endoclamp.

Robotic assistance in minimal access

Currently the two commercially available systems – Zeus®/Aesop® (Computer Motion, California) and Da Vinci® (Intuitive Surgical, California) provide multiple robotic arms, controlled remotely by a surgeon using a console incorporating manual commands and visual display. Software miniaturization of the surgeon's movements and elimination of natural tremor enable the robot to 'improve' operative manipulation. Stereoscopic 3-D visualization improves depth perception in an otherwise 2-D image. This technology allows a distant surgeon to conduct or mentor trainees in robotic surgery. Totally Endoscopic Coronary Artery Bypass Grafting (TECAB) has been performed on both the arrested and beating heart using such technology. Multi-vessel revascularization using pedicled ITA grafts has been reported as well as single LITA-LAD bypass. Early angiographic results of robotic anastomoses are acceptable but TECAB is currently very expensive and time-consuming. The ultimate goal of routinely performing off-pump multi-vessel TECAB is still remote. The benefits of TECAB over endo-ACAB are currently marginal, although improved stabilization and visualization may improve the TECAB procedure. The development of conduit-coronary and aorta-conduit anastomotic devices should also aid TECAB development. Alternatively, 'hybrid' revascularization combining TECAB LITA-LAD grafting with coronary stenting may become a reality for multi-vessel disease.

Conduit harvest

Conduit harvesting leaves long scars causing discomfort, wound complications and prolonged hospitalization. Various endoscopic devices are commercially available for harvesting saphenous vein and radial artery conduits. Some involve endoscopic cameras and video assistance (Endosaph®, Endopath®) whilst others resemble laryngoscopes enabling dissection up to 15 cm from the entry incision (Autosuture Mini-Harvest®). Endoscopic techniques are best suited to the thigh where the perivenous plane is easier to develop. This approach has been shown to reduce postoperative pain and wound infection.

Further reading

1. Diegeler A, Thile H, Falk V et al. Comparison of stenting with minimally invasive bypass surgery for stenosis of the left anterior descending coronary artery. *N Engl J Med* 2002; **347:** 561–6.
2. Stanbridge D, Hadjinikolau LK. Technical adjuncts in beating heart surgery. Comparison of MIDCAB to off-pump sternotomy: a meta-analysis. *Eur J Cardiothorac Surg* 1999; **16:** S24–S33.
3. Gillinov AM, Banbury MK, Cosgrove DM. Hemisternotomy approach for aortic and mitral valve surgery. *J Card Surg* 2000; **15:** 15–20.
4. Falk V, Jacobs S, Gummert JF et al. Computer-enhanced endoscopic coronary artery bypass grafting: the da Vinci experience. *Semin Thorac Cardiovasc Surg* 2003; **15:** 104–11.

Related topics of interest

16.7 Percutaneous coronary intervention

Keith D Dawkins

Development

Percutaneous coronary intervention (PCI) was pioneered in Switzerland in 1977 by Andreas Gruentzig who coined the term PTCA (percutaneous transluminal coronary angioplasty). Retrograde transfemoral passage of a balloon-tipped catheter aided by guide-wire positioning under fluoroscopy before inflation ensures precise deployment. Due to technical limitations, early experience related to the treatment of short, proximal, discrete, non-calcified lesions that were remote from branch points.

Barotrauma from balloon inflation results in localized vessel injury and distal embolism. Histological assessment of coronary arteries following PTCA demonstrated so much mechanical disruption and thrombosis that it is surprising the technique works at all.

Early reports confirmed that PTCA could improve coronary stenoses and symptoms of myocardial ischemia. There was no evidence that the procedure improved survival. Furthermore, PTCA was associated with significant early complications (abrupt vessel closure due to arterial spasm, dissection, thrombus formation, acute myocardial infarction precipitating emergency surgery). Angiographic restenosis occurred in 10–50% of patients usually within 6 months. Among the postulated mechanisms of restenosis (early) elastic recoil and (late) fibromuscular hyperplasia from an exaggerated 'healing' response to balloon trauma are probably the major culprits.

As PTCA gained popularity it was supplemented by other devices including atherectomy (directional, extraction and rotational) and facilitated laser angioplasty (excimer and holmium: YAG). Randomized controlled trials showed scanty evidence that these developments improved either short- or long-term results with the restenosis rate remaining unaltered.

Currently over 500 000 PCI procedures are undertaken annually in the USA (estimated >1 000 000 procedures worldwide).

Intracoronary stents

The first intracoronary stent was implanted in 1986. Since then early complications of PTCA are virtually abolished although in-stent restenosis remains a significant problem. In the UK (2001), intracoronary stents were used in 87% of PTCA and the need for emergency CABG had fallen to 0.4%.

Stents need to be biocompatible with low thrombogenicity. Currently there is no perfect stent and >55 varieties are available commercially.

Early clinical observations confirmed the feasibility and safety of coronary stenting. Subsequent randomized trials (e.g. BENESTENT and STRESS) have demonstrated its superiority over PTCA: acute complications were reduced; the lumen diameter achieved was larger in the stented vessels; and late angiographic restenosis was approximately halved. However, these trials were limited to 'simple' de-novo lesions in native vessels; it is clear that complex anatomy (e.g. bifurcations), small vessels, long lesions, vein graft lesions, in-stent restenosis, and treatment of diabetic disease are all associated with more restenosis.

Adjunctive pharmacology

Stent thrombosis was initially reported in approximately 5% of patients frequently culminating in death or major myocardial infarction within the first few days. Antithrombotic therapy evolved from anticoagulants and thrombolytics to antiplatelet agents (aspirin, ticlopidine/clopidogrel) with concomitant reduction of stent thrombosis rate to <0.5%. A series of trials with abciximab (CAPTURE, EPIC, EPILOG, EPISTENT) have demonstrated the efficacy of this platelet IIb/IIIa inhibitor as an adjunct to PCI, particularly in high-risk patients by reducing the impact of platelet microemboli during the procedure.

Early complications

The 'routine' use of intracoronary stents has significantly reduced the frequency of early complications. Ostial dissection of coronary artery, loss of a major side-branch, coronary perforation and balloon detachment are occasionally seen and mostly dealt with by an experienced interventionist without the need for surgical revascularization. The outcomes of CABG following failed PCI are less favorable than elective CABG, with an increase in mortality and perioperative myocardial infarction, and less frequent use of arterial conduits. In some patient subsets including primary PCI for acute myocardial infarction, rescue PCI after failed thrombolysis, salvage PCI for cardiogenic shock, and possibly failed PCI in a patient who has undergone previous CABG, emergency CABG is unlikely to benefit.

Late complications (restenosis)

Stent deployment during PTCA has significantly late outcome. Nevertheless, angiographic restenosis occurs in 15–20% of patients, clinical restenosis in 10%, and target vessel reintervention in 5–10%.

Stent implantation results in platelet activation, a local inflammatory response, triggering intimal hyperplasia and late restenosis (usually <6 months). Diabetics have exaggerated intimal hyperplasia and tend to have small coronaries where this process has a greater impact. Thus recurrence rates of 40–50% have been reported in diabetics.

Drug eluting stents

Recently, it has transpired that neointimal hyperplasia following stenting can be prevented. Using the stent as the local delivery device has led, via in-vitro and pre-clinical animal data, to randomized clinical trials which demonstrated the benefit of such devices over bare metal stents.

Two drugs have been extensively studied: sirolimus (rapamycin) and paclitaxel (Taxol). Both are immunosuppressants with varying effects on the cell cycle with cytotoxic and anti-inflammatory properties (paclitaxel). Other modalities under evaluation include rapamycin derivatives (tacrolimus), anti-inflammatory agents (dexamethasone) and anti-sense gene delivery.

Data from the 'First in Man' registry confirmed the potential of sirolimus which are recently confirmed in the RAVEL and the SIRIUS trials (multicenter, randomized, double blind). Relatively simple lesions were recruited and the angiographic restenosis rate was reduced dramatically in the drug eluting stent arm from 26% to 0% (p < 0.0001) in RAVEL and from 35.4% to 3.2% (p < 0.001) in the SIRIUS trial. These were reflected in the 6-month event-free survival of 96.7% in the treated arm versus 72.9% in the control arm (RAVEL). Both trials demonstrated substantially less restenosis in diabetics with small vessels, a hitherto challenging group for PCI.

Early results from the ELUTES, ASPECT and DELIVER II trial similarly confirmed efficacy for paclitaxel.

These trials have intensive follow-up including angiography and intravascular ultrasound searching for late aneurysm formation and late stent thrombosis. It is clear that both the choice of drug and dosing are important for maintaining patency. Clinical follow-up is presently limited to 3 years and it remains to be seen whether restenosis is arrested completely or merely delayed. If the results of the early drug eluting trials are confirmed in high-risk patients (e.g. long lesions, small vessels, multivessel disease, left mainstem), drug eluting stents may profoundly influence the number and nature of candidates for surgical revascularization.

Primary PCI for acute myocardial infarction

Primary PTCA has been shown to be superior to fibrinolytic therapy for the treatment of acute myocardial infarction (higher acute vessel patency rates, higher grades of coronary flow, less reinfarction, better preservation of LV function, more durable vessel patency and lower mortality). Intracoronary stenting improves all aspects of primary angioplasty. Non-randomized prospective data confirm that systematic stenting is superior to a bailout stenting strategy. Randomized trials of primary PTCA versus systematic primary stenting demonstrated a reduction in major adverse cardiac events and better event-free survival for up to 24 months.

New technology

With lessons learned in carotid stenting, embolic protection devices are now available for high-risk PCI patients. As plaque temperature may reflect inflammatory activity, interrogating a plaque with an intraluminal thermometer coupled with endovascular ultrasound may identify characteristics of a high-risk lesion.

Further reading

1. Kutryk MJB, Serruys PW (eds). *Coronary Stenting: Current Perspectives.* Martin Dunitz Ltd: London, 1999.
2. Joint Working Group on Coronary Angioplasty of the British Cardiac Society and British Intervention Society. Coronary angioplasty: guidelines for good practice and training. *Heart* 2000; **83:** 224–35.
3. National Institute for Clinical Excellence Technology Appraisal Guidance No. 4. *Guidance on Coronary Artery Stents in the Treatment of Ischaemic Heart Disease.* May 2000.
4. ACC/AHA Guidelines for Percutaneous Coronary Intervention (Revision of the 1993 PTCA Guidelines): A Report of the American College of Cardiology/American Heart Association Task Force on Practice Guidelines. *J Am Coll Cardiol* 2001; **37:** 2239 i–xvi.
5. Gray HH, Callum KG. NCEPOD. Percutaneous Transluminal Coronary Angioplasty: a report of the National Con

Related topics of interest

16.8 Surgery versus percutaneous coronary intervention

David Taggart

Surgery

The current rationale for surgical treatment of coronary artery disease (CAD) is based on the results of three large multi-center and several single-center randomized trials of coronary artery bypass grafting (CABG) and medical therapy conducted in the late 1970s. A meta-analysis of these studies by Yusuf and colleagues identified those patients most likely to benefit from CABG. Briefly, these were patients with severe angina and objective evidence of ischemia with certain anatomic patterns of coronary disease (especially left main stem and triple-vessel disease involving the proximal left anterior descending coronary artery) and particularly in the presence of left ventricular impairment.

It should be noted that the trial patients were low-risk by current standards and included few elderly or female patients. Furthermore, both medical and surgical therapies have improved significantly since the trials. There was no use of statins or ACE inhibitors and few patients received an internal thoracic artery. The meta-analysis also emphasized that patients at low risk of death (i.e. predominantly patients with normal ventricular function and two-vessel disease) had little to be gained by surgery.

Percutaneous coronary intervention (PCI)

Gruntzig introduced percutaneous transluminal coronary angioplasty (PTCA), now called percutaneous coronary intervention (PCI) for CAD in 1977. Initial studies comparing PCI versus medical therapy for single-vessel coronary disease suggested a greater symptomatic benefit with PCI, albeit at increased risk of early complications. Furthermore, the best medical therapy at that time did not include statins and ACE inhibitors. Even so, the indications for PCI have increased widely.

The first description of the use of stents during PCI was by Sigwart and colleagues in 1987. In 1994 two trials reported that the use of intracoronary stents was superior to angioplasty alone in reducing angiographic restenosis (from 32% in the angioplasty group to 22% in the stent group: p = 0.02). This was accompanied by a reduction in the need for re-intervention by more than one-third at 6 months. Stents are particularly effective for dealing with dissection of the coronary artery and/or abrupt closure during angioplasty. In practice this has reduced the need for emergency surgery to less than 1%.

Further advances in stent technology along with more invasive interventional techniques and more potent anti-thrombotic drugs such as ticlodipine and clopidogrel have increased the deployment of stents in over 75% of current PCI procedures. Most recently, platelet glycoprotein IIb/IIIa receptor antagonists, such as abciximab and eptifibatide, have been shown to suppress pro-thrombotic activity in the stent, leading to improved short-term outcome.

Nevertheless, restenosis remains the 'Achilles heel' of stents. Pathophysiologically the process is typified by neointimal hyperplasia causing circumferential stenosis. The current rate of in-stent restenosis is in the region of 20%, but appears to be higher in small vessels, in longer or bifurcating lesions and particularly in diabetic patients. The initial promise of brachytherapy to reduce this problem has been unfulfilled while the role of drug eluting stents remains to be defined.

CABG versus PCI

Several trials have attempted to compare CABG and PCI in patients with 'multi-vessel' disease. The major limitation of these trials continues to be the definition of 'multi-vessel' disease. In most trials fewer than 10% of potentially eligible patients have been included and this has resulted in predominantly patients with two-vessel disease and normal left ventricular function. However, this is the very group of patients who were already known not to benefit prognostically from CABG. Consequently, failure to show a survival advantage for CABG over PCI was therefore predictable. The usual reasons for excluding patients from these trials were angiographic demonstration of left main coronary disease, chronic total occlusion and diffuse coronary artery disease, i.e. the typical CABG population who are known to benefit from CABG.

1. CABG versus PCI (without stents)

Two meta-analyses have examined randomized trials comparing CABG and PCI (without stents). The trials showed fairly consistent results. There was no overall survival benefit of CABG, but far better symptomatic relief and a significantly lower rate of need for re-intervention (from 33% in the PCI group to 3% in the CABG group). At 3 years there was a trend towards increased mortality in the PCI group (odds ratio 1.2, 95% confidence interval (CI) 0.97–1.48). At 7 years follow-up in the BARI trial the overall mortality was 16% in the CABG group and 19% in the PCI group ($p = 0.04$). This finding was predominantly due to the difference ($p = 0.001$) in 7-year mortality rates in 353 diabetic patients undergoing CABG (24%) and PCI (44%). In the remaining non-diabetic patients in the BARI trial there was no difference in mortality rates (13% at 7 years for both procedures).

2. CABG versus PCI (with stenting)

A number of randomized controlled trials have compared CABG with stent-supported PCI including the ARTS, ERACI II and SoS trials which recruited patients with multi-vessel CAD. Again, however, most patients actually had two vessel coronary disease and normal left ventricular function. In all studies the need for additional revascularization procedures was greater with PCI, but there was a marked reduction when compared to previous studies using simple balloon angioplasty. In the SoS Trial PCI group, at a median follow-up of 2 years, the observed rate was 21% compared to 6% in the CABG arm (hazard ratio 3.85, 95% CI 2.56–5.79, $p < 0.001$). Similar findings have been reported by the ARTS investigators (1-year repeat revascularization rate 21% PCI versus 4% CABG) and from the ERACI II trial (18-month repeat revascularization rate 17% PCI versus 5% CABG). In SoS patients initially managed with PCI, crossover to subsequent CABG revascularization was reported in 9% of cases. This also represents a 50% reduction from values reported with balloon angioplasty. There were no significant differences in the rates of composite clinical outcomes of death or non-fatal myocardial infarction (combined in some studies with cerebrovascular accident).

In patients with multi-vessel disease, death rates in the PCI group were as expected and comparable between studies (1 year all-cause mortality: SoS 2.5%, ARTS 2.5%).

Surgical mortality in SoS was very low. To some extent this is a reflection of the nature of the trial population with favorable coronary anatomy and surgical risk profile. The mortality rates in the surgical group at 1 year (0.8%) and 2 years (1.6%) remained very low and were below that reported in the ARTS and ERACI II trials. This resulted in an apparent reduced mortality with CABG (PCI 4.5%, CABG 1.6%: hazard ratio 2.91, 95% CI 1.29–6.53, p=0.01). As the absolute number of events is low this could represent the play of chance (of nine cancer deaths in SoS, eight were in patients managed with PCI). A planned meta-analysis will provide more information. When evaluating these trials, it is important to realize that the study populations are highly select and do not truly represent a contemporaneous surgical cohort (e.g. of the 1200 patients enrolled into ARTS, >2/3 of patients had two-vessel disease and normal LV function, a group known not to benefit prognostically from surgery).

Cost benefit analyses from SoS and ARTS have suggested that initial management with PCI is associated with marked cost saving, sustained to 1 year of follow-up (by which time most repeat revascularizations have occurred). However, such cost-saving potential of stenting is undermined by the need for multiple stent deployments, re-interventions and antiplatelet therapies.

Future prospects

To date, the highly select nature of the patients entered into trials of CABG versus PCI has served to illustrate that the two procedures deal with a different spectrum of ischemic heart disease. In appropriately chosen patients (primary PCI for acute coronary syndrome, stenosed vein grafts, unfit for surgery), PCI is an extremely valuable and effective treatment. Significant advances in interventional cardiology over the last decade are now being challenged by the surgical concepts of total arterial revascularization and beating heart CABG.

Further reading

1. Yusuf S, Zucker D, Peduzzi P et al. Effect of coronary artery bypass graft surgery on survival: overview of 10-year results from randomised trials by the Coronary Artery Bypass Graft Surgery Trialists Collaboration. *Lancet* 1994; **344:** 563–70.
2. Pocock SJ, Henderson RA, Rickards AF et al. Meta-analysis of randomised trials comparing coronary angioplasty with bypass surgery. *Lancet* 1995; **346:** 1184–9.
3. Rihal CS, Yusuf S. Chronic coronary artery disease: drugs, angioplasty, or surgery? *Br Med J* 1996; **312:** 265–6.
4. Serruys PW, Unger F, Sousa JE et al. Comparison of coronary-artery bypass surgery and stenting for the treatment of multivessel disease. *N Engl J Med* 2001; **344:** 1117.
5. Gunn J, Taggart DP. Revascularization for acute coronary syndromes: PCI or CABG? *Heart* 2003; **89:** 967–70.

Related topics of interest

16.9 Biological bypass

Rachel H Cohn, Todd K Rosengart

Introduction

For over a century, myocardial revascularization techniques have been developed in an attempt to reperfuse the myocardium. In the 1930s Beck attempted to increase blood supply by grafting omentum to the surface of the heart. This was followed by the Vineberg procedure, which grafted the ITA directly into the myocardium. Pifarré and associates modified the Vineberg procedure by implanting autogenous vein grafts anastomosed to the descending aorta into the myocardium. Since the 1960s the techniques of CABG, angioplasty, and intracoronary stenting have been refined, while direct revascularization techniques have largely been abandoned. With an increase in patients with severe coronary disease which is refractory to medical treatment and unamenable to surgery, direct myocardial revascularization was recommended in the 1990s using laser energy to create myocardial channels to perfuse the heart – transmyocardial revascularization (TMR). The administration of growth factors to stimulate new blood vessel growth (therapeutic angiogenesis) represents a corollary of this strategy. In reality, these 'new' therapies actually represent modifications and enhancements of older needle acupuncture and poudrage techniques.

TMR utilizes laser energy to create channels in the myocardium that can direct oxygenated blood from the LV cavity into ischemic myocardium, bypassing the coronary vasculature altogether. Therapeutic angiogenesis describes the strategy of administering growth factors via a variety of delivery techniques in order to enhance myocardial revascularization. It is debatable whether TMR actually induces the formation of patent channels or whether the injury induced by TMR causes an increase in endogenous growth factors, known to be a natural response to injury, and thereby induces angiogenesis.

Preclinical data and TMR mechanisms of action

Both the holmium:YAG and CO_2 lasers use infrared light to thermally ablate myocardial tissue to create transmyocardial channels. The YAG laser requires multiple cardiac cycles to create a single channel, while the CO_2 laser creates a transmural channel with a single pulse. Both experimental and clinical studies have found no evidence for patency of TMR channels, which has led to the hypothesis that TMR induces inflammation and neoangiogenesis. Although several authors have speculated that laser energy is irrelevant to these effects of TMR, and a needle acupuncture is sufficient, others have shown that only laser and not needle therapy induces changes in vascularization and perfusion.

Animal models have found a relationship between the number of channels created by the excimer laser and perfusion using Tc-99 m-sestamibi, with corresponding increased vessel density. Similar animal work with a CO_2 laser found significant increase in the number of blood vessels per high-powered field (200×) in the ischemic zone of the TMR group compared to the nonischemic zone of the same group. Furthermore, there was more than two-fold increase in the amount of vascular endothelial growth factor (VEGF) mRNA in the ischemic zone of the laser-treated pigs versus control. Further animal work using a model of chronic ischemia has confirmed improvements in myocardial blood flow to the lased region and a trend towards improved resting wall motion with YAG or the CO_2 lasers that was absent in the excimer laser and sham groups.

Although such perfusion data appear to represent a compelling mechanistic explanation underlying TMR effects, an alternative hypothesis proposes that the laser-induced myocardial damage may involve local neuronal tissue. This hypothesis suggests that there is a decrease in anginal symptoms due to cardiac nerve fibers being destroyed during the TMR procedure. Support for this hypothesis has been found in a canine model in which TMR- and phenol-treated areas of myocardium failed to demonstrate a reflex response to bradykinin. However, other studies demonstrating regeneration of nerve endings tend to contradict these findings and fail to explain changes in perfusion seen after TMR. At best, neuronal changes may explain early symptomatic improvement, while angiogenic mechanisms may play a more important chronic role.

TMR clinical trials

Since the early 1990s more than 6000 TMR procedures have been reported worldwide. The most consistent finding in clinical trials thus far has been that TMR decreases anginal symptoms and increases exercise tolerance in the majority of patients, with some evidence for improvement in myocardial perfusion. No difference was found in the 1-year mortality between TMR and medically managed patients. Long-term outcome has been evaluated by Horvath et al. who reported a 7-year follow-up after TMR with a CO_2 laser. Of the 78 patients followed, 81% reported having no angina or being in CCS class I or III at 1-year post-operation. There was no significant change in anginal class levels, with 80% of patients reporting no angina or being in CCS class I or II at 5 years post-operation.

Percutaneous transmyocardial revascularization (PTMR)

PTMR is a catheter-based myocardial revascularization laser procedure. Because of its fiberoptic capabilities, the holmium: YAG laser is preferentially used for this technique. In this technique, light energy is transmitted through an optical fiber contained in a catheter introduced through the femoral artery and directed to the LV cavity, contacting the myocardium, allowing the controlled creation of non-transmural laser channels. Despite initial enthusiasm, recent studies have shown that the outcomes of PTMR were inferior to those of TMR and not statistically distinct from placebo controls. In the only randomized, blinded clinical trial of PTMR (the DIRECT trial), 298 patients were assigned to one of the following treatment groups: LV mapping without channel creation (placebo), 10–15 channels per treatment zone, and 20–25 channels per treatment zone. Of 298 patients, only 10 major adverse cardiac events (3.4%) occurred within 30 months. This study also demonstrated that there was no significant improvement in anginal status or exercise duration following PTMR compared to medical therapy alone (placebo procedure). These findings highlight the importance of placebo effect in angina improvements. This study led to the abandonment of PTMR, but should not undermine the efficacy of TMR, which functions at a higher point on the 'dose–response' curve.

Therapeutic angiogenesis

The classical model of therapeutic angiogenesis is the migration of fully differentiated endothelial cells, migrating from native vessels to generate new collateral vessels. New evidence is emerging which suggests that circulating bone marrow-derived endothelial progenitor cells (EPC) may also migrate when stimulated to ischemic areas, a process referred to as vasculogenesis, which was previously only recognized during embryonic development. There is evidence from animal models to suggest that EPC are mobilized by growth factors such as vascular endothelial growth factor (VEGF).

Animal models of both acute and chronic myocardial infarction have found that a variety of growth factors play an important role. These include acidic fibroblast growth factor (α-FGF), basic fibroblast growth factor (β-FGF), VEGF and platelet-derived growth factor (PDGF). Other factors which are released subsequent to an inflammatory response such as transforming growth factor beta (TGF-β) and interleukin 6 (IL-6) also increase VEGF expression. Both VEGF and β-FGF when delivered by epicardial injection or intra-arterially have been found to limit infarction and restore myocardial perfusion in animal models of ischemia. The mode of delivery and whether direct delivery of the protein or gene transfer should be employed is currently under evaluation, together with the potential long-term toxicity of gene therapy (retinopathy in diabetics and tumor growth).

Both β-FGF and VEGF either as a protein or gene transfer have been utilized in clinical studies involving patients with ischemic heart disease (IHD) and peripheral vascular disease. In patients with peripheral vascular disease, the gene for VEGF has been introduced to initiate angiogenesis and improve perfusion in ischemic areas. Similar findings have been obtained following direct injection of VEGF or of naked DNA carrying VEGF in patients with IHD. Symes et al., in a phase I clinical trial in 20 patients using plasmid DNA coding for VGEF-165, found a reduction in ischemic defects with 7 patients angina-free at 6 months. More recent 3-year follow-up of patients who had undergone FGF injection has found that the early angiographic increase in collateral circulation is permanent. Therapeutic angiogenesis may extend therapeutic options and be utilized alone or as an adjunct to CABG or percutaneous coronary intervention.

Further reading

1. Horvath KA, Arnaki SF, Cohn LH et al. Sustained angina relief 5 years after transmyocardial laser revascularization with a CO_2 laser. *Circulation* 2001; **104**: I81–4.
2. Stone GW, Teirstein PS, Rubenstein R et al. A prospective, multicenter, randomized trial of percutaneous transmyocardial laser revascularization in patients with nonrecanalizable chronic total occlusions. *J Am Coll Cardiol* 2002; **39**: 1581–7.
3. Ware JA, Simons M. Angiogenesis in ischemic heart disease. *Nature Med* 1997; **3**: 158–64.
4. Simons M, Banno RO, Chronos N et al. Clinical trials in coronary angiogenesis: issues, problems, consensus. *Circulation* 2000; **102**: E73–E86.

Related topic of interest

25.7   Cellular cardiomyoplasty

17 Surgery for complications of ischemic heart disease

17.1 Post-infarction ventricular septal rupture

Malcolm Dalrymple-Hay, James L Monro

Introduction

Rupture of the ventricular septum (ventricular septal defect or VSD) following myocardial infarction (MI) was first described in 1845 by Latham. The first successful surgical repair was performed over a century later by Cooley in 1957. Necrosis of septal muscle and subsequent perforation complicates 1–2% of MI and accounts for approximately 5% of early deaths after MI. There is a suggestion that increasing use of thrombolysis and primary angioplasty has decreased the incidence of post-infarct VSD.

Anatomy

Septal rupture is usually associated with complete occlusion of a coronary artery: most commonly anteroapical (60–80%) in location as a result of full-thickness infarction following occlusion of LAD; alternatively, postero-septal rupture (20–40%) following inferoseptal infarction associated with occlusion of a dominant RCA or circumflex coronary artery. In 5–10% of cases the defects are multiple.

Pathophysiology

Two factors contribute to the development of heart failure:

(1) the site and size of infarction
(2) the magnitude of the left to right shunt across the defect.

Clinical presentation and diagnosis

The patients present at a variable time following MI (most commonly 2–4 days) with a deterioration in hemodynamics. This is associated with further chest pain in 50% of patients. There is a new harsh pansystolic murmur heard loudest over the left sternal edge of the 4–5th intercostal space. A precordial thrill may be present and some degree of pulmonary edema is usually present.

An ECG may show new right axis deviation, right bundle branch block or AV block. The chest x ray confirms pulmonary edema. Echocardiography is the most useful investigation. It differentiates post-infarct VSD from acute papillary muscle rupture, demonstrates left to right shunt and documents mitral and tricuspid regurgitation and left and right ventricular function. A Swan-Ganz catheter may provide useful hemodynamic information such as the magnitude of the shunt and measurement of right-sided pressures.

The value of coronary angiography is controversial. It is usually performed if the patient is stable enough to tolerate it. The decision rests between a balance of the benefit associated with documenting the coronary disease and the disadvantages of undertaking angiography in a compromised patient. There is mixed evidence that CABG at the time of repair of the defect improves either early mortality or survival.[1]

Management

Emergency surgical closure of the defect offers the best chance of survival. Percutaneous device closure either as definitive treatment or to improve pre-operative condition has not been widely reported. Treated medically, 40% of patients will die within 48 hours and only 7% are alive at 1 year.

Pre-operative management

The aim is to decrease systemic vascular resistance and therefore left to right shunt, to maintain cardiac output and peripheral perfusion and increase coronary perfusion. This is best accomplished by an intra-aortic balloon pump (IABP), which we advocate in nearly all cases. Where necessary inotropic support and diuretic therapy is started. The patient is hemodynamically optimized without delaying surgery.

A few patients self-select when the VSD is found several weeks or months after the infarct. In these cases prompt surgical correction is not critical.

Patients with cardiogenic shock and multiple end-organ failure, in whom the risk of surgery is very high, represent a difficult challenge. There are some centers that administer a trial of intensive non-operative therapy to try and decrease the operative risk; however, there is little evidence to support this stance in the literature, and each case therefore should be treated on its own merit.

Operative

Surgical repair is undertaken with cardiopulmonary bypass, moderate systemic hypothermia and antegrade blood cardioplegia for myocardial protection. Trans-infarct approach to the VSD is used, with the site of the ventriculotomy dictated by the site of infarction. There is no evidence to support infarctectomy. Complete visualization of the defect may be very difficult in inferior defects and some surgeons divide the IVC to improve exposure.

There are two common methods of repair. The defect may be closed without tension using a pericardial patch. The patch is sewn in with a continuous suture to viable muscle. The patch is deliberately large and lies loosely over the defect. Left ventricular pressure is relied on to hold the patch over the VSD during systole.[2] The patch is brought out through the infarctotomy and the ventricle closed in two layers with Teflon strips. Alternatively, a patch is sewn into left ventricular endocardium to exclude necrotic muscle and the VSD from the left ventriculotomy. This is a repair technique described as infarct exclusion.[3]

In chronic cases the edge of the defect is fibrous and thus readily accepts and holds sutures. In these cases the sutures may be placed through the edge of the defect. Left ventricular aneurysms may accompany these chronic ischemic post-infarct VSDs and the indications for excision/LV tailoring remain the same as for isolated LV aneurysms.

Prior to weaning from CPB patients should be monitored and supported using sequential pacing, RA and LA lines. Following surgical repair left ventricular cavity and stroke volume are proportionally reduced, which therefore requires a higher heart rate to maintain any given cardiac output. Intraoperative TEE is useful for confirming closure of the defect and assessing de-airing and cardiac function in the peri-operative period. An IABP is usually required. Where available, centers may consider the use of mechanical assist devices.

Results

Operative mortality
Depending on the series, 30-day/in-hospital mortality of between 20 and 50% is reported. Factors associated with higher operative mortality include increasing age, presence of pre-operative cardiogenic shock, and site of defect (posterior is worse than anterior). Proponents of the infarct exclusion repair technique report no significant difference in mortality between posterior and anterior defects.

Survival and follow-up
Survival is 75% at 5 years. It is controversial whether CABG at time of repair confers a survival benefit. Many survivors attain a good functional result – 80% NYHA functional class I or II.[4]

Residual shunts across the defect are not uncommon. They usually do not require redo surgery and closure, but each case with its associated morbidity must be carefully considered. Successful percutaneous and operative closure have been reported.

References

1. Dalrymple-Hay MJR, Langley SM, Sami SA et al. Should coronary artery bypass grafting be performed at the same time as repair of a post infarction ventricular septal defect? *Eur J Cardiothorac Surg* 1998; **13**: 286–92.
2. Skillington P, Davies R, Luff A et al. Surgical treatment for infarct-related ventricular septal defects. Improved early results combined with analysis of late functional status. *J Thorac Cardiovasc Surg* 1990; **99**: 798–808.
3. David TE, Dale L, Sun Z. Postinfarction ventricular septal rupture: repair by endocardial patch with infarct exclusion. *J Thorac Cardiovasc Surg* 1995: **110**: 1315–22.
4. Davies R, Dawkins K, Skillington P et al. Late functional results after surgical closure of acquired ventricular septal defect. *J Thorac Cardiovasc Surg* 1993; **106**: 592–8.

Related topic of interest

17.2 Left ventricular aneurysm surgery

Vincent M Dor

Introduction

In the majority of cases LV aneuryms are caused by ischemic heart disease (IHD). Although surgical treatment has been described since the 1950s, the last decade has seen significant changes in its definition and management.

Definition
The classical definition of the LV aneurysm is transmural infarction with dyskinesis (paradox) of the LV. The aneurysmal segment is indicated by an area that puckers and collapses when the LV is vented at surgery. The modern definition has been extended to include akinesia and the term of asynergic LV wall is more accurate.

Surgical technique
The original surgical approaches of Beck (1944), Likoff and Bailey (1955) and Cooley (1958) described resection of exteriorized scarred tissues followed by a long linear suture. This is an easy and safe technique which may be undertaken on a beating or arrested heart but results in sub-optimal LV geometry and hemodynamics in most cases. Consequently, other techniques emerged: Jatene (1985) presented a large experiment using an external circular reconstruction of the LV wall with plication of akinetic septum (10% of patients had patch closure and 20% underwent CABG). Concurrently, Dor (1985) proposed a repair involving a patch inserted inside the ventricle on contractile muscle and excluding all akinetic areas, thus restoring LV geometry. Similar techniques were published such as 'endoaneurysmorrhaphy' by Cooley (1989), or 'tailored scar incision' by Mickleborough (1994). These techniques, termed LV reconstruction (LVR), aim to improve upon results of linear repair.

Post-infarct LV remodeling

Although right coronary occlusion is the most common cause of infarction, the antero-apical-septal area is the most frequently affected. In contrast the posterior/postero-lateral area (RCA and circumflex) is involved in 12–15%; 3–4% have a bifocal localization.

After transmural infarction the affected area undergoes necrosis, fibrosis and subsequent calcification. Remaining unaffected muscle initially hypertrophies but ultimately the LV dilates. With transmural infarction there is often delineation between viable muscle and scarred tissue, which is usually dyskinetic.

Gorlin (1967) demonstrated when >20% of LV wall infarcts LV progressively develops global akinesia. MI triggers a complex and interrelated sequence of events termed post-infarction LV remodeling. This describes the compensatory response of the CVS to infarction, ultimately resulting in progressive spherical dilatation. LV dilatation is initially beneficial as it maintains stroke volume (Frank–Starling Law), but further dilatation increases wall tension (Laplace Law). Neurohormonal adaptations, although initially beneficial, eventually lead to adverse remodeling and progressive ventricular failure.

It is unknown if these deleterious secondary processes occur only when <20% of the ventricular mass is infarcted. Long-term LV volume is a marker of post-infarction ventricular dysfunction and LV end-systolic volume index (LVESVI) is a very important predictor of post-MI prognosis.

With the advent of thrombolysis for MI, early restoration of coronary perfusion prevents transmural infarction. Although the sub-epicardial muscle is salvaged, sub-endocardial muscle may still undergo necrosis. These partially salvaged LV walls show a mixture of viable and scarred myocardium at surgery with evidence of viability during thallium testing, but akinesia with echocardiography/angiography. MRI may define the presence of both scarred and viable myocardium within the same akinetic segment.

The impact of early arterial recanalization to limit infarction and secondary responses to injury is known, but the benefit of a surgical approach and its timing to prevent LV dilation needs further investigation.

LV reconstruction

Circular reorganization of the LV is termed endoventricular circular patch plasty (EVCPP).

Surgical technique

The mitral valve is assessed by TEE. Surgery is conducted with a totally arrested heart. CABG is undertaken, then the LV wall is opened in the center of the depressed area; clots are removed, the endocardial scar is dissected and resected. If the scar is calcified or if spontaneous or inducible ventricular tachycardia (VT) exists, cryotherapy is applied to the edge of the resection margins. In case of mitral insufficiency, the valve is assessed by atrial and ventricular approach and either repaired or replaced. The rebuilding of the LV cavity is initiated by continuous monofilament purse-string suture passed on the junction between scarred and normal muscle and tied over an endoventricular balloon inflated at the calculated diastolic capacity for the patient (50–60 ml/m² of BSA). This endoventricular circular suture restores LV geometry to pre-infarction state and aids selection of patch shape, size and orientation. For antero-septo-apical infarcts, the septum and apex are more involved than the lateral wall. The sutures are placed deeply in the septum, totally excluding the apex, a small part of posterior wall below the root of the posterior papillary muscle and a small portion of lateral wall, above the antero-lateral papillary muscle root. The orientation of this new neck follows the direction of the septum. A patch of Dacron or pericardium is modeled to the size of this neck. Excluded areas are either resected or sutured above the patch.

Alternative techniques

(1) Autologous tissue may be used instead of a synthetic patch: a semi-circle of fibrous endocardial scar mobilized with a septal hinge (when not calcified and free of thrombi), or autologous pericardium.
(2) In cases of posterior or postero-lateral localization: a triangular patch, with its base fixed on posterior or postero-lateral mitral annulus and on the posterior or antero-lateral

papillary muscle root. This allows normal mitral and LV posterior wall geometry to be restored after large endocardectomy. If the posterior papillary muscle is totally involved in the resected scar, the mitral valve has to be replaced and this is undertaken via the trans-ventricular approach.

(3) Necrotic tissues: When repair is undertaken after an acute mechanical complication of MI (septal or free wall rupture), the patch is inserted at the limit between sound and necrotic tissue by transmural U sutures reinforced with Teflon pledgets. The patch is anchored above the septal rupture which is excluded from the LV cavity.

Concomitant surgical procedures

CABG
Revascularization of all diseased coronaries of the contractile area is mandatory. Revascularization of the infarcted area is almost always possible, even when the LAD is not easily opacified on angiography. At 1-year follow-up, >80% of LITA to LAD grafts are patent. CABG was accomplished in 97% of our patients with 90% ITA usage.

Mitral insufficiency
When mitral insufficiency is grade II or more, and mitral annular size is >35 mm, an annuloplasty is mandatory.

Ventricular arrhythmias
Spontaneous ventricular tachycardia (VT) (13% in our series) or inducible VT (25% in our series) is frequent. In such circumstances we have performed sub-total non-guided endocardectomy of the endoventricular scar with cryotherapy to the resection margins.

Applicability of technique for large areas of LV akinesia

This technique may be applied to selected cases with large areas of dyskinesia/akinesia. The latter can be objectively measured by the centerline method and considered as large when >50% of the LV circumference.

Patients with this type of lesion are in congestive heart failure (CHF) with mean PAP >25 mmHg, EF <30%, end-diastolic volume index (EDVI) >150 ml, and end-systolic volume index (ESVI) >60 ml. VT is present in nearly 50% and mitral insufficiency often requires repair (>30%). Simple exclusion of all scarred areas would result in inadequate LV cavity with subsequent LV diastolic incompliance. Surgical technique needs to be appropriately modified to preserve LV dimension (larger patch and more distal purse-string).

Results

Patients with post-infarct LV aneurysm form a heterogenous population with varying mortality. The hospital mortality over a 15-year period for more than 1000 patients who underwent LVR was 7.5%, which has fallen to 4.8% for the last 6-year period, but rises to 8% for patients who had a large area of LV akinesia. EVCPP improves ventricular morphology, systolic and diastolic function and reduces ventricular arrhythmias (controlled in 90% at 1 year).

In long-term follow-up those with a pre-operative ESVI <90 ml and NYHA class II-III, 10-year survival is 80%, compared to 50% for patients in NYHA class IV and ESVI >120 ml.

Further reading

1. Cooley DA, Collins HA, Morris GC et al. Ventricular aneurysm after myocardial infarction: surgical excision with use of temporary cardiopulmonary bypass. *JAMA* 1958; **167**: 557.
2. Jatene AD. Left ventricular aneurysmectomy resection or reconstruction. *J Thorac Cardiovasc Surg* 1985; **89**: 321–31.
3. Cooley D. Ventricular endoaneurysmorrhaphy: a simplified repair for extensive postinfarction aneurysm. *J Cardiac Surg* 1989; **4**: 200–5.
4. Dor V. Left ventricular reconstruction by endoventricular circular patch plasty repair: a 17-year experience. *Semin Thorac Cardiovasc Surg* 2001; **13**: 435–47.

Related topics of interest

17.3 Surgery for ischemic mitral regurgitation

A Marc Gillinov, Delos M Cosgrove

Introduction

Ischemic mitral regurgitation (IMR) is caused by coronary artery disease (CAD) with result-ant myocardial ischemia. In most cases, IMR is a consequence of myocardial infarction (MI). IMR must be distinguished from organic mitral valve disease with coexisting CAD; the latter combination requires different treatment strategies and carries a favorable prognosis. In con-trast, IMR portends a poor prognosis (approximately 50% survival at 5 years irrespective of surgical modality).

Etiology

IMR is caused by myocardial ischemia. As such, this condition is a disease of the left ventric-ular muscle rather than the mitral apparatus itself. In IMR, the valve leaflets and chordae appear normal. Although IMR is most often the result of a completed myocardial infarction, left ventricular dysfunction caused by transient ischemia may also cause IMR. There are four mechanisms responsible:

(1) *Transient myocardial ischemia.* Temporary ischemia causes regional left ventricular dys-function and intermittent mitral regurgitation.
(2) *Functional ischemic mitral regurgitation.* This is the most common form of IMR. MI causes changes in left ventricular, papillary muscle, and mitral annular geometry. In iso-lated annular dilatation (Carpentier Type I), there is lack of central coaptation with otherwise normal leaflets. In Carpentier Type IIIb the mitral leaflets become tethered and restricted (apical tenting), preventing proper systolic coaptation. Echocardiography fre-quently demonstrates restricted leaflet motion and a central jet of mitral regurgitation.
(3) *Ruptured papillary muscle (Carpentier Type II).* Occasionally acute MI causes papillary muscle rupture. This causes acute IMR and intractable pulmonary edema.
(4) *Infarcted papillary muscle without rupture (Carpentier Type II).* Infarcted but unrup-tured papillary muscles may elongate with time, causing leaflet prolapse and mitral regurgitation.

Clinical presentation

The presentation of patients with IMR is quite variable because they have both CAD and mitral regurgitation. Symptoms of myocardial ischemia (angina) or mitral regurgitation (heart failure) may predominate. The presentation depends upon the extent of CAD, left ventricular function, and, to a large extent, upon the mechanism and degree of IMR.

Transient myocardial ischemia

In these patients, chest pain is the most common presenting symptom. The degree of heart failure and pulmonary edema varies with the degree of mitral regurgitation.

Functional ischemic mitral regurgitation

In these patients, symptoms of heart failure generally predominate. However, it is not uncommon to identify asymptomatic 2 or 3+ functional IMR in patients presenting for CABG.

Ruptured papillary muscle

These patients present with pulmonary edema complicating acute MI. The pulmonary edema and new murmur of mitral regurgitation generally occur 2–8 days after MI.

Infarcted papillary muscle without rupture

These patients present with heart failure. Frequently there is some angina related to CAD in viable territories.

Investigations

All patients with suspected IMR should have pre-operative echocardiography to document the degree of mitral regurgitation and quantify left ventricular function under physiologic conditions. Accurate objective measures of regurgitation include regurgitant volume (Rvol >50 ml/beat = severe) and effective regurgitant orifice (ERO >20 mm^2 = severe).

In addition, intraoperative transesophageal echocardiography is essential to determine the precise mechanism of mitral regurgitation and the results of valve repair or replacement. Patients with IMR require cardiac catheterization to assess the coronary anatomy and determine the need for revascularization. In patients with left ventricular ejection fraction less than 30%, positron emission tomography (PET) scanning may be used to determine prognosis and the extent to which myocardial revascularization will improve myocardial function. Patients with more than 40% scar by PET scan have a particularly poor prognosis.

Surgical management

Myocardial revascularization alone

Patients with transient IMR in the setting of active myocardial ischemia usually in the inferior territory are treated by myocardial revascularization alone.

Mitral valve repair

Mitral valve repair is most applicable to patients with functional IMR. Annular dilatation without leaflet restriction is corrected by annuloplasty alone. Circumferential and posterior annuloplasties are equally effective. The use of interrupted sutures and ring-support offers superior outcome to sutures alone. There is a belief that a more rigid ring would maintain the reduction in the septolateral diameter better although the evidence is weak. Repair of ruptured or infarcted and elongated papillary muscles is more difficult.

Mitral valve replacement

Mitral valve replacement with chordal preservation is an acceptable strategy for selected patients with IMR. These include the seriously ill, hemodynamically unstable patients requiring emergency operation and those with a complex regurgitant jet. The latter is often associated with established lateral wall infarct or excessive apical leaflet tenting resulting in pseudo-anterior leaflet prolapse. Furthermore, patients with papillary muscle infarction, with or without rupture, should generally undergo mitral valve replacement. Bioprostheses should be employed, as most of these patients will not survive long enough to experience structural valve deterioration.

Left ventricular remodeling procedures

Patients with severe left ventricular dysfunction and IMR may be candidates for a left ventricular remodeling procedure (e.g. LV volume reduction) in conjunction with mitral valve repair or replacement.

Heart transplantation

Given the poor prognosis in patients with IMR, heart transplantation may be considered in younger patients with severe left ventricular dysfunction.

Surgical results

Operative mortality for IMR is currently 5–13%. Five-year survival is 55%. In the most severely ill patients, results are uniformly poor with mitral valve repair or mitral valve replacement. However, in better risk, elective patients, mitral valve repair confers a survival advantage.

Further reading

1. Dion R. Ischemic mitral regurgitation: when and how should it be corrected? *J Heart Valve Dis* 1993; **2**: 536–43.
2. Gillinov AM, Wierup PN, Blackstone EH et al. *J Thorac Cardiovasc Surg* 2001; **122**: 1125–41.
3. Miller DC. Editorial: ischemic mitral regurgitation: to repair or replace? *J Thorac Cardiovasc Surg* 2001: **122**: 1059–62.

Related topics of interest

18.1 Aortic valve replacement: stented prostheses

R Scott Stuart, William Baumgartner

Aortic valve replacement (AVR) with a prosthetic valve for aortic stenosis and/or aortic insufficiency is well established.

Etiology

Aortic stenosis and/or aortic insufficiency. The major causes of aortic stenosis include:

- congenital bicuspid valve
- calcific or senile degeneration
- rheumatic heart disease.

The pathophysiology of aortic stenosis may be mimicked by supravalvular stenosis or sub-valvular stenosis including idiopathic hypertrophic subaortic stenosis (IHSS) and systolic anterior motion of the mitral valve (SAM). AVR alone will not correct these latter causes.

Major causes of aortic insufficiency requiring valve replacement include all of the above factors with aortic stenosis, since any disease process which restricts leaflet opening may also impair normal valve closure. Additional causes include idiopathic, endocarditis and connective tissue disorders.

Clinical presentation

In valve lesions which are predominantly regurgitant in nature, patients classically present with signs and symptoms of congestive heart failure. In predominantly stenotic lesions, patients complain of the classic triad of angina, syncope, or dyspnea. Investigating these symptoms is particularly important in aortic stenosis since the average life expectancy after onset of these symptoms is only 3 years. Patients who present with symptoms of congestive heart failure alone have an average survival of 1–2 years. Patients with aortic insufficiency who are in heart failure have estimated survival of 75% at 5 years and 60% at 10 years. Regardless of presenting symptomatology, patients with aortic valve disease will invariably have a significant murmur.

Diagnosis

This usually begins with echocardiography (TTE/TEE). Ultimately patients will require cardiac catheterization to investigate:

- valvular pathology
- pulmonary artery hemodynamics
- coronary artery disease.

Indications for surgery for isolated aortic stenosis include:

- peak systolic gradient >50 mmHg with normal LV function.
- aortic valve area <0.75 cm^2/m^2 (adults) and <0.5 cm^2/m^2(children)
- significant symptoms.

Any one of the above indications is sufficient alone to refer the patient for surgery. Peak systolic gradient >25 mmHg with abnormal leaflet motion in patients requiring concomitant cardiac procedure should also be considered for AVR. LVEF <25% need not exclude patients for AVR as their prognosis may improve following surgery although operative risk is increased. The transvalvular gradient in this group is usually apparently low (<30–40 mmHg).

Patients with aortic insufficiency are referred for surgery if they have:

- increasing symptoms of congestive heart failure despite medical treatment
- decreasing LV function despite medical treatment, even without worsening symptoms
- ventricular enlargement (LV end-diastolic diameter >55 mm)
- severe regurgitation in endocarditis.

Evidence shows that early surgery before onset of ventricular dysfunction (EF >50%) improves long-term prognosis.

Treatment

Surgical technique

Standard approach is through median sternotomy (minimally invasive techniques utilize limited parasternal incisions).

Standard cannulation techniques are employed and right superior pulmonary venous venting may be used. CPB is established and the patient is cooled (28–32°C).

Cardioplegia is administered. The route may be antegrade, retrograde, or directly into the coronary ostia after aortotomy. The valve is approached through the aortotomy. An oblique aortotomy is made approximately 4 cm above the root curving towards the non-coronary sinus. This can be extented across the aortic annulus and into the LA should aortic root enlargement become necessary (e.g. Manouguian procedure). This should be considered with the indexed effective orifice area of the intended prosthesis <0.85 cm^2/m^2. The leaflets are excised whilst preserving aortoventricular continuity. Annular debridement may be done with scissors or small rongeurs. It is important to remove virtually all annular calcium. After debridement is completed the aortic annulus, sinuses, and LV are copiously irrigated with saline. Care must be taken to avoid retained calcium particles either in the ventricle or around the coronary ostia. The annulus is then sized with the appropriate prosthetic sizer.

Suturing techniques include:

- simple interrupted
- interrupted horizontal mattress (with or without pledgets)
- continuous
- horizontal everting mattress (with or without pledgets).

The everting technique will reduce the size of the effective orifice and thus one should err towards a smaller prosthesis. With the horizontal mattress technique adjacent sutures should be positioned in close proximity, with each mattress suture spanning no more than 5 mm. Non-everting (simple interrupted) techniques are also acceptable for all prosthetic valves as long as care is taken in the placement of the annular sutures. A supra-annular position may often gain an additional size for a prosthetic valve. Pledgets may be used to reinforce a friable annulus. Great care is taken during suture placement at the commissure between the right and non-coronary cusps. This is to avoid damaging the atrioventricular bundle within the membranous septum. The sutures are subsequently passed through the annulus of the prosthetic valve. The valve is seated onto the annulus and the sutures are tied. With mechanical valves in particular, it is important to ensure that leaflet motion is not impinged by subannular tissue. This is especially true of bi-leaflet valves.

The aortotomy is then closed with a running suture. The aorta is then unclamped with the patient in the Trendelenburg position and de-airing is undertaken from the ascending aorta at the highest point. Additional de-airing maneuvers may be undertaken. Adequacy of de-airing and confirmation of normal valve function are evaluated by TEE.

Postoperative care

Unique aspects include:

- preservation of sinus rhythm and cardiac output
- avoid systolic hypertension (>120 mmHg)
- anticoagulation therapy for mechanical prosthesis.

Some surgeons advocate systemic anticoagulation and others antiplatelet therapy for tissue valves for the first 6 weeks (to allow endothelialization of the Dacron sewing ring). There is no strong data to favor either approach.

Late results

Regardless of the valve type, operative mortality for isolated AVR should be less than 5% in patients with good LV function. Major determinants for late mortality include decreased LV function and advancing age. Long-term freedom from re-operation is lowest with mechanical valves. Mechanical valve deterioration/dysfunction is rare (less than 0.1%). Late prosthetic endocarditis, thromboembolism, and bleeding complications occur at a rate of approximately 1% per patient year. Bioprosthetic valves do not carry the need, nor risk, of Coumadin, and its bleeding complications; however (warfarin) thromboembolic rates are still in the 0.5–1% range per year. Bioprosthetic valves will deteriorate with porcine valves averaging 8–12 years longevity and newer pericardial valves 12–15 years (structural valve deterioration is accelerated in younger patients <70 years at the time of implantation).

Long-term survival is approximately 80–85% at 5 years and 65–80% at 10 years, with the vast majority of patients being NYHA class I or II. Mechanical valve longevity should be unlimited. For stented porcine valves, freedom from re-operation at 10 years is 80% and for stented pericardial valves, 83% at 14 years.

Further reading

1. Boucher CA, Bingham JB, Osbakken MD et al. Early changes in left ventricular size and function after correction of left ventricular volume overload. *Am J Cardiol* 1981; **47**: 991–1004.
2. Bonow RO, Picone AL, McIntosh CL et al. Survival and functional results after valve replacement for aortic regurgitation from 1976–1983: impact of preoperative left ventricular function. *Circulation* 1985; **72**: 1244.
3. Czer LS, Gray RJ, Stewart ME et al. Reduction in sudden late death by concomitant revascularization with aortic valve replacement. *J Thorac Cardiovasc Surg* 1988; **95**: 390–401.
4. Lund O, Pilegaard HK, Magnussen K et al. Long-term prosthesis-related and sudden cardiac-related complications after valve replacement of aortic stenosis. *Ann Thorac Surg* 1990; **50**: 396–406.
5. Aupart MR et al. Edwards aortic pericardial valves. *Ann Thorac Surg* 1996, **60**: 615–20.

Related topics of interest

18.2 Aortic valve replacement: stentless prostheses

Ani C Anyanwu, Asghar Khaghani

Introduction

Stentless valves encompassing xenografts, autografts and homografts are implanted directly to the recipient annulus without use of a rigid sewing ring. Autografts are procured from the same individual (e.g. pulmonary to aortic), homografts (allografts) from the same species, and xenografts from different species. By eliminating a rigid sewing ring these prostheses have increased effective orifice area (EOA) and lower transvalvular gradients than comparable stented counterparts. Furthermore, they preserve natural annular motion better and incorporate less non-biological material. Stentless valves provide the closest anatomical and hemodynamic match to the native valve.

Although homograft replacement of atrioventricular valves has been undertaken, clinically stentless valves are largely restricted to aortic valve replacement (AVR) and pulmonary valve/RVOT reconstruction. In the 1960s, Ross and Barratt-Boyes pioneered homografts as an alternative to the ball-and-cage valve and its associated prosthesis-related complications (thromboembolism and anticoagulation). In the autograft (Ross) operation, the pulmonary valve is excised and transposed into the aortic position, employing a homograft to restore pulmonary artery continuity. With subsequent development of disk valves and stented xenografts, technically demanding homograft insertion was abandoned by many surgeons. Some however, persisted with the technique and their cumulative experience since the 1970s rekindled interest in homografts/autografts and catalyzed commercial development of stentless xenografts through the 1990s.

Valve procurement

Homografts are procured from three sources – autopsies, multi-organ brain dead donors (heart unsuitable for transplantation), and hearts explanted during orthotopic transplantation. Donors should be free from hepatitis and HIV. Valves are 'sterilized' in an antibiotic solution and thereafter either kept fresh in tissue culture and antibiotic solution for use within weeks or cryopreserved for longer-term use. Cryopreservation preserves cellular viability whereas the antibiotic-sterilized valves lose all viability unless used within a few days. Alternatively, explanted valves are kept in an antibiotic-free culture medium immediately after harvest for early implantation. Such 'homovital' valves retain significantly more cellular viability and may equate to a live valve if implanted within 24 hours. A pulmonary autograft is explanted as a cylinder before its immediate transfer to the aortic position without chemical treatment. Stentless xenografts are commercially available as whole roots or isolated valves.

Indications

(1) Younger patients who wish to pursue an active life. Superior hemodynamics allow recipients to engage in strenuous activities with less valve-related limitations.
(2) Small aortic roots. Implanting a stented valve here invariably results in significant residual gradient. A stentless valve root replacement produces satisfactory hemodynamics without further annular/outflow tract enlargement.
(3) Prosthetic and native valve endocarditis. Homografts may be more resistant to infection and are regarded as the prosthesis of choice for aortic endocarditis. Homograft root replacement is particularly useful for excluding aortic root abscess and reconstructing the mitral valve.
(4) Congenital heart disease. Stentless valves can reconstruct ventricular outflow tracts which are congenitally narrow/deficient. They offer further advantages of technical flexibility, growth potential and freedom from anticoagulation.
(5) Surgeon preference as an alternative to stented tissue valves.

Disadvantages

- An appropriate homograft (size, position, preservation) may not be available immediately.
- Implantation can be technically demanding with a steep learning curve. Prolonged CPB and global myocardial ischemia may be detrimental to outcome in some instances.
- Structural valve deterioration (SVD) is more rapid in children/young adults but degeneration rate is slower than the stented counterparts in similar age groups. The likelihood, risk and acceptance of re-operations should be considered carefully. In all but the elderly, it should be assumed that the patient would require re-operation. If the patient rejects re-operation, or the risk of re-operation is prohibitive, a mechanical prosthesis is preferable.

Surgical techniques

(a) Subcoronary
The inflow suture line follows a single plane at the ventriculoaortic junction. The outflow suture line follows the coronet shape along the scalloped margins of the stentless prosthesis so that the implanted valve sits in a subcoronary position. The need for correct graft size and precise alignment renders this technique more technically demanding and prone to valve distortion with resultant aortic regurgitation.

(b) Miniroot
The prosthesis is implanted as an inclusion cylinder within the aortic root with subsequent coronary artery re-implantation. There is less risk of valve malalignment but potential exists for prosthesis compression and distortion if blood accumulates between the miniroot and native aortic wall.

(c) Root replacement
In the modified Bentall technique the valve is inserted as a full root with re-implantation of coronary buttons. As the valve-root complex remains intact, there is virtually no potential

for valve distortion. Size matching is less crucial as even moderate graft–annulus mismatch can be accommodated during implantation. Consequently, it is technically the most forgiving. The major complications include coronary distortion/obstruction and bleeding. This technique is also applicable to repair of aneurysm and dissection of the ascending aorta. Long-term freedom from SVD is reduced compared to subcoronary implantation.

Structural valve deterioration

Viable homografts (cryopreserved or homovital) contain living cells which may elicit an immune response. Without immunosuppression, tissue rejection ensues. Analysis of explanted and post-mortem valves shows that most homografts become acellular within a year of implantation. It is theoretically possible that immunosuppression may improve longevity of homografts as other forms of living valve transplantation where the immune response is either non-existent (pulmonary autograft) or attenuated (heart transplantation) do not suffer from donor cell destruction and late SVD. The toxicity of current immunosuppressive agents, however, precludes routine immunosuppression of homograft recipients.

Prosthetic calcification is a major cause of late SVD in stentless valves despite their superior hemodynamics. Improvements in tissue engineering and anti-calcification treatments specifically addressed this problem but long-term data are awaited.

Operative mortality

In experienced hands, this should match figures for stented AVR (<5%) and is largely determined by the etiology of valve disease, LV function, concomitant procedures performed, age and co-morbidity rather than the choice of prosthesis or technique of implantation. There is, however, a selection bias as most surgeons opt for stented AVR in high-risk patients where a complex procedure may compromise outcome.

Follow-up

Annual echocardiography should identify the onset of significant valve degeneration. Moderate aortic regurgitation or LV dilatation mandate re-operation regardless of symptoms. Less commonly, calcific aortic stenosis may be the indication. Re-operations following autograft implantation are usually related to degeneration of the pulmonary homograft (autograft degeneration is rare).

Long-term outcome

Freedom from SVD was 62% at 10 years and 18% at 20 years. The corresponding 15-year figure was 71% for the homovital homografts (versus 32% for non-vital) suggesting improved long-term results. Freedom from endocarditis and thromboembolism was 93% and 89% at 10 years, respectively. Anticoagulant-related bleeding was rare. Freedom from re-operations was 81% and 35% at 10 and 20 years, respectively. Most valve failures occurred in the second decade following implantation. A second homograft operation can be undertaken with low mortality (3.4%) and good long-term outcomes (10-year freedom from SVD 80%). For patients keen to avoid another re-operation, a mechanical prosthesis can be implanted even when a root replacement was initially performed. Severe homograft root calcification, however, mandates root re-replacement.

Homograft or autograft?

Echocardiography in a randomized trial detected early signs of subclinical dysfunction in some homografts but none in autografts, which could translate into superior long-term outcomes with autografts. However, with increased surgical complexity and risk of re-operation for pulmonary homograft failure, autograft procedures are likely to be confined to children and young adults.

Homograft or stentless xenograft?

Three-year follow-up data in a randomized study have not revealed any clinical or echocardiographic differences between the groups. However, cusp calcification detected by electron beam tomography appears more accelerated in the homografts compared to the xenografts although the implication of this currently remains unclear.

Further reading

1. Aklog L, Carr-White GS, Birks EJ, Yacoub M. Pulmonary autograft versus homograft for aortic valve replacement: interim results from a prospective randomised trial. *J Heart Valve Dis* 2000; **9**: 176–88.
2. Hasnat K, Birks EJ, Liddicoat J et al. Patient outcome and valve performance following a second aortic valve homograft replacement. *Circulation* 1999; **100**: II42–7.
3. Khaghani A, Dhalla N, Penta S et al. Patient status 10 years or more after aortic valve replacement using antibiotic sterilized homografts. In: *Biologic and Bioprosthetic Valves*. Bodnar E, Yacoub M (eds). Yorke Medical Books: New York, 1986: pp 38–46.
4. Melina G, Mitchell A, Amrani M, Khaghani A, Yacoub MH. Transvalvular velocities after full aortic root replacement: results from a prospective randomised trial between homograft and the Medtronic Freestyle prosthesis. *J Heart Valve Dis* 2002; **1**: 54–8.
5. O'Brien MF, Harrocks F, Stafford EG et al. The homograft aortic valve: a 29-year, 99.3% follow-up of 1022 valve replacements. *J Heart Valve Dis* 2001; **10**: 334–45.

Related topics of interest

18.3 Aortic valve repair

Carlos Duran

The first aortic valve commissurotomy was performed by Tuffier in 1913. With the advent of cardiopulmonary bypass, the techniques of bicuspidization, circumclusion and cusp extension were applied with limited success. Further progress was encouraged by successful repair of the atrioventricular valves, awareness of the long-term problems inherent to artificial prostheses and significant improvements in myocardial protection.

Aortic valve conservation is very similar to mitral valve repair in its advantages (avoid anticoagulation) and disadvantages.

Patient selection

The indications for aortic valve repair are determined by:
(1) etiology
(2) valve pathology
(3) degree of regurgitation
(4) patient characteristics.

While the decision to repair a valve with a simple pathology (e.g. annulus dilatation, commissural fusion, single prolapse) is easy, heavily calcified valves must be replaced. Moderate rheumatic or degenerative aortic lesions associated with a repaired mitral valve are the ideal cases for repair. Similarly, repair will at least delay re-operation while avoiding the long-term problems of prosthesis in ischemic patients requiring revascularization who have a moderate stenotic or regurgitant lesion, and where either ignoring or replacing the aortic valve is unsatisfactory. Young patients with severe regurgitation, where permanent anticoagulation is unreliable, can be offered cusp extension with glutaraldehyde-treated autologous pericardium.

Intraoperative transesophageal echocardiography

As in mitral repair, intraoperative transesophageal echocardiography (TEE) is an essential tool for pre- and post-repair evaluation. Long- and short-axis views should be used to determine the degree of annulus and sino-tubular dilatation, the location and degree of cusp prolapse or fusion, the location of calcific nodules, and leaflet mobility and coaptation. These data should serve as a roadmap for the selection of the appropriate conservative surgical maneuvers. Although there are a number of indirect indicators of the success of surgical repair (such as pulse pressure, absence of diastolic thrill and murmur, and left ventricular vent return), if available, TEE is the gold standard.

Surgical pathology and techniques

Aortic valve lesions are traditionally classified as stenotic, regurgitant or mixed. This clinically useful classification, however, fails to facilitate planning of conservative surgery. Grouping of pathologies based on cusp mobility should be used because it can better determine the type of repair required. Basically, lesions can be classified as normal, increased or decreased mobility (Figure 1).

1. Normal mobility

Normal mobility is found with aortic regurgitation due to cusp perforation, rupture or, more often, lack of leaflet coaptation. Perforations usually from healed endocarditis are treated with patch closure with glutaraldehyde-treated pericardium. Leaflet rupture cannot be resuspended because of the resulting lack of tissue. Lack of leaflet coaptation can be due to isolated dilatation of the annulus, the sino-tubular junction or, more frequently, involves aneurysmal dilatation of the whole aortic root. Isolated aortic annulus dilatation is rare. Several techniques are being used today:

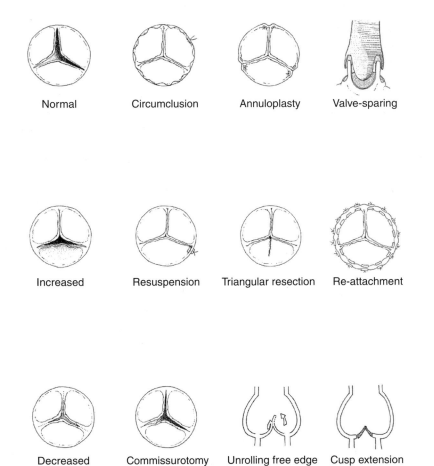

Normal   Circumclusion   Annuloplasty   Valve-sparing

Increased   Resuspension   Triangular resection   Re-attachment

Decreased   Commissurotomy   Unrolling free edge   Cusp extension

Figure 1 Aortic valve repair techniques according to leaflet mobility.

1.1 Circumclusion

The aortic lumen is reduced by passing circumferentially an intraluminal suture that, crossing the commissures, follows the lower aspect of each sinus of Valsalva and is tied outside the aorta, opposite the non-coronary sinus. We do not favor this technique because, being in a single plane, it ignores the scalloped configuration of the aortic annulus and distorts the sinuses. It is, however, being used successfully in the Ross procedure to compensate for significant disparity between the patient's aortic orifice and the pulmonary autograft.

1.2 Commissural annuloplasty

A constricting pledgeted 'U' suture is passed through the aortic wall on either side of each commissure. The suture and pledgets should not come into contact with the adjacent cusp. When tied, it plicates the aorta, reducing its circumference and displacing the commissures medially. This often complements other repair techniques in rheumatic or congenital cases. It reduces a non-dilated annulus to compensate for deficient leaflet tissue.

1.3 Sino-tubular constriction

A pericardial or Dacron band surrounding the aorta at the level of the junction reduces its diameter. This simple maneuver can often abolish mild-to-moderate regurgitation.

1.4 Root replacement

Aortic root dilatation from various pathologies (e.g. Marfan syndrome) is the most common cause of pure aortic regurgitation. The entire aortic root and ascending aorta become aneurysmal, thus predisposing to dissection. To avoid increased operative mortality associated with non-elective presentation, surgery is indicated when aortic diameter exceeds 5 cm. Standard treatment is with aortic root replacement utilizing either the conventional (Bentall–DeBono procedure) or a variety of 'valve-sparing' techniques. In the hands of its author, the results of the Yacoub technique have been excellent with an overall operative mortality of less than 5% and nil in elective cases. The 10-year actuarial survival rate was 94% for aneurysms, 75% for chronic dissections and 63% for acute dissections. Recently, a number of technical modifications have been introduced particularly directed towards supporting the aortic valve annulus.

2. Increased mobility

These lesions result from cusp prolapse due to either aortic dissection or elongation of the cusp free edge with sagging of the leaflet body.

2.1 Commissural reattachment

A strip of Teflon felt is placed between the dissected aortic wall layers, which are closed with pledgeted sutures. The advent of biological glues that are placed between the layers has significantly simplified this technique.

2.2 Leaflet resuspension

This is probably one of the oldest and most successful repair techniques. Resuspension of the free edge is simplified by temporarily joining the three nodules of Arantius with a suture so that the amount of redundant free edge can be determined. A small pledgeted suture placed in the elongated free edge anchors it to the aortic wall close to the commissure. Although this technique is mostly applied to regurgitations due to an unsupported leaflet above a ventricular septal defect, it can also be used in other pathologies where there is free-edge elongation such as bicuspid valves.

2.3 Leaflet triangular resection
The base of the triangle is the free edge with its apex directed towards the leaflet base. The resulting gap is closed with interrupted sutures. Although some authors have described good results with this technique, the difficulty of determining the amount of resection and the friability of the cusp tissue has severely limited its popularity.

3. Reduced cusp mobility
Reduced cusp mobility is most often secondary to rheumatic fever. Variable degrees of commissural fusion and leaflet thickening, retraction and calcification are present. Advanced lesions, usually in the elderly, appear macroscopically very similar, irrespective of whether the underlying pathology was sclerotic, rheumatic or congenital. In most cases, no single surgical maneuver will solve the problem. The following techniques are used:

3.1 Commissurotomy
Since the main objective is to increase leaflet mobility, any degree of cusp fusion must be treated. While holding the two leaflets, the incision is made and extended into the thick collagenous area of the aortic wall. In some cases, the commissure is the only calcified area of the entire valve. Surprisingly, good results can be achieved by incising through the calcium and shaving it from both cusps. Aortic commissurotomy is particularly useful in the young patient with congenital stenosis. Although the majority of cases are now treated with balloon dilatation, re-intervention is virtually unavoidable. An open commissurotomy will significantly delay the eventual (but always problematic) prosthetic valve replacement in a young patient. Significant reduction in transvalvular gradient can be achieved with median delay to redo surgery of 12 years. Aortic valve replacement with an adult size prosthesis can usually be done for recurrent stenosis and less commonly for severe regurgitation. This same attitude of delaying valve replacement applies to the young patient with rheumatic disease as well as to the elderly ischemic patient requiring revascularization in the presence of moderate stenosis where valve replacement seems unwarranted. Operative mortality in children is low (<2%), with somewhat higher risks in neonates (approximately 10%).

3.2 Free-edge mobilization
In young rheumatic patients the cusp free edge is bent towards the sinuses, reducing the height of the cusps. Unfolding of the free edge is possible by careful incisions parallel and 2–3 mm from the edge. In older patients, this free-edge folding results in a fibrous band that can be shaved, increasing leaflet mobility.

3.3 Cusp extension
In the presence of very severe cusp retraction, the above maneuvers cannot be used and the leaflets need to be extended with glutaraldehyde-treated autologous pericardium. Single cusp extension is simpler but the results of triple extension have been shown to be superior. The results of this technique have not been reported beyond 10 years.

Further reading

1. Choo SJ, McRae G, Olomon JP et al. Aortic root geometry: pattern of differences between leaflets and sinuses of Valsalva. *J Heart Valve Dis* 1999; **8:** 407–15.
2. Duran CMG. Aortic valve repair and reconstruction. *Operative Techniques Cardiothorac Surg* 1996; **1:** 15–29.

Related topics of interest

18.4 Mitral valve repair and replacement

Eric Lim, Francis Wells

The mitral valve is a complex structure that plays a significant part in the normal function of the LV. The chordae tendinae act as tie rods supporting the complex cone shape of the LV. Breaking this connection between the base of the heart and the LV free wall causes the LV to become globular and highly inefficient as a result of loss of the twisting motion in systole. Since this interaction has been better understood, surgeons have modified repair and replacement techniques in such a way as not to interfere with LV function.

Mitral regurgitation (MR)

Competence of the mitral valve may be compromised by disease affecting any component of the mitral apparatus: namely, the annulus, leaflets, chordae, papillary muscles and the LV. The increase in end-diastolic volume (and later end-systolic volume) results in compensatory dilatation of the LV. Initially, ventricular contractility is hyperdynamic with preserved EF. The LV offloads into the low-pressure pulmonary circuit and when valvular competence is restored true LV function becomes manifest.

Etiology

Degenerative
Myxomatous degeneration is the most common cause of MR in developed countries. Defective fibroelastic tissue results in annular dilatation and posterior leaflet prolapse. Ruptured chordae frequently occur and may precipitate the catastrophic onset of pulmonary edema.

Ischemic
The acute effect of MI with papillary muscle rupture, chronically ischemic papillary muscle or ventricular dysfunction will produce MR. Papillary muscle rupture will produce instant and often catastrophic pulmonary edema usually followed by sudden death.

Rheumatic
The acute effects of rheumatic fever can result in mitral annular dilatation. Late effects are leaflet thickening, chordal disease, commissural fusion with annular and leaflet calcification. Although mitral stenosis (MS) is a common end result, a fixed orifice can produce combined stenosis and regurgitation.

Endocarditis
Endocarditis can result in valve destruction with leaflet perforation and chordal rupture leading to MR.

Other causes
Marfan syndrome and trauma.

Natural history

The overall mortality rate for untreated patients with MR is 6% per year. This increases to 34% per year following the onset of NYHA functional class III/IV dyspnea.

Indications for surgery

Current indications for surgery have expanded, as better results are obtained for operative intervention at a much earlier stage of disease. Until recently, the indications for surgery have been:

(1) NYHA class III/IV symptoms.
(2) Left ventricular impairment
    (a) ejection fraction of less than 60%
    (b) LVESD more than 55 mm.

As valve repair has become more established, the present indications for surgery are severe mitral regurgitation with or without symptoms, before the onset of LV impairment, atrial fibrillation or pulmonary hypertension.

Mitral stenosis (MS)

The normal mitral valve orifice area ranges from 4 to 5 cm^2. Symptomatic MS usually occurs after the valve orifice area decreases to <2.5 cm^2 and corresponds to a diastolic pressure gradient developing across the mitral valve. Obstruction to forward flow may result in LA dilatation, atrial fibrillation and pulmonary hypertension.

Etiology

Rheumatic

Leaflet thickening, commissural or chordal fusion are the principal causes of MS. The majority of patients will have a history of rheumatic fever during childhood.

Congenital

This is rare, and can be part of hypoplastic left heart syndrome and often presents in infancy.

Natural history

The 10-year survival for patients with MS is 60%. This decreases sharply to <15% following the onset of significant symptoms.

Indications for surgery

- NYHA class III/IV symptoms
- Systemic embolism despite adequate anticoagulation
- severe MS (mitral valve area <1.5 cm^2)
- atrial fibrillation, symptoms of pulmonary venous congestion and pending pregnancy are relative indications.

Surgical techniques

Operative assessment

The ability to identify all coexisting lesions of the mitral apparatus is critical to surgical success. TEE provides useful information on the morbid anatomy and function of the valve. Together with careful operative assessment, this holds the key to complete surgical correction. The functional classification (Carpentier) helps with intraoperative decision making:

- **Type I.** Normal leaflet motion

  Annular dilatation or leaflet perforation

- **Type II.** Excess leaflet motion

  Papillary muscle or chordal elongation and/or rupture

- **Type III.** Restricted leaflet motion

  IIIa – restricted opening; IIIb – restricted closure (rheumatic valve disease and IHD)

Mitral valve repair

Where possible, mitral valve repair is preferable to replacement. Established benefits are prolonged survival, improved ventricular function and avoidance of long-term anticoagulation for patients in sinus rhythm. Surgical techniques vary according to the etiology of MR.

(1) Leaflet procedures

(a) Quandrangular resection
The prolapsing portion of the posterior leaflet is resected as a quadrangle (with the longer side at the annulus) defined by radial lines drawn from the center of the septal portion of the annulus.

(b) Patch repair
Simple patch repair is undertaken for isolated perforations using either bovine pericardium or native pericardium soaked in 4% glutaraldehyde.

(2) Chordal procedures

(a) Chordal shortening
This can be achieved by invaginating elongated chord into the papillary muscle. This is then secured with 5–0 monofilament non-absorbable suture. This technique is now rarely used as a result of early failure.

(b) Chordal replacement
This can be performed with pledgetted PTFE sutures attached to the papillary muscle and then to the leading edge of the leaflet.

(c) Chordal transfer
Prolapsing portions of the leaflet can be supported by transferring secondary chordae to the leading edge of the leaflet.

(d) Leaflet transfer
Resection of the opposing portion of the leaflet with retention of the chordal attachment allows it to be flipped over and sutured to the prolapsing portion.

(3) Procedures on the annulus

(a) Simple annular plication

This plicates the annulus with 2–0 sutures. It often accompanies quadrangular leaflet resection to repair the annular defect and ring annuloplasty.

(b) Ring annuloplasty

The function of an annuloplasty ring is to restore the size and shape of the annulus. It also confers stability to the repair and prevents further annular dilatation. A selection of rigid and flexible rings may be used. The perceived benefit of a flexible ring is minimal hindrance to annular motion, although the benefit in man are yet to be proven.

(c) Sliding annuloplasty

This is used when excessive posterior leaflet tissue is present. Following a quadrangular resection the posterior leaflet remnant is detached from the posterior annulus which is plicated with interrupted horizontal mattress sutures. Excessive leaflet height is eliminated by triangular resection of the leaflet base or by incorporating excessive tissue into the suture line. The leaflets are then reapproximated to each other and to the annulus. This technique has been developed to avoid systolic anterior motion (SAM) of the anterior mitral valve leaflet following repair and ring annuloplasty.

Mitral valve replacement

Selection of valve prosthesis depends on age, clinical status (renal failure) and contraindications to anticoagulation. Early structural valve deterioration is the principal disadvantage of bioprosthesis in the mitral position (median 7–14 years), perhaps due to higher closing pressure.

The importance of preserving the subvalvular apparatus is established for maintenance of normal LV function and reduction in the risk of atrioventricular disruption. Often the whole posterior leaflet can be retained. Excision of the majority of the anterior leaflet with reattachment of the principal chords is usually achievable. If chordae cannot be preserved, chordal replacement to reattach the papillary muscle to the annulus may be undertaken.

Interrupted or continuous suture techniques are acceptable. Special techniques have been described for intraoperative management of a heavily calcified posterior mitral annulus. Knowledge of the anatomy of the mitral annulus is essential to avoid complete heart block, inferobasal ischemia (circumflex artery injury) or obstruction to the coronary sinus.

Results

Mitral valve repair

Operative mortality is low (<4%). The 5- and 10-year survival rates are 83% and 68%, respectively. LV function remains the strongest predictor of long-term survival. In patients with EF >40%, 8-year survival is 98%. Freedom from re-operation at 10 years is 93%. Freedom from thromboembolism at 10 years is 68%; 33% of patients require anticoagulation. Overall, 17% of patients with atrial fibrillation convert to sinus rhythm within 3 years.

Mitral valve replacement

Overall operative mortality is 5% but depends on pre-operative functional status, age, gender and LV function. The 5- and 10-year survival rates are 69% and 52%, respectively. Freedom from re-operation at 10 years is 80%. Freedom from thromboembolism at 10 years is 70%.

Further reading

1. Bonow RO, Carabello B, de Leon AC Jr et al. ACC/AHA guidelines for the management of patients with valvular heart disease: a report of the American College of Cardiology/American Heart Association Task Force on Practice Guidelines (Committee on Management of Patients with Valvular Heart Disease). *J Am Coll Cardiol* 1998; **32**: 1486–588.
2. Carpentier A, Deloche A, Dauptain J et al. A new reconstructive operation for correction of mitral and tricuspid insufficiency. *J Thorac Cardiovasc Surg* 1971; **61**: 1–13.
3. Grossi EA, Galloway AC, Parish MA et al. Experience with twenty-eight cases of systolic anterior motion after mitral valve reconstruction by the Carpentier technique. *J Thorac Cardiovasc Surg* 1992; **103**: 466–70.
4. Enriquez-Sarano M, Schaff HV, Orszulak TA et al. Valve repair improves the outcome of surgery for mitral regurgitation: a multivariate analysis. *Circulation* 1995; **91**: 1022–8.
5. Wells FC, Shapiro LM. *Mitral Valve Disease.* Butterworth-Heinemann: Oxford, 1996.

Related topics of interest

18.5 Tricuspid valve surgery

Augustine TM Tang, Christopher M Feindel

Pathology and etiology

Surgically significant tricuspid valve disease, particularly in isolation, is uncommon. The pathological lesions and etiology include:

Tricuspid stenosis (TS)
- rheumatic (commonest cause, left heart valves invariably more affected)
- carcinoid (± pulmonary valve involvement)
- right atrial tumor and collagen vascular disease (rare).

Tricuspid regurgitation (TR)
- Functional (secondary to left heart valve lesions, pulmonary hypertension, RVOTO, RV dysfunction, congenital heart defects, e.g. Ebstein's anomaly).
- Organic:
  (1) infective (intravenous drug abuse and pacemaker leads)
  (2) traumatic (percutaneous intervention, penetrating and blunt chest injury)
  (3) myxomatous (± mitral valve prolapse).

Mixed lesions
- Rheumatic, carcinoid and collagen vascular disease.

Rheumatic tricuspid stenosis demonstrates identical but milder pathology to those affecting left-heart valves (thickening and fusion of leaflet/chords with calcification). Functional TR invariably reflects right-heart failure/volume overload. As the septal leaflet is part of the central fibrous skeleton, annular dilatation naturally involves the anterior and posteroinferior portions.

Clinical assessment

Presentation
As isolated tricuspid valve disease is rare, symptoms may also reflect left-heart pathology. Dyspnea and lethargy occur commonly. Systemic venous hypertension (jugular venous distention, pulsatile hepatomegaly, ascites and peripheral edema) may accompany any valve lesion. Characteristic diagnostic features include:

- Tricuspid stenosis – loud S1, mid-diastolic rumble, accentuated A wave in distended JVP.
- Tricuspid regurgitation – pansystolic murmur (lower sternum), large V wave in distended JVP.

Investigations

- Blood: liver function test (hepatic dysfunction) and coagulation screen (↑INR) for right-heart failure.
- EKG: mostly in AF. If in SR a prominent right atrial P wave may exist in TS. RBBB.
- Echocardiography: TS diagnosed on 2-D. TR conventionally graded from I to IV on color Doppler depending on size of jet, percent RA filled by jet and systolic flow blunting/reversal in systemic veins. Other relevant features include tricuspid annular dimension, tricuspid valve area, right-heart size, function and pressures as well as left-heart valve pathology.
- Cardiac catheterization: raised RA pressure and presence of giant A or V waves. Transvalvular pressure gradient >5 mmHg diagnostic of TS. Evaluate pulmonary hypertension. Left-heart catheterization is indicated if aortic/mitral pathology is suspected.
- Angiography: exclude coronary disease in at-risk patients. Right ventriculography offers a visual impression of overall RV function and TR severity.

Surgery

Surgical approach

Tricuspid valve is exposed through an oblique right atriotomy with snaring of bicaval venous cannulae. Mitral valve may be approached through a trans-septal, superior septal or standard left atrial incision. Tricuspid surgery may be performed after completion of left-heart procedures and aortic cross-clamp removal on a beating heart. Some surgeons advocate performing tricuspid valve repair (TVr) before mitral surgery to avoid tricuspid annular distortion.

Tricuspid valve repair

When to repair

Decision on TVr is simpler when instrinsic valvular pathology is present and is feasible for most lesions (TR more suitable). Criteria for repairing functional TR remain controversial with recent trends towards early repair. This stems from the significant incidence of need for subsequent isolated TVr if functional TR was ignored during previous aortic/mitral surgery. Furthermore, experience shows that it is difficult to predict the extent of functional TR regression on individual basis following left-heart valve correction. Current recommendations for TVr during left-heart valve surgery include:

- Moderate/severe TR on preoperative echocardiography.
- Any grade of TR with the following.
  - (1) symptoms from systemic venous hypertension
  - (2) dilated tricuspid annulus (>70 mm excluding septal portion)
  - (3) right ventricular dysfunction
  - (3) PA systolic pressure >60 mmHg.

How to repair

Bicuspidization/plication: running sutures placed along the posteroinferior tricuspid annulus are shortened to eliminate the corresponding leaflet and produce a bicuspidized valve. An annuloplasty ring may be added.

de Vega annuloplasty: the two arms of a running suture are weaved along the tricuspid annulus from the anteroseptal to the posteroseptal commissures. When shortened, this reverses the annular dilatation typically found in functional TR. Many modifications exist including the use of pledgets, 'segmental' repair, exteriorization of suture ends to allow for adjustment on a full beating heart and a 'vanishing' repair using absorbable sutures.

Ring annuloplasty: though increasingly popular, the choice of flexible versus rigid rings remains controversial. Inserted using interrupted mattress sutures, some rings feature a gap (e.g. Carpentier-Edwards) to spare the AV node whilst complete rings are implanted in a supra-coronary sinus position to avoid heart block.

Intraoperative assessment
Echocardiography performed with near-physiological hemodynamics on a full beating heart offers reliable assessment of residual TR. More than mild TR mandates further repair or replacement.

Tricuspid valve replacement (TVR)
TVR is necessary when TVr fails primarily or during follow-up and when repair is unlikely to succeed (e.g. advanced rheumatic or carcinoid valve). Some surgeons advocate TVR for severe TR associated with grossly dilated annulus and/or attenuated leaflets (e.g. infection and Ebstein's). Interrupted and/or running sutures can be used. Preservation of the leaflets and subvalvular apparatus may preserve RV function. Placement of sutures through the septal leaflet reduces the risk of heart block from stitching through the triangle of Koch. The optimal prosthesis remains unclear. Biological valves are believed to be sufficiently long-lasting (low RV pressures) and less prone to late prosthetic thrombosis. However, redo TVR primarily from structural valve deterioration becomes significant after 10 years follow-up. The anticoagulant-sparing benefit of a bioprosthetic TVR is lost when mechanical aortic/mitral valves are used. Anticoagulation was found to confer a survival advantage in a large series of TVRs. These prompted some surgeons to shift towards bi-leaflet mechanical prosthesis for TVR.

Tricuspid valvectomy
This interim measure followed by delayed TVR is advocated for treating infective endocarditis associated with intravenous drug abuse, and potentially avoids early prosthetic valve reinfection. However, some patients may not tolerate sudden/acute massive TR following valvectomy. Use of homografts (stented/unstented) and xenografts may represent a compromise in this difficult situation, although the type of prosthesis chosen seems not to be a major determinant of outcome.

Outcome

Mortality
The operative mortality of 14% for tricuspid surgery (TVR = TVr) relates not to its technical complexity but predominantly reflects the fact that emergence of significant tricuspid pathology, particularly functional TR, denotes advanced RV cardiomyopathy. Over two-thirds of deaths occur from myocardial failure with bleeding, sepsis and arrhythmia responsible for the rest. Late postoperative survival values at 1, 5, 10 and 20 years are approximately 85%, 70%, 45% and 10%, respectively. Valve conservation does not confer survival advantage.

Morbidity

Need for permanent pacing (approximately 1%) represents the major early postoperative complication with equal incidence following TVR and TVr. Paraprosthetic leak, prosthetic infection and intrinsic valve failure occur more commonly during late follow-up after TVR. Interestingly, more thromboembolism has been observed after TVr, although anticoagulant-related hemorrhage was more common following TVR. Actuarial freedom from redo TVR/r at 1, 5, 10 and 20 years are approximately 95%, 90%, 60% and 30%, respectively. Valve-sparing surgery did not mitigate need for redo operations.

Further reading

1. Antunes MJ, Girdwood RW. Tricuspid annuloplasty: a modified technique. *Ann Thorac Surg* 1983; **35**: 676.
2. McGrath LB, Gonzalez-Lavin L, Bailey BM et al. Tricuspid valve operations in 530 patients. *J Thorac Cardiovasc Surg* 1990; **99**: 124.
3. Arbulu A, Holmes RJ, Asfaw I. Surgical treatment of intractable right-sided infective endocarditis in drug addicts: 25 years experience. *J Heart Valve Dis* 1993; **2**: 129.
4. Nakano K, Koyanaji H, Hashimoto A et al. Tricuspid valve replacement with the bileaflet St. Jude Medical valve prosthesis. *J Thorac Cardiovasc Surg* 1994; **108**: 888.
5. Carrier M, Hebert Y, Pellerin M et al. Tricuspid valve replacement: an analysis of 25 years of experience at a single center. *Ann Thorac Surg* 2003; **75**: 47–50.

Related topics of interest

18.6 Surgery for endocarditis

Larry W Stephenson, Daniel N Gwan-Nulla

Infective endocarditis is an important cause of cardiac valvular problems. The definitive diagnosis is established by demonstrating microorganisms by culture or histology in a valvular vegetation or intracardiac abscess. The clinical criteria for diagnosis are based on the demonstration of bacteremia and echocardiographic evidence of valvular vegetation with or without valve destruction and/or perivalvular abscess. Most patients are managed with antibiotics only. Surgery is indicated when antibiotic treatment is ineffective and/or significant hemodynamic deterioration occurs secondary to valve destruction. Operations include radical debridement of infected tissue followed by valve repair or replacement. Valve excision is an option in selected cases of right-sided endocarditis. Non-infective causes of endocarditis such as Libman–Sacks disease (SLE) and antiphospholipid syndrome are much less common. Diagnosis is by exclusion of infection and demonstration of appropriate auto-antibodies.

Etiology

Infective endocarditis is the result of:

(1) bacteremia
(2) endothelial injury
(3) altered hemodynamics
(4) valvular injury.

Any microorganism may cause endocarditis. Gram-positive bacteria predominate, with *Staphylococcus aureus* and alpha-hemolytic streptococci (especially *Streptococcus viridans*) being the most frequently cultured organisms in native and late (>60 days postop) prosthetic valvular infections. Coagulase-negative staphylococcus is the most common cause of early (<60 days postop) prosthetic valve endocarditis (Table 1).

Table 1 Microorganisms causing endocarditis.

Bacteria	Frequency of colonization (%)
Streptococci	25–40
Staphylococci	15–35
Gram-negative bacilli	5–10

Pathophysiology

The initiating event is the formation of a sterile fibrin–platelet thrombus at a site of endothelial disruption. Platelet–fibrin thrombus becomes a nidus for bacterial colonization.

Subsequent cycles of bacterial infection and repetitive thrombus formation lead to the development of valvular vegetations. The vegetation grows, sheds organisms, fragments and embolizes. Infective valvular vegetations result in local tissue destruction which may result in valvular regurgitation, pericarditis, formation of paravalvular abscess, aneurysm or fistula. Immune complexes may result in polyarteritis and glomerulonephritis. Most patients with endocarditis have a history of underlying valvular disease, congenital heart disease, a prosthetic valve (incidence 1% per year) or intravenous drug abuse (IVDA). The elderly and immunocompromised patients are particularly vulnerable. However, around 20–30% of patients have no known predisposing risk factors. *Staphylococcus aureus* occurs in greater than 50% of cases associated with IVDA. The pathogen's portal of entry is often difficult to ascertain. Any condition leading to bacteremia can cause endocarditis. Commonly reported portals of entry include dental infection and dental procedures, surgery, endoscopy, indwelling intravenous catheters, IVDA and infection of skin, lungs, bowel and genitourinary tract.

Clinical presentation

Fever is the most ubiquitous presenting symptom, occurring in more than 90% of cases. Finding of a new or changing cardiac murmur on examination is common. However, a murmur is absent in approximately 15% of patients with endocarditis. Murmurs are most likely to be absent in endocarditis caused by a virulent organism associated with an acute course and in right-sided endocarditis. Congestive heart failure (CHF) is the most common cardiac complication as well as the leading cause of death. It is often the result of aortic insufficiency or myocarditis. Emboli to the coronary arteries can lead to myocardial infarction (MI). Infective endocarditis is the most common cause of embolic MI. Neurologic findings, often the result of cerebral embolizaton, are present in 15% of patients. Several peripheral vascular phenomena and cutaneous signs bear a well-known association with infective endocarditis. These include splinter hemorrhages, Janeway lesions (erythematous non-tender lesions on palm or sole), Osler's nodes (tender subcutaneous nodules in pulp of digits) and Roth's spots (retinal hemorrhage with white center). These 'classic' lesions are late sequelae of infective endocarditis and are rarely seen in modern practice.

Diagnostic investigation

Blood tests (complete blood count, culture, biochemical screen and inflammatory markers), ECG and echocardiogram are essential. For a definitive diagnosis see Duke's criteria for diagnosing infective endocarditis (Table 2).

Transthoracic echocardiography (TTE) provides a limited view of posterior cardiac structures or fine anatomic detail but can be better than transesophageal echocardiography (TEE) for evaluating tricuspid and pulmonary valve lesions. TEE offers superior image quality of the posterior structures of the heart and prosthetic valves and readily identifies local complications such as paravalvular abscess, aneurysm and fistula.

Table 2 Duke's criteria for diagnosing infective endocarditis.

Major
- Positive blood cultures (3 positive sets each taken 12 hours apart from 2 different sites)
- Endocardial involvement (positive echocardiogram for vegetation, abscess, new dehiscence or valvular regurgitation)

Minor
- Predisposition (e.g. cardiac lesion, IVDA)
- Pyrexia (>38°C)
- Embolic/immunological phenomena
- Positive blood culture not meeting major criteria
- Positive echocardiogram not meeting major criteria

> Definitive diagnosis = Either 2 major, or 1 major + 3 minor, or 5 minor criteria

Medical management

All patients should be hospitalized and monitored for signs of changing murmurs, ongoing sepsis, hemodynamic compromise, evidence of embolization, signs of myocardial abscess or extracardiac infection. Treatment requires the use of bactericidal antibiotics over a sustained period of time (usually 6 weeks minimum) to sterilize vegetations. Effective standard regimens have been established for the more common etiologies of endocarditis.

Surgical therapy

When medical management is ineffective surgery is indicated. The failure of medical management is manifested by persistent sepsis, worsening valvular function and/or heart failure. Large vegetations (>10 mm) may have higher embolic potential. Some surgeons have lower thresholds to operate for certain pathogens such as fungus and *Staphylococcus*. Left-sided endocarditis more typically requires surgical therapy than right-sided lesions. Right-sided endocarditis is more often treated successfully with antibiotics, and complications from endocarditis such as valve disruption and emboli are usually more tolerable.

Prosthetic valve endocarditis carried a high mortality (100% in 1960s) despite treatment, but recent results are much improved (approximately 15%). Prosthetic valve infection occurring early (within 3 months) after valve replacement usually requires surgery.

Patients with recent neurological injury should be prompty investigated (CT of brain) prior to surgery. Following exclusion of cerebral hemorrhage and extensive infarction, early surgery is associated with improved outcome. However, some surgeons advocate delaying surgery until the patient emerges from coma.

Surgical technique

The basic operative principles are removal and debridement of infected tissues, closure of cardiac defects and repair or replacement of the valve(s).

Operative technique depends principally on the degree of valvular dysfunction and local complications as well as the age and compliance of the patient. Repair is the preferred operation by some surgeons for mitral and tricuspid valve lesions. Success is more likely if the area of infected leaflet tissue is relatively small. In most cases of successful repair, the amount of damaged valve leaflet is less than 50% of the total valve area. Although some aortic valve lesions can be treated with valvuloplasty, replacement is generally preferred. The operative technique for valve replacement is identical to that used in uninfected cases. The decision of whether to select mechanical, bioprosthetic or homograft valves is based on the usual selection criteria for valve replacement. Homograft valves and pulmonary autografts may be less prone to recurrent bacterial endocarditis than stent-mounted xenograft or mechanical valves. It may be necessary to excise and reconstruct the intervalvular fibrous body between the aortic and mitral valves if it is destroyed by infection. Valve excision without replacement has been performed for tricuspid valvular endocarditis in patients with IVDA, especially those with drug-resistant strains. In selected IVDA patients with normal heart function, normal right-sided pressures and hemodynamics who are likely to be noncompliant, valve excision may be the preferred therapy. As long as there is no pulmonary hypertension, it is possible to have acceptable hemodynamics.

Outcome (Table 3)

Table 3 Outcomes for native valve versus prosthetic valve endocarditis.

	Native valve endocarditis (%)	Prosthetic valve endocarditis (%)
Operative mortality	10	20
Redo surgery for infection	5	15
5-year survival	80	60

Further reading

1. Ferguson E, Reardon MJ, Letsou GV. The surgical management of bacterial valvular endocarditis. *Curr Opin Cardiol* 2000; **15**: 82–5.
2. Vlessis AA, Boiling SF. *Endocarditis: A Multidisciplinary Approach to Modern Treatment*. Futura Publishing Company, Inc: Armonk, NY, 1999.
3. David TE, Kuo J, Armstrong S. Aortic and mitral valve replacement with reconstruction of the intervalvular fibrous body. *J Thorac Cardiovasc Surg* 1997; **114**: 766–71.

Related topics of interest

19 Aortic surgery

19.1 Aortic root surgery

Derlis Martino, Frank A Baciewicz

Introduction

Understanding the structure and function of the aortic root is essential to the assessment of its pathology and surgical treatment. Aortic root pathology has been identified as a major cause of aortic incompetence in the USA. Some patients undergoing aortic valve replacement have small aortic roots relative to their body surface area (BSA) which requires surgical root modification to accommodate an appropriately sized prosthesis.

Despite an established track record of valve replacement, there is a trend towards repairing the native valve.

Anatomy

See Chapter 1.1.

Pathophysiology

Pathology affecting predominantly valve leaflets is described elsewhere. However, it is important to mention that with endocarditis of the native or prosthetic valve, root abscesses may coexist. Root enlargement may be necessary in some cases of aortic stenosis. Other conditions include:

- **Acute aortic dissections** – aortic incompentence complicates 40–60% of type A dissections from distortion of the sinotubular ridge and the sinuses, along with the commissures and the interleaflet triangles, created by the retrograde dissection.
- **Annuloaortic ectasia** – defined as dilatation of the aortic root, also known as aortic root aneurysm. It may be idiopathic, or associated with Marfan syndrome, Marfan 'forme fruste', aortic dissection, aortitis, and connective tissue disorders (Ehlers–Danlos syndrome, osteogenesis imperfecta, and pseudoxanthoma elasticum). It is also common in patients with bicuspid aortic valve and aortic insufficiency. These patients may have normal or mildly diseased valve leaflets, with important surgical implications.
- **Aneurysm of the sinus of Valsalva** – commonly involves the non-coronary sinus. They can be congenital or acquired. Complications include infection, space-occupying effect, e.g. obstruction of RVOT, rupture and fistula formatia (often into a cardiac chamber). Aortic incompetence develops as the sinotubular ridge dilates.

With some ascending aortic aneurysms, the sinotubular ridge is dilated. This stretches the leaflet commissures, causing failure of coaptation and valve regurgitation.

Surgical indications

- **Endocarditis with aortic root abscess formation** – radical debridement is the only means of preventing abscess recurrence.
- **Small aortic root** – enlargement by various techniques is indicated to avoid patient-prosthesis mismatch (PPM), particularly in patients with LV dysfunction.
- **Type A aortic dissection** – with or without involvement of the aortic root.
- **Annuloaortic ectasia/ascending aortic aneurysm** – when accompanied by valve incompetence and/or annular diameter >50 mm.
- **Sinus of Valsalva aneurysms** – simple or complicated.

Surgical options

1. Ascending aortic aneurysms with dilatation of the sinotubular ridge

In these cases, aortic insufficiency is caused by outward displacement of the commissures, which prevents leaflet coaptation. The annular size and leaflets are relatively normal. Aortic insufficiency can be corrected by normalizing the sinotubular ridge. This is accomplished by replacing the ascending aorta with a tubular Dacron graft with a diameter slightly smaller than the average length of the free margins of the three leaflets, and suturing the graft at the sinotubular ridge. In addition to a dilated sinotubular ridge, one or more of the sinuses of Valsalva may also be aneurysmal. The non-coronary sinus is the most commonly affected. The proximal end of the graft is then tailored to replace the aneurysmal sinus(es). If one of the coronary sinuses is affected, the corresponding coronary artery needs to be reimplanted to the 'neo-sinus'.

2. Annuloaortic ectasia

Several options exist. If the leaflets are normal, the remodeling procedure (Yacoub) can be used, combined with correction of the dilated annulus. The ascending aorta and the sinuses of Valsalva need to be replaced together with coronary reimplantation. An annuloplasty procedure, if considered necessary, can be accomplished by passing multiple horizontal mattress sutures through the fibrous component of the LVOT immediately below the lowest level of leaflet insertion, through a single horizontal plane reinforced with a strip of felt.

Alternatively in aortic valve 'reimplantation' (David), all three dilated sinuses are excised, leaving small coronary buttons and a thin strip of juxta-annular aorta. Multiple mattress sutures are passed from inside out of the LVOT. This suture line follows the scalloped shape of the aortic annulus in its muscular component, and runs in a horizontal plane along the fibrous component. A tubular Dacron graft of diameter equal to the average length of the free margins of the three leaflets is selected. The sutures in the LVOT are then passed from inside out of the graft. Annular reduction is mainly accomplished underneath the sub-commissural triangle between the left and non-coronary leaflets. The native aortic valve is then resuspended inside the graft ensuring optimal leaflet coaptation. The coronary buttons are then reimplanted.

The standard option is replacement of the aortic valve and ascending aorta with a valved conduit, as described by Bentall. The prosthetic valve is usually mechanical. The ascending aorta is opened and the leaflets excised; a tubular composite Dacron graft is anastomosed to the aortic annulus. The coronary buttons are then reimplanted directly onto the graft. When the ostia are laterally displaced by a large aneurysm, an interposition graft (prosthetic in Cabrol) may be needed to avoid tension on the coronary anastomoses.

Risks and benefits of each approach should be calculated for each patient. The use of mechanical valve prostheses requires lifelong anticoagulation and introduces an increased potential for endocarditis. The valve-sparing options are subject to potential late valve deterioration requiring re-operation, and ongoing annular dilatation, especially in Marfan syndrome.

Other surgical options include aortic homografts/stentless roots and the Ross procedure.

3. Type A aortic dissection with aortic valve involvement

In these cases, aortic insufficiency may be due to pre-existing annuloaortic ectasia, or detachment of one or more commissures of the aortic valve. If the leaflets are normal, remodeling of the root can be performed as described above. In the case of a type A dissection the detached commissures can be resuspended and the ascending aorta replaced with a tubular Dacron graft of appropriate diameter. The graft is sutured right at the sinotubular ridge, which restores normal valve function. In cases of extensive dissection of the sinuses, reimplantation of the aortic valve or aortic valve replacement with a composite graft should be performed.

Further reading

1. Underwood MJ, El Khoury G et al. The aortic root: structure, function and surgical reconstruction. *Heart* 2000; **83**: 376–80.
2. Pessotto R, Santini F, Pugliese P et al. Preservation of the aortic valve in acute type A dissection complicated by aortic regurgitation. *Ann Thorac Surg* 1999; **67**: 2010–13.
3. David TE. Annuloaortic ectasia. In: *Mastery of Cardiothoracic Surgery.* Kaiser LR, Kron IL et al. (eds). Lippincott-Raven: Philadelphia, PA, 1998: pp. 453–8.
4. David TE, Armstrong S, Ivanov J et al. Results of aortic valve-sparing operations. *J Thorac Cardiovasc Surg* 2001; **122**: 39–46.
5. David TE. Surgery of the aortic valve. *Curr Problems Surg* 1999; **36**: 424–501.
6. Doty DB. Aortic aneurysm. In: *Cardiac Surgery: Operative Technique.* Mosby: St. Louis, MO, 1997: pp 324–9.

Related topics of interest

19.2 Surgery of the aortic arch

Michael A Borger

Epidemiology

Aortic arch surgery is uncommon (<1% of adult cardiac operations). The primary indications include aneurysm and aortic dissection. The aortic arch is involved in approximately 10% of aortic aneurysms and approximately 70% of Stanford type A dissections.

Arch aneurysm
- Incidence: approximately 6/100 000 person-years.
- Peak age: 7th decade of life.
- Male-to-female ratio: 1.5:1.
- Etiology: medial degenerative disease (elderly hypertensive smokers with diffuse atherosclerosis), Marfan syndrome and other connective tissue disorders, infection (mycotic aneurysms), previous aortic trauma, aortitis (Takayasu's syndrome, Behçet's syndrome, syphilis), localized medial defect (saccular aneurysm) and congenital lesions.

Aortic dissection
- Incidence: approximately 5/1 000 000 person-years, with a 2.5:1 male-to-female ratio.
- Peak age: 6th and 7th decades of life but also in very young patients.
- Etiology: hypertension, connective tissue disorders, aortic stenosis (bicuspid valve), pregnancy, and iatrogenic trauma. Aortic dissections usually present acutely, but infrequently become chronic – this important distinction has practical significance.

Anatomy

The aortic arch extends from the brachiocephalic artery to the left subclavian artery. Its normal diameter should not exceed 30 mm in women and 35 mm in men. Congenital lesions and anatomic variations of the aortic arch are discussed elsewhere.

Pathophysiology

The pathophysiology of aortic aneurysm and dissection is discussed in detail in separate chapters.

Diagnosis and evaluation

Arch aneurysm

- Non-invasive imaging: CT, MRI, or TEE. Echocardiography (TEE or TTE) also detects cardiac ± valvular dysfunction.
- Cardiac catheterization with concomitant aortography: to assess significant coronary artery disease and arch anatomy, respectively.

Aortic dissection

For acute dissection:

- Non-invasive imaging: as arch aneurysm above, but only echocardiography could reveal regional wall motion abnormalities (particularly inferior hypokinesis related to RCA dissection). This is equally useful for both acute and chronic dissection.
- Cardiac catheterization and aortography: should be omitted pre-operatively in acute dissection to avoid delaying surgery and risk of aortic rupture. This is safer in chronic dissection and may be useful for delineating the pattern of vital organ perfusion.

Indications for surgery

Arch aneurysm

Commonly asymptomatic, surgery aims to prevent rupture (usually fatal) as operation for acute rupture rarely results in survival. The most important predictors of rupture are size (indexed to adjacent normal aorta), rate of expansion, and symptomatology. Current indicators include:

(1) aortic diameter >5.5 cm in low-risk candidate
(2) aortic diameter >8.0 cm in a high-risk candidate
(3) saccular aneurysm >5.0 cm
(4 aneurysm expansion >0.5 cm/year
(5 symptoms related to the aneurysm (chest pain, hoarseness, cough).

Aortic dissection

Emergency surgery is indicated for all acute dissection involving the ascending aorta ± arch (Stanford type A or DeBakey type I and II lesions) as soon as the diagnosis is made because without operative intervention 50% die within 48 hours.

Chronic arch dissection, i.e. diagnosed >2 weeks after initial presentation, is much less life-threatening. Surgery is reserved for aneurysmal dilation (>5.5 cm) or new symptom related to the dissection. In assessing chronic dissection, both true and false lumens must be included since the risk of rupture relates to total vessel diameter.

Intraoperative management

Patients should be monitored with a PA catheter, as well as a central temperature probe. The right radial artery should always be monitored to verify cerebral perfusion during CPB. Antifibrinolytics may reduce bleeding although the prothrombotic risk of aprotinin and circulatory arrest concerns some surgeons. Methylprednisolone is given prior to circulatory arrest and hyperglycemia should be avoided.

The right atrium is the preferred route of venous drainage for aortic arch operations. The arterial line should have a 'Y' connection in place. For aortic aneurysm surgery, arterial inflow is performed via the ascending aorta. Femoral artery inflow may generate retrograde embolization from descending aortic atherosclerosis. In aortic dissection, cannulation is performed via the femoral artery or preferably the right axillary artery. Cardiopulmonary bypass (CPB) is started slowly to prevent movement of intimal flaps. Loss of the right radial artery tracing signifies cerebral malperfusion. Immediate options include redirecting arterial inflow to: (1) the right axillary artery or (2) transection of the ascending aorta with direct cannulation of the true lumen.

Systemic cooling should be performed over 20 min to a target termperature dependent upon adoption of adjunctive cerebral protective measures. Flow rate is gradually decreased during cooling. Ventricular fibrillation will occur during core cooling necessitating LV venting. Cardioplegia is only necessary for concomitant coronary artery bypass. Aortic cross-clamping should be avoided with acute dissection to prevent pressurizing the false lumen and causing multiple re-entry tears.

The Achilles' heel of arch surgery is interruption of the arch vessels producing cerebral ischemia. Three related techniques have been developed for cerebral protection:

Deep hypothermic circulatory arrest (DHCA)
See Chapter 10.

Retrograde cerebral perfusion (RCP)
RCP is predominantly an effective method of brain cooling, but may also supply some nutritive flow and flush out arterial emboli. RCP reduces dependence on DHCA and the associated coagulopathy.

Circulation is arrested after cooling to 20–25°C, depending on complexity of the arch pathology. The superior vena cava (SVC) is cannulated (24F straight cannula) and attached to the 'Y' connection in the arterial line. The SVC/RA junction is temporarily occluded. Cold (10°C) blood is infused at ≤500 ml/min. to keep CVP below 25 mmHg. When the distal arch anastomosis is completed, the SVC cannula is redirected into the Dacron graft and antegrade systemic perfusion instituted. This technique allows for safe circulatory arrest up to 40 min.

Antegrade cerebral perfusion (ACP)
ACP may offer the most effective cerebral protection during aortic arch surgery although its applicability is limited by technical difficulty. ACP allows for moderate hypothermia (20–28°C), thereby lowering the risk of coagulopathy.

After cooling and circulatory arrest, the aortic arch is opened and the cerebral vessels transected at their origin. Separate cannulae are inserted into the innominate artery (18F) and the left carotid artery (14F). After de-airing, the proximal arteries are snared and cold blood is infused at 800 ml/min or to achieve a right radial pressure of 40 mmHg. A specially designed Dacron graft with three side-branches is anastomosed to the aorta, with each branch subsequently attached to the arch vessels.

Alternatively, ACP involves cannulation of the distal innominate or right axillary artery with occlusion of the proximal arch vessels. The left carotid artery can be cannulated separately if EEG suggests cerebral ischemia. Standard Dacron tube grafts can be used with this technique.

The aortic arch may be replaced with a 26–30 mm gelatin-impregnated Dacron graft. In hemi-arch replacement the beveled distal anastomosis involving descending aorta and arch vessels is performed first using running 3–0 Prolene. Teflon strips and biologic glue are useful adjuncts in aortic dissection. The graft is then cannulated to restore antegrade systemic perfusion (starting at 1000 ml/min and slowly increasing with rewarming). In total arch replacement, the cerebral vessels are reimplanted to the graft before subsequent cannulation. In chronic aortic dissection, the distal anastomosis must incorporate both true and false lumens ± septation procedure to avoid subsequent organ malperfusion. Proximal anastomosis to native ascending aorta is performed during rewarming on antegrade perfusion.

Results and long-term follow-up

Surgical outcomes have steadily improved over time. Current operative mortality is approximately 9% and stroke risk is approximately 7%. Ten-year survival is 60–70%. Aneurysm and dissection should be followed with annual CT/MRI to assess the remaining aorta. Lifetime beta-blockade is necessary for aortic dissection or connective tissue disorders.

Further reading

1. David TE, Armstrong S, Ivanov J, Barnard S. Surgery for acute type A aortic dissection. *Ann Thorac Surg* 1999; **67**: 1999–2001.
2. Moshkovitz Y, David TE, Caleb M, Feindel CM, de Sa MPL. Circulatory arrest under moderate systemic hypothermia and cold retrograde cerebral perfusion. *Ann Thorac Surg* 1998; **66**: 1179–84.
3. Reich DL, Uysal S, Ergin MA, Griepp RB. Retrograde cerebral perfusion as a method of neuroprotection during thoracic aortic surgery. *Ann Thorac Surg* 2001; **72**: 1774–82.
4 Kazui T, Washiyama N, Muhammad BAH et al. Total arch replacement using aortic arch branched grafts with the aid of antegrade selective cerebral perfusion. *Ann Thorac Surg* 2000; **70**: 3–9.

Related topics of interest

19.3 Thoracoabdominal aortic surgery

Joseph S Coselli, Lori D Conklin, Scott A LeMaire

Thoracoabdominal aortic aneurysms (TAAs) involve both the descending thoracic and abdominal aorta in continuity. Advances in vascular imaging combined with an aging population have led to an increase in the diagnosis and treatment of TAAs. Since Etheredge and Rob reported the first successful TAA repairs in 1955, advances in preoperative management, anesthesia, surgical techniques, blood conservation, and postoperative care have reduced morbidity and mortality. However, TAAs remain among the most significant challenges faced by cardiovascular surgeons.

Classification

TAAs were classified by Crawford according to the extent of aortic involvement in order to evaluate survival and complications. Extent I involves most of the descending thoracic aorta, usually beginning near the left subclavian artery, and extending into the suprarenal abdominal aorta. Extent II aneurysms also arise near the left subclavian artery, but extend into the infrarenal aorta and often reach the aortic bifurcation. Extent III aneurysms originate in the lower descending aorta (below the sixth rib) and extend into the abdomen. Extent IV aneurysms begin at the level of the diaphragm and often involve the entire abdominal aorta. Extent II, III, and IV aneurysms may have associated iliac artery aneurysmal disease and/or renal artery occlusive disease.

Etiology

Most TAAs are the result of nonspecific medial degenerative disease (approximately 82%) or aortic dissection (17%). Less common causes include connective tissue disorders, such as Marfan syndrome and Ehlers–Danlos syndrome; infections of the aortic wall; aortitis, as seen in Takayasu's disease; and trauma.

Clinical presentation

Approximately 50% of patients are identified while asymptomatic. The most common symptom is pain resulting from expansion of the aortic wall or erosion of the spine. The pain is classically described as sharp or stabbing in nature and is usually located in the upper to mid-back region, posterior thorax, abdomen, or flanks. Compression of adjacent structures can cause hoarseness from left recurrent laryngeal nerve paralysis, dyspnea from airway obstruction, or dysphagia from esophageal compression. Patients may also present with distal venous stasis secondary to compression of the inferior vena cava (IVC). Erosion of the aneurysm into the lung or gastrointestinal tract is a late consequence of expansion and causes catastrophic hemoptysis or hematemesis, respectively. Acute severe pain and/or syncope can be associated with rupture or acute dissection superimposed upon a pre-existing aneurysm.

Diagnosis

Abnormalities serendipitously discovered on chest x ray performed for unrelated reasons are often the first indication of aortic pathology. The most important diagnostic modalities include CT or MRI scans of the chest and abdomen to delineate the extent of aortic involvement. Aortography is reserved for patients in whom branch vessel stenosis is suspected, such as those with symptoms of iliac occlusive disease. Careful attention must be paid to minimizing the nephrotoxic effects of intravenous contrast material, especially in patients with pre-existing renal insufficiency, diabetes mellitus, and hypertension. Echocardiography or ultrasonography do not provide sufficient anatomic information in TAAs.

Indications for operation

Patients with symptomatic aneurysms undergo operative repair regardless of aneurysm size, provided they do not have severe medical co-morbidities that preclude surgery. Ruptured TAAs are treated immediately. Patients with asymptomatic aneurysms should undergo surgical repair when the diameter of the aneurysm reaches 5.0–6.0 cm, exceeds twice the diameter of an adjacent normal aortic segment, or expands at >1 cm/year, regardless of size. Patients with Marfan syndrome, aortic dissection, and saccular aneurysms are evaluated and treated more aggressively.

Pre-operative evaluation

Due to their advanced age (average age at repair 65–70 years), patients with TAAs have predictable operative risk factors that can be evaluated and potentially modified to decrease postoperative complications. All elective patients should undergo cardiac evaluation. Patients without significant risk factors for ischemic heart disease (IHD) may require only TTE/TEE to evaluate LV and valvular function. Patients with EF <30% or with symptoms or signs of IHD, such as angina or EKG findings, should undergo a non-invasive evaluation of myocardial perfusion (e.g. thallium scan or dobutamine echocardiography). Findings consistent with significant IHD warrant cardiac catheterization. Pulmonary function tests are carried out routinely, and patients with an FEV_1 >1.0l and a $PaCO_2$ <45 mmHg are considered surgical candidates. Renal status is evaluated using CT and/or MRI scans and pre-operative biochemistry. Coagulation and liver function tests are routinely performed. Carotid Dopplers are performed selectively in patients at high risk for carotid artery disease, including those with advanced age, history of CVA/TIA, or carotid bruits.

Surgical treatment

Surgical management varies according to aneurysm extent. The procedure involves aneurysm replacement with a Dacron tube graft via a left thoracoabdominal approach. Single lung ventilation, permissive mild hypothermia to 32–34°C, and moderate heparinization (1 mg/kg) are performed routinely, regardless of extent. We also advocate aggressive reattachment of patent segmental intercostal and lumbar arteries, particularly those between T8 and L1, as well as sequential aortic clamping whenever possible. The renal arteries are perfused with Ringer's lactate solution (with mannitol (12.5 g/l) and methylprednisolone (125 mg/l)) cooled to 4°C if the aneurysm extends into the infrarenal aorta. Patients with extent I or II TAAs undergo cerebrospinal fluid (CSF) drainage and left-heart bypass (LHB) without a heat exchanger; these techniques are associated with a decreased incidence of postoperative neurological dysfunction. The celiac axis and superior mesenteric artery are selectively perfused with normothermic blood from the LHB pump in patients with extent I or II aneurysms.

Complications

The most devastating complication is paraplegia or paraparesis caused by spinal cord ischemia. The most common postoperative complication is pulmonary dysfunction which is often attributed to pre-existing chronic obstructive pulmonary disease and tobacco abuse. Other complications include renal failure, stroke, cardiac dysfunction, sepsis, bleeding, and left vocal cord paralysis due to injury of the left recurrent laryngeal nerve.

Postoperative management

CSF drainage is continued in extent I and II repairs with a target CSF pressure of 10–12 mmHg. The drain is removed 24–48 hours after surgery unless paraplegia or paraparesis is present. Lower extremity movement is assessed as soon as the patient awakens from anesthesia and prior to the administration of further sedatives. If concern exists regarding postoperative paralysis, the mean arterial pressure (MAP) is increased to 90–100 mmHg, a CSF drainage catheter is inserted (if not already present), and mannitol and steroids are administered. To protect fragile suture lines, strict blood pressure control is implemented (MAP 80–90 mmHg) for the initial 24–48 hours. Peripheral pulses are followed closely. Whenever possible, the patient is weaned from the ventilator and extubated within the first 24–36 hours, and aggressive pulmonary toilet is initiated. Chest tubes are removed when the total output <300 ml/24 hours. Renal-dose dopamine is administered to enhance urine output. A rising creatinine level is treated aggressively. The abdominal drain is usually removed within 24 hours. To minimize the risk of graft infection, intravenous antibiotics are administered until all central venous access lines, chest tubes, and abdominal drains are removed. Oral antibiotics are continued through hospital discharge.

Results

Our experience with 1609 consecutive patients undergoing repair of TAAs is summarized in Table 1. Extent II aneurysms remain a major risk factor for adverse outcomes and are associated with the highest levels of mortality, paraplegia or paraparesis, renal failure, and postoperative bleeding. Interestingly, we have found no difference in mortality, neurological dysfunction, or renal failure in patients with dissection versus those without dissection. As

Table 1 Thoracoabdominal aortic aneurysm repair in 1609 consecutive patients.

Extent	Number of patients	30-day survival	In-hospital survival	Paraplegia/ paraparesis	Renal failure*	Reoperation for bleeding
I	533	478 (89.7%)	467 (87.6%)	17 (3.2%)	11 (2.1%)	6 1 (1%)
II	512	452 (88.3%)	436 (85.2%)	34 (6.6%)	37 (7.2%)	17 (3.3%)
III	264	241 (91.3%)	241 (91.3%)	8 (3.0%)	15 (5.7%)	5 (1.9%)
IV	300	274 (91.3%)	267 (89.0%)	6 (2.0%)	20 (6.7%)	8 (2.7%)
Total	1609	1445 (89.8%)	1411 (87.7%)	65 (4.0%)	83 (5.2%)	36 (2.2%)

*Patients requiring hemodialysis.

expected, mortality and morbidity following surgery in patients presenting acutely – i.e. TAAs with rupture, acute dissection, or acute pain – are higher than following elective repair. Although current morbidity and mortality in specialist centers is 2–4 times higher for acute cases than for elective cases, repair is associated with a reasonable long-term survival and is justified given the fatal course without treatment. The relatively poor outcome following emergency repair of ruptured TAAs justifies an aggressive approach to treat these aneurysms earlier.

Further reading

1. Coselli JS, LeMaire SA. Surgical techniques: thoracoabdominal aorta. *Card Clin N Am* 1999; **17**: 751–65.
2. Svensson LG, Crawford ES, Hess KR, Coselli JS, Safi HJ. Experience with 1509 patients undergoing thoracoabdominal aortic operations. *J Vasc Surg* 1993; **17**: 357–70.
3. Coselli JS, LeMaire SA, Miller CC III et al. Mortality and paraplegia after thoracoabdominal aortic aneurysm repair: a risk factor analysis. *Ann Thorac Surg* 2000; **69**: 404–14.
4. Panneton JM, Hollier LH. Nondissecting thoracoabdominal aortic aneurysms: part I. *Ann Vasc Surg* 1995; **9**: 503–14.
5. Panneton JM, Hollier LH. Dissecting descending thoracic and thoracoabdominal aortic aneurysms: part II. *Ann Vasc Surg* 1995; **9**: 596–605.

Related topics of interest

10   Hypothermic circulatory arrest
19.2   Surgery of the aortic arch
19.4   Aortic dissection

19.4 Aortic dissection

Steven A Livesey

In aortic dissection the aortic wall splits or dissects along its length between the internal and external elastic laminae. This may progress both proximally and distally along the whole length of the aorta creating true and false lumens. This usually presents as an acute surgical emergency.

Classification

Common systems in usage include the DeBakey and the Stanford Classifications (Table 1). The Stanford classification is preferred by surgeons as it indicates the need for urgent surgery when the ascending aorta is involved.

Table 1 Classification of aortic dissection.

	Classification	Region of aorta affected
DeBakey	I	Whole aorta
	II	Ascending aorta
	III	Descending aorta
Stanford	A	Ascending aorta (± any other region)
	B	Ascending aorta **not** involved

Incidence and etiology

The incidence is 10–20/million. It occurs more commonly in men (male:female: 2:1–5:1), and peaks in their 60s. Recognized risk factors include hypertension, connective tissue diseases (e.g. Marfan syndrome), bicuspid aortic valve, coarctation, atherosclerosis and pregnancy. Dissection can also occur following aortic manipulation, e.g. cardiac catherization, aortic cannulation and cross-clamping. The dissecting process begins with an intimal tear and is propagated along the length of the aorta by the ingress of blood. There may then be multiple re-entry tears, usually in the descending aorta. The most common entry site is in the ascending aorta (65%) approximately 2 cm above the sinotubular junction. The aortic arch (opposite the innominate artery – 10%) and the upper descending aorta (20%) are the next most common entry sites. The dissection then progresses anteriorly, often stripping off the commissures either side of the non-coronary cusp and the right coronary ostium and then spiraling around the aortic arch into the thoracoabdominal aorta. The inter-coronary commissure and the left coronary artery are usually spared.

Presentation

Chest pain is typically severe and acute in onset, often described as sharp or tearing in nature and subsequently settling in the inter-scapular region. Symptoms can often be vague and related to tissue malperfusion (cardiac, cerebral, visceral or peripheral) causing ischemia. The patient may be breathless if either aortic regurgitation or tamponade has occurred.

Clinical signs

Patients are often in extreme discomfort. Findings depend on the effects of the dissection. The patient may be hypotensive (due to tamponade), or hypertensive (autoregulatory processes are disturbed if baroreceptors in the arch are stripped off by the dissection). There may be peripheral pulse deficit(s). There may be the early diastolic murmur of aortic regurgitation and a variety of signs as a result of end-organ ischemia.

Investigations

EKG may show LV hypertrophy or acute ischemia/bundle branch block (from coronary dissection). A widened mediastinum on chest x ray may be the first clue to the diagnosis which can be confirmed by TTE/TEE, CT or MR imaging. Angiography is not recommended unless CAD is suspected.

The dissection flap may be seen on TTE but the images are rarely of diagnostic quality. TEE provides much better definition and high levels of diagnostic accuracy are reported, but hypertension and the Valsalva effect associated with passing the probe may have deleterious effects. MR scanning gives excellent images of the aorta but the practicality, rapidity and image quality of spiral CT makes this the current imaging modality of choice.

Medical management

Hypotensive patients should be resuscitated with volume/inotropes. Commonly, patients are hypertensive and, following adequate analgesia, this should be controlled, aiming for a systolic pressure of 110–120 mmHg. Beta-blockers are preferred since they reduce aortic shear stress. A combined alpha- and beta-adrenergic antagonist (e.g. labetalol) infusion is often used for effective blood pressure control. Nitrates and nitroprusside should not be used without prior beta-blockade to avoid tachycardia.

Surgical management

Type A dissection

This requires immediate surgery. The aim of surgery is to prevent fatal complications of intrapericardial aortic rupture, severe aortic regurgitation and myocardial ischemia.

Operative methods include:

(1) interposition graft replacement of the ascending aorta
(2) method 1 with resuspension of the aortic valve (structurally normal valve dissected)

(3) method 1 with aortic valve replacement (abnormal aortic valve)
(4) aortic root replacement (dissection of sinuses and coronary ostia)
(5) valve-sparing root replacement (Yacoub/David techniques).

The key surgical decisions are:

(1) *Site of arterial cannulation.* This can be guided by imaging but irrespective of which femoral artery is chosen it is important that the true lumen is cannulated and that the perfusion line pressure is checked. Alternative sites include the axillary artery and as a last resort through the apex of the left ventricle and across the aortic valve (transventricular cannulation).

(2) *Resuspend the valve or replace the root.* There is some evidence that aortic root replacement results in fewer subsequent interventions (e.g. for severe AR)

(3) *Open or closed distal technique.* The advantage of being able to inspect the aortic arch and total replacement of the intrapericardial aorta using circulatory arrest must be weighed against its adverse effects.

(4) *Should the aortic arch be replaced?* This may be necessary if the entry site in the ascending aorta extends into the arch. Prophylactic replacement of the whole ascending aorta and arch has the theoretical advantage of eliminating more diseased aorta. Acceptable results are reported but it is technically challenging.

(5) *Should the ascending aorta be clamped?* It has been suggested that the avoidance of aortic clamping prior to the restoration of antegrade flow may reduce the propagation of the dissection.

The femoral artery is cannulated prior to sternotomy. If there is significant tamponade, opening the sternum and pericardium can precipitate a hypertensive surge. After sternotomy the RA is cannulated for venous drainage. The degree of core cooling depends on the extent of intimal tear and operative repair. The aorta may be cross-clamped, opened and the heart arrested with a combination of antegrade and retrograde cold blood cardioplegia. If the aortic valve is structurally abnormal, it is excised and root replacement undertaken. If it is structurally normal, the commissures are resuspended with pledgetted sutures, the proximal dissection is repaired with surgical glue and re-enforced with Teflon collars on both the luminal and adventitial aspects. A non-porous woven Dacron graft (with a side arm for re-institution of antegrade flow following distal repair) is then sewn end-to-end to the proximal aorta. If circulatory arrest is indicated, profound hypothermia (18°C) is used and retrograde cerebral perfusion commenced via the superior vena cava (SVC) at 500 ml/min to a maximum SVC pressure of 30 mmHg. The aortic arch can then be inspected and either replaced or the distal anastomosis performed, again reinforced with surgical glue and Teflon. The circulation is restored with antegrade flow and the patient is rewarmed.

Type B dissection

The initial management is medical with adequate analgesia, control of hypertension and maintenance of urine output. Indications for urgent operation are evidence of rupture (hemothorax), malperfusion or persistent pain. The aim of surgery is to resect the entry intimal tear, which is usually in the proximal descending aorta and to ensure distal perfusion. Fenestration of the intimal flap may be needed to prevent distal ischemia. If distal ischemia persists, either endovascular stenting or local surgery may be required (e.g. femoro–femoral crossover graft).

Results

The majority of patients with acute type A aortic dissection die within 48 hours without surgery, whereas with appropriate medical treatment the majority of patients with type B dissection survive. With modern techniques, 80–90% of patients can be expected to survive surgery for type A dissection. The majority (95%) of patients have a persistent distal false lumen whatever surgical approach is taken. This is prone to dilatation and lifelong follow-up (regular CT/MRI) is required. Hypertension should be rigorously controlled with beta-blockade to minimize aortic dilatation/redissection.

Chronic dissection

Remarkably, not all patients with aortic dissection present acutely. Some are seen only when the effects of aneurysm or aortic regurgitation cause symptoms. They should be operated on according to the size of the aneurysm or severity of the aortic regurgitation, and not simply because a chronic dissection is identified.

Intra-mural hematoma of the aorta

This is a curious condition that is being increasingly recognized with better imaging techniques. Patients present with pain and are usually elderly hypertensives. The etiology is uncertain but may be due to penetration of an atherosclerotic plaque or rupture of vasa vasora. If a penetrating ulcer is seen in the ascending aorta the treatment should be surgical, otherwise treatment of any hypertension and serial scans may be more appropriate in these often frail patients.

Further reading

1. Elefteriades JA, Tittle SL, Kopf GS. Management of aortic intramural hematoma. *J Am Coll Cardiol* 2002; **39**: 180–1.
2. Kuroczynski W, Dohmen G, Hake U et al. Aortic valve preservation in acute type A dissection: mid-term results. *J Heart Valve Dis* 2001; **10**: 779–83.
3. Westaby S, Saito S, Katsumata T. Acute type A dissection: conservative methods provide consistently low mortality. *Ann Thorac Surg* 2002; **73**: 707–13.

Related topics of interest

20 Surgery for atrial fibrillation

Geoffrey M Tsang

Background

Atrial fibrillation (AF) affects 1% of the general population and 6% of those aged >65 years. Patients with AF become symptomatic from palpitations, limited cardiac output from loss of atrial transport and chronotropism as well as systemic thromboembolism. Although generally well tolerated, long-term complications of AF are increasingly recognized. AF increased the risk of stroke five-fold and doubled the risk of death despite rate-control therapy and anticoagulation (the Framingham Study). This rekindled interest in catheter ablation and surgery for AF to restore sinus rhythm (SR) and atrioventricular synchrony. The surgical approach has been revived with newer energy sources becoming available to create atrial lesions, which were previously only feasible with incisions and/or cryotherapy. The purported advantages of such energy sources including microwave, radiofrequency (unipolar, bipolar, irrigated) and laser include more rapid creation of reliable lesions which will permit AF surgery to be combined with routine valve and CABG surgery. An off-pump approach using microwave energy to isolate the pulmonary veins has been described which may be particularly beneficial for paroxysmal AF. A similarly minimal access approach to the maze procedure has been reported in large cohorts encompassing both isolated AF surgery and combined cardiac operations.

Pathophysiology

AF is a highly disorganized arrhythmia whereby multiple, random and simultaneous macro re-entrant circuits cause the atrium to contract at 300–500 bpm. The ventricular response is governed by AV nodal conduction. The principles of the maze procedure are to create lesions within the atria which act as electrical blocks and hence disrupt the macro re-entrant circuits (Figure 1). Furthermore, these lesions guide impulses generated from the sinoatrial node to propagate in an orderly fashion to activate the atrial mass before progressing through the AV node to activate the ventricles (Figure 1).

Surgical treatment

Initial surgical treatment of AF was reported in 1980 with left atrial isolation. This isolated the LA from the AV node so that the RA alone was responsible for sinus rhythm. However, the isolated LA could still fibrillate and pose thromboembolic risk. In 1985, Guiraudon introduced the corridor operation with similar pitfalls and this was later abandoned. The Cox maze procedure reported in 1987 has become the cornerstone of AF surgical treatment. Subsequent introduction of the maze III procedure (Figure 2) in 1992 substantially improved both short- and long-term outcome.

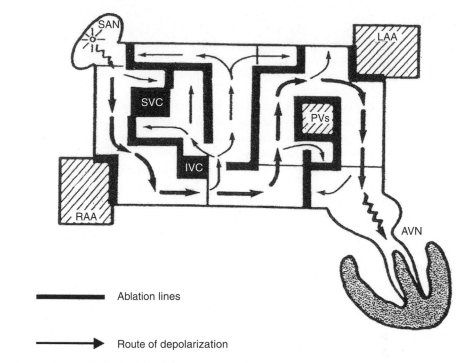

Ablation lines

Route of depolarization

Figure 1 Anatomical principle of the maze procedure.

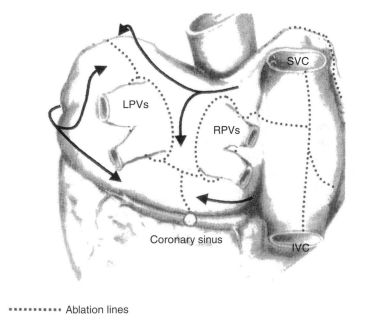

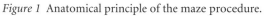 Ablation lines

Route of depolarization from SA node

Figure 2 Surgical lesion pattern set in Cox maze III procedure.

Outcome

Percutaneous catheter-based radiofrequency approaches to replicate the maze III are currently more time-consuming and less successful. However, catheter-based pulmonary vein isolation for patients with lone or paroxysmal AF appears more promising with freedom from AF rates >60%.

Surgical ablation can be done with acceptable CPB and aortic cross-clamp times. Cox's operative mortality is <3% with short- and long-term freedom from AF and maintenance of sinus rhythm reported in 60–80% of patients. Overall, patients undergoing maze and mitral valve surgery have a higher rate of relapse into AF. This may be due to patient heterogeneity and variations in surgical technique/ablation lesion sets used by individual surgeons. More impressive are the consistent results of long-term freedom from thromboembolism (<1%). Restoration of SR is important, but LA appendagectomy and LA reduction (when LA >7 cm) also play important roles in preventing thromboembolism. It is unclear why Cox's series demonstrated a 5% incidence of permanent pacemaker implantation; this may be due to underlying sick sinus syndrome rather than the lesion pattern created. It is important to note that these results derive from a retrospective cohort and no randomized data exist.

The incidence of early postoperative AF following maze procedure can reach 35% and may be related to lesion healing and surgically induced inflammation. Small macro re-entry circuits underlying such arrhythmia usually respond well to short-term anti-arrhythmic drugs.

The newer energy sources have enabled endocardial application on the arrested heart cases as well as an epicardial approach to create limited lesions in off-pump cases. Pulmonary vein isolation alone offers a quicker and simpler option for patients unsuitable for the full maze procedure but has a 10–15% lower success rate. Current debate surrounds which is the optimal lesion set as many modifications of the original maze III procedure generate apparently comparable results. Data from forthcoming trials will elucidate this further.

Further reading

1. Benussi S, Pappone C, Nascimbene OG et al. A simple way to treat atrial fibrillation during mitral valve surgery. The epicardial radiofrequency approach. *Eur J Cardiothorac Surg* 2000; **17**: 524–9.
2. Cox JL, Ad N, Palazzo T. Current status of the Maze procedure for the treatment of atrial fibrillation. *Sem Thorac Cardiovasc Surg* 2000; **12**: 15–19.
3. Grossi EA, Galloway AC, LaPietra A et al. Minimally invasive mitral valve surgery: a 6-year experience with 714 patients. *Ann Thorac Surg* 2002; **74**: 660–4.
4. Mohr FW, Fabricus AM, Falk V et al. Curative treatment of AF with intraoperative RF ablation: Short term mid term results. *J Thorac Cardiovasc Surg* 2002; **123**: 919–27.

Related topics of interest

21 Surgery for pericardial disease

David G Cable, Richard C Daly

Diastolic dysfunction is the predominant etiology in 15–50% of clinically overt congestive cardiac failure (CCF). Diastolic heart failure is characterized by elevated cardiac filling pressures despite preserved ejection fraction. This occurs when diastolic ventricular filling is restricted by impaired ventricular relaxation ± compliance, thereby limiting stroke volume and cardiac output. Common causes include hypertrophic cardiomyopathy, restrictive cardiomyopathy, pericardial constriction and cardiac tamponade. Amongst these, pericardial constriction stands out as being potentially correctable by surgery. Cardiac encasement by a rigid noncompliant pericardium restricts ventricular filling exclusively to during early diastole.

Etiology

- Postoperative: incidence 0.2–0.3%; identified risk factors – anticoagulation and early postoperative pericardial effusions.
- Mediastinal radiation: incidence (5–8%) has been rising over time and is dependent on the radiation dose with mantle-field therapy for lymphoproliferative diseases at highest risk.
- Infections: tuberculosis is uncommon in Western societies (<5%) but a major cause in developing countries (38–83%); increasing in HIV patients.
- Idiopathic: major cause (30%) in the developed world.

Diagnosis

Differentiation between pericardial constriction and restrictive cardiomyopathy is challenging but crucial in view of the therapeutic and prognostic implications. Clinical symptoms and hemodynamic and echocardiographic findings may be similar. Pericardial constriction causes restricted ventricular diastolic filling with characteristic respiratory variation and ventricular interdependence as both ventricles share the limited space in the thickened noncompliant pericardium. These findings are absent in restrictive cardiomyopathy with a stiff and noncompliant ventricular myocardium.

Clinical assessment

Symptoms of right/left-sided heart failure include dyspnea, fatigue, weakness, anorexia and peripheral edema. Presentation with abdominal symptoms attributable to hepatosplenomegaly and ascites may confuse initial diagnosis. Signs may include distended neck veins, ascites, peripheral edema, pleural effusions, diffuse/indistinct apex beat, muffled heart sounds, loud pericardial knock (resembling S₃ gallop) and narrowed pulse pressure. Pulsus paradoxus and Kussmaul's sign are typically absent in chronic pericardial constriction. The arterial pressure is normal/slightly reduced.

Investigations

- EKG: low voltage ± atrial arrhythmias.
- Blood: increased atrial natriuretic peptide levels with CCF.
- Chest x ray (CXR): pericardial calcification.
- MRI: quantifies pericardial thickening and demonstrates impaired RV diastolic filling.
- CT: as MRI, and demonstrates pericardial/myocardial calcification.
- Cardiac catheterization: indicated when noninvasive imaging fails to clinch the diagnosis and for endomyocardial biopsy. The position and course of all patent grafts from previous CABG must be evaluated by pre-operative angiography. The classic findings are:
  - 'square root sign' – representing a 'dip-plateau' pattern of ventricular pressure during diastole. Pericardial constriction causes the bulk of ventricular filling to occur in early diastole, which is abnormally rapid due to elevated venous pressures. This halts abruptly in mid-diastole when total cardiac volume fills the entire pericardial sac.
  - prominent 'y' descent of the RA pressure tracing – due to rapid equalization of RA and ventricular pressures in early diastole, followed by a steep 'a' wave and 'x' descent as the RA attempts to eject blood into a full RV.
  - equalization of RVEDP and LVEDP – the fixed pericardial volume and the rapid early diastolic ventricular filling accentuate the normal diastolic coupling of the ventricles via the pliable interventricular septum.

These findings could be masked by hypovolemia and therefore reversed with rapid transfusion. Hemodynamic data favoring the diagnosis include:

- >5 mmHg gradient between RVEDP and LVEDP
- RVSP <50 mmHg
- RVEDP:RVSP >1:3.
- Echocardiography: cardinal features identified by analysis of pulmonary and hepatic venous flow and the mitral inflow include:
  - dissociation of intrathoracic and intracardiac pressures during respiration
  - interdependence of the right and left ventricles
  - impaired diastolic ventricular filling.

Surgery

Approach

Anterolateral left thoracotomy permits ventricular pericardiectomy to be accomplished off-pump. Both ventricles are accessible, including the LV posterior to the left phrenic nerve. This approach may be preferred with previous CABG as it avoids patent anterior grafts. If CPB is required, the incision can be extended across the sternum and bilateral thoracotomies performed. Median sternotomy facilitates concomitant cardiac procedures to be performed. CPB is often required to complete a posterior pericardiectomy and cardioplegic arrest is advantageous when widespread adhesions are present with extensive epicarditis. Postoperative bleeding aggravated by CPB may be ameliorated by aprotinin.

Complete pericardiectomy

This removes thickened pericardium and epicardium from both ventricles over the diaphragmatic, anterior and lateral surfaces. The phrenic nerves are carefully preserved with a window created between the left-sided phrenic nerve and pulmonary veins. Incomplete pericardiectomy risks residual constrictive hemodynamics. Removal of densely adherent, often calcified, atrial pericardium is unnecessary since the pathophysiology affects only ventricular filling.

The dissection plane between the pericardium and heart is difficult to define. Two techniques are helpful:

- Initiate dissection along the diaphragmatic surface, as for redo sternotomy, as minimal epicardial fat in this region facilitates visualization of the correct surgical plane. The entire pericardium must be resected posteriorly to the level of the central tendon of the diaphragm.
- Make a full-thickness cruciate incision through the pericardium on the most accessible aspect of the LV. Subsequently, traction on individual flaps allows appreciation of the correct plane of decortication.

Large calcifications may enter the myocardium, resembling an iceberg, with the risk of ventricular perforation if completely excised. These are debrided with rongeurs ± Cavitron ultrasound aspirator down to the epicardial surface. Residual islands of calcification are not constrictive provided the associated pericardial thickening is completely excised. It is essential that any fibrous epicardial peel is also excised to avoid a risky re-operation for residual constriction. If the epicardium is densely adherent to coronary arteries/myocardium without a clear dissection plane, sequential perpendicular releasing incisions to create multiple boxes may be undertaken ('waffle' procedure). In cases with extremely dense adhesions, islands of thickened pericardium surrounding patent grafts may be left.

Outcome

Mortality

Overall operative mortality has remained constant (approximately 12.8%) at the Mayo Clinic (1936 to 1996). Risk is reduced with idiopathic constriction (7.8%). Factors predisposing to early death include previous cardiac surgery (23.1%), prior mediastinal radiation (17.2%), worse NYHA class, low-voltage EKG, low serum albumin, old age and calcification on CXR.

Morbidities

Common problems are:

- Infection, bleeding, stroke, prolonged intubation, ventricular arrhythmias (7%) and re-exploration (7%).
- Low cardiac output (12%) is a major contributor to perioperative death. Causes include primary myocardial damage (e.g. mediastinal radiation) and myocardial atrophy from longstanding constriction. Sudden removal of the supporting pericardium may allow the ventricles to overdistend. Avoiding cardiac overfilling throughout the perioperative period may be important.
- Re-operations for residual constriction are required in <10% usually from failure to remove epicardial sclerosis.

Late survival

Late survival is reduced in advanced CCF, old age and those with a history of malignancy, pericardial procedure, and mediastinal radiation. The 5- and 10-year survival is approximately 70% and 50%, respectively.

Further reading

1. McCaughan BC, Schaff HV, Piehler JM et al. Early and late results of pericardiectomy for constrictive pericarditis. *J Thorac Cardiovasc Surg* 1985; **89**: 340–50.
2. Arsan S, Mercan S, Sarigul A et al. Long-term experience with pericardiectomy: analysis of 105 consecutive patients. *Thorac Cardiovasc Surgeon* 1994; **42**: 340–4
3. Tsang TS, Barnes ME, Hayes SN et al. Clinical and echocardiographic characteristics of significant pericardial effusions following cardiothoracic surgery and outcomes of echo-guided pericardiocentesis for management: Mayo Clinic experience, 1979–1998. Chest 1999; **116**: 322–31.
4. Ling LH, Oh JK, Schaff HV et al. Constrictive pericarditis in the modern era: evolving clinical spectrum and impact on outcome after pericardiectomy. *Circulation* 1999; **100**: 1380–6.

Related topic of interest

22 Surgery for cardiac tumors

Charles R Bridges

Cardiac tumors can be classified as primary or secondary. The incidence ranges from 0.002% to 0.3% in postmortem series. Approximately three-quarters of primary cardiac tumors are benign and most are amenable to surgical resection. Secondary (metastatic) tumors are 30 times more common. Surgery for cardiac metastases is palliative and involves the management of recurrent pericardial effusions.

Primary benign tumors

Myxoma

1. Incidence

Myxomas represent 41% of benign primary tumors in adults and 15% in children. They are more common in women than in men. Most patients are between 30 and 60 years of age. Seventy-five percent originate in the LA, usually from the interatrial septum. The next most common sites, in order, are the RA, RV and LV. A familial form (Carney complex) is more common in males, occurs at an earlier age and is more often biatrial or multicentric.

2. Pathology

Grossly, most tumors are ovoid, pedunculated, have a smooth or granular appearance and are somewhat friable. They are often mucoid and gray-white in color. Histologically myxomas contain an acid mucopolysaccharide matrix with polygonal cells, capillary-like structures and areas of hemorrhage.

3. Presentation

Specific presenting complaints relate to the obstruction of blood flow, interference with valvular function or systemic embolization. The vast majority of patients also have constitutional symptoms or laboratory abnormalities such as fever, weight loss, malaise, myalgias, arthralgias, anemia and elevations in inflammatory markers.

4. Clinical examination

Physical examination findings are nonspecific. Left atrial myxomas may mimic the auscultatory findings of mitral stenosis or an early diastolic 'tumor plop' can be confused with a third heart sound or an opening snap. The pulmonic component of the second heart sound 'P$_2$' may be accentuated. Right atrial myxomas may cause similar auscultatory findings and are more often associated with a murmur of tricuspid regurgitation due to valvular destruction by a 'wrecking ball' mechanism. Signs of pulmonary hypertension and right-sided heart failure may be present. Left ventricular myxomas may cause findings typical of left ventricular outflow tract obstruction. Any of these auscultatory findings is often a function of position, providing a clue to its origin.

5. Diagnostic studies

The most useful diagnostic modality is TTE or TEE. Both are highly sensitive for detection of atrial tumors. TEE may be more useful for planning intraoperative strategy since more precise localization is often possible. Chest x ray (CXR) and EKG findings may include signs of LA enlargement but are nonspecific.

6. Surgery and results

Surgery is performed via a median sternotomy or right thoracotomy. CPB is performed with bicaval cannulation and snares to divert venous return away from the RA. Manipulation of the heart is minimized at all times and particularly prior to placement of the aortic cross-clamp. Left atrial myxomas can be approached via a longitudinal left atriotomy incision. For larger LA or biatrial myxomas, particularly when a portion of the interatrial septum must be resected, the addition of a second incision parallel to the first in the RA is recommended. The latter incision is convenient for patch closure of the septum that is usually required. For large RA myxomas, direct, more distal cannulation of the vena cavae may be required. Occasionally, a brief period of hypothermic circulatory arrest is necessary to perform a complete resection safely.

Ventricular myxomas are usually approached via an atrial incision via the mitral or tricuspid valves. Occasionally, outflow tract tumors can be approached via the semilunar valves.

The results of surgical resection are excellent, with mortality rates of approximately 5% and recurrence rates of 0–5% in the sporadic type of myxoma.

Non-myxomatous, benign primary tumors

Excluding cysts, these tumors comprise 59% of benign primary cardiac tumors. Lipoma, papillary fibroelastoma, and rhabdomyoma account for approximately two-thirds of non-myxomatous tumors in roughly equal proportions.

1. Lipoma

Lipomas are well-encapsulated tumors that occur in all locations in the heart. Most are solitary. They are frequently subendocardial and may be quite large, causing obstructive symptoms. Tissue characterization by MRI or direct biopsy usually allows for pre-operative diagnosis. Symptomatic lipomas or asymptomatic lipomas encountered during surgery should be excised. The long-term results are excellent.

2. Fibroelastoma

Fibroelastomas arise from the cardiac valves and ventricular endothelium. They are seen most commonly in patients over the age of 50. Grossly, the tumors have been described as resembling a sea anemone with frond-like projections. Involvement of the mitral and aortic valves is most common. These lesions, which can mimic vegetations on echocardiography, may cause symptoms due to obstruction or embolization and should be resected even if asymptomatic. Valve repair should accompany resection if indicated.

3. Rhabdomyoma

Rhabdomyomas are the most common benign primary cardiac tumors in infants and children. The majority are multicentric, often pedunculated, originating from either ventricle and projecting into the ventricular lumen. Histologically, they contain large glycogen-filled cells containing bundles of myofibrils and hyperchromatic nuclei. These tumors are thought to represent fetal hamartomas rather than true neoplasms. Clinically they are associated with obstructive symptoms, valvular regurgitation, arrhythmias and sudden death; 30–50% are associated with a diagnosis of tuberous sclerosis. The surgical approach is generally conservative and directed toward alleviation of symptoms. Rarely is radical excision of these lesions indicated.

4. Other tumors

Other benign tumors are relatively rare, including fibroma, hemangioma, teratoma and mesothelioma of the AV node. Exceedingly rare tumors include neurofibroma, granular cell tumor and lymphangioma.

Primary malignant tumors

Primary malignant tumors of the heart are relatively rare, accounting for 25% of all primary cardiac neoplasms. Nearly all are sarcomas and nearly all are incurable. Surgery is usually aimed at obtaining definitive histological diagnosis. Cardiac transplantation should be considered for those without evidence of metastatic spread. These tumors typically occur in adults older than 40 years. The two most common types are angiosarcoma and rhabdomyosarcoma.

1. Angiosarcoma

These tumors are three times more common in men than women and most arise in the RA or pericardium. These intensely vascular tumors are often bulky and partially intracavitary. Signs of vena caval or valvular obstruction predominate. Distant metastases are usually present at the time of diagnosis. Almost all tumors are inoperable. Median survival is approximately 6 months from the time of diagnosis.

2. Rhabdomyosarcoma

These tumors, mostly multicentric in nature, arise with equal frequency in all areas of the heart. There is a slight male predominance. Most patients have symptoms resulting from valvular obstruction. Resection combined with radiation and chemotherapy has been advocated for small tumors in the absence of signs of distant metastasis. However, the results have generally been poor with greater than 50% mortality within the first year.

3. Other primary malignant tumors

These include fibrous histiocytoma, fibrosarcoma, leiomyosarcoma, liposarcoma, osteosarcoma, plasmacytoma and chondromyxocytoma and sarcomas involving other cell types.

Secondary tumors

Metastatic tumors

These tumors are 30 times more common than primary cardiac tumors. In patients with widely metastatic tumors 10–12% have cardiac involvement. Common cancers include leukemia, breast, lung, lymphoma, melanoma and sarcoma. Surgical therapy is palliative, most commonly for treatment of recurrent pericardial effusions. The subxiphoid approach is preferred. With direct extension of renal cell carcinoma to the RA, hypothermic circulatory arrest with atriotomy and cavotomy usually allows for gentle tumor extraction.

Further reading

1. Hall RA, Anderson RP. Cardiac neoplasms. In: *Cardiac Surgery in the Adult*. Edmunds LH, (ed). McGraw Hill: 1997: New York, pp 1345–63.
2. Reynen K. Cardiac myxomas. *N Engl J Med* 1995; **333**: 1610–17.
3. Schaff HV, Mullany CJ. Surgery for cardiac myxomas. *Sem Thorac Cardiovasc Surg* 2000; **12**: 77–88.

23 Surgery for trauma

23.1 Blunt aortic trauma

Robert F. Wilson, James G. Tyburski

Approximately 80–90% of patients with blunt trauma to thoracic great vessels, particularly the aorta, die at the scene and up to 50% of the remaining patients die within 48 hours if not properly treated. Of the blunt injuries to the great vessels in patients reaching the hospital alive, 80–90% involve the isthmus of aorta between the left subclavian artery and ligamentum arteriosum, about 5–15% involve branches of the aortic arch and about 5–10% involve more than one area.

Although emphasis has generally been to get the patient with such injuries to the operating room as soon as possible, it is probably much more important to diagnose and treat other life-threatening injuries first. If the patient's systolic pressure is kept <120 mmHg, it is unlikely that a partially torn aorta will rupture prematurely. Surgery should be performed on such lesions only if uncontrolled bleeding is present or if the conditions for repair are optimal.

Pathophysiology

Blunt trauma generally distributes energy over a much larger area than penetrating trauma. It is usually associated with high-speed motor vehicle accidents or falls. Due to the differential inertia, extreme strains are put onto points of anatomical fixation such as the ligamentum arteriosum. Further deformation of tissue occurs at the point of impact. The resulting strain may produce a stretch or compressive deformity. Consequently, major cardiovascular injury can occur in the absence of any overt external chest wall trauma.

Signs and symptoms

One should suspect traumatic rupture of the aorta (TRA) in anyone who has had sudden, severe deceleration, including high-speed motor vehicle accidents. Patients with TRA usually complain primarily of their associated injuries and generally have few or no symptoms related to the aortic injury itself. The most common symptom that may be due to the aortic injury itself is retrosternal or interscapular pain from 'stretching' or dissection of the aortic adventitia. Less common symptoms, due to pressure from the hematoma on adjacent structures, include dysphagia, stridor, dyspnea, voice change, or hoarseness. Physical findings that suggest aortic injury include upper extremity hypertension, decreased pulsations or blood pressure in the lower extremities, and presence of a harsh systolic murmur over the upper chest or posterior interscapular area.

Radiographic studies

The diagnosis of TRA is usually suspected from the findings on routine chest radiography. The most notable finding is widening of the superior mediastinum, usually to more than 8.0–8.5 cm. However, AP films taken with the patient supine will tend to make the mediastinum look wider. The optimal chest radiograph is a PA view with the patient in an upright position from a distance of 1.5 m and leaning forward at 15 degrees.

The most reliable chest radiographic sign of TRA is deviation of the esophagus (highlighted by nasogastric tube) or trachea greater than 1–2 cm to the right of the spinous process of T4. In several series, none of the patients with the esophagus less than 1.0 cm from the midline had TRA.

The value of CT in screening for TRA remains controversial. In stable patients with equivocal chest radiographs, but with a low clinical suspicion of vascular injury, CT can reliably differentiate mediastinal hematoma from other causes of mediastinal widening and also reveal concomitant injuries. The newer spiral CT scanner is even more accurate.

The newer generations of magnetic resonance imaging (MRI) scanners should be ideal for posttraumatic studies of thoracic vessels if the patient: (a) is hemodynamically stable, (b) does not require mechanical ventilation, (c) can lie still for full duration of study and (d) does not have a pacemaker or other metallic objects susceptible to the magnetic field.

Thoracic aortography is still considered the gold standard for diagnosing TRA, and most trauma surgeons believe that it should be done on all patients who are suspected of having a TRA.

If transesophageal echocardiography (TEE) is readily available, it can detect blunt injuries to the aorta with a high sensitivity and specificity in the hands of a skilled operator.

Treatment

If the systolic blood pressure of a patient with TRA can be kept <120 mmHg, surgery should be delayed to optimize outcome. This may be particularly important in patients with other multiple severe injuries, especially to the brain.

The clamp/repair technique should not be used if the surgeon is unaccustomed to thoracic aortic surgery or if the repair is likely to require more than 30 min of aortic clamp time (because of the increased risk of paraplegia). With the clamp/repair technique, the proximal clamp is usually placed on the arch between the left common carotid and left subclavian arteries. A clamp is also placed on the left subclavian artery and on the descending aorta just distal to the hematoma to avoid interference with the upper intercostal arteries.

Critics of the clamp/repair technique have noted that aortic cross-clamping may result in high mortality and morbidity rates, especially if the aorta is clamped for more than 30 min. In addition, significant hemodynamic and metabolic changes can occur in patients without a shunt or bypass to the distal aorta.

Heparin-bonded tubing as a shunt from the ascending aorta or the apex of the left ventricle (Gott shunt) either to the descending aorta or to a femoral artery can reduce the danger of distal ischemia to the spinal cord and abdominal viscera. It can also prevent proximal hypertension causing cardiac and cerebral injury and has the benefit of avoiding systemic heparinization in a traumatized patient.

Repair of trauma rupture of the thoracic aorta is often performed under partial CPB because it allows increased time for a meticulous repair. Total CPB offers the advantage of systemic hypothermia with additional spinal/cerebral protection during surgery and is mandatory in repairing tears of the ascending aorta or arch.

One form of partial CPB use is femoral vein to femoral artery bypass with vacuum-assisted venous drainage. This involves use of an oxygenator and requires heparinization, which can be a significant risk in patients with multiple trauma.

If a vortex pump (e.g. BioMedicus) is used with left atrial-femoral artery bypass, an oxygenator is not needed, reducing heparin requirement and the risk of excessive bleeding. This may be particularly important in patients with associated injuries to the brain, eyes, or retroperitoneum. In most series in which this technique was used, few deaths (5%) and no paraplegia have been reported. This is increasingly becoming the technique of choice in these multiply injured patients. However, it is important to maintain distal aortic flow at greater than 1.0 l/min to prevent clotting and to maintain adequate distal perfusion.

Endovascular stenting is currently being investigated as an alternative treatment for this condition in selected candidates.

Complications

The most serious complications in patients who survive surgery for blunt trauma to thoracic great vessels are paraplegia and renal failure. Certainly an inadequate blood flow to the lower spinal cord for more than 30 min greatly increases the risk of this complication, especially if the patient is hypotensive before, during, and/or after aortic clamping.

Renal failure is usually proportional to the duration and severity of any hypoperfusion of the kidneys. The degree of renal damage can probably be assessed most accurately by calculating creatinine clearance from directly measured urine creatinine levels.

Further reading

1. Fujekawa T, Yukioka T, Ishimaru S et al. Endovascular stent grafting for the treatment of blunt thoracic aortic injury. *J Trauma* 2001; **50**: 223–9.
2. Mattox KL, Wall MJ Jr, Lemaire SA. Injury to the thoracic great vessels. In: *Trauma. 4th Edn.* Mattox KL, Feliciano DV, Moore EE (eds). McGraw-Hill: New York, 2000: pp. 559–82.
3. Wilson RF. Trauma to intrathoracic great vessels. In: *Handbook of Trauma: Pitfalls and Pearls.* Wilson RF (ed). Lippincott, Williams & Wilkins: Philadelphia, 1999: pp 275–88.
4. Wilson RF, Stephenson LW. Trauma to intrathoracic great vessels. In: *Management of Trauma: Pitfalls and Practice.* Wilson RF, Walt AJ (eds). Williams & Wilkins: Philadelphia, 1996: pp 373–87.
5. Wilson RF, Tyburski JG. Penetrating trauma to the aortic arch, innominate and subclavian arteries. In: *Current Therapy in Vascular Surgery.* Ernst CB, Stanley JC (eds). Mosby: St. Louis, 1995: pp 608–13.

Related topics of interest

23.2 Penetrating mediastinal trauma

Robert F Wilson, James G Tyburski

Patients who survive the initial penetrating trauma to mediastinal vessels and reach hospital alive generally do so because of local tamponade. The formation of an arteriovenous fistula or an injury in the pericardial cavity may also avoid exsanguination, thus prolonging survival.

Pathophysiology

Common causes include knives, firearms and motor vehicle accidents producing fragments. The extent of injury depends on kinetic energy (KE) transfer delivered by the projectiles where $KE = mv^2/2$ (m = mass of projectile; v = velocity; g = gravity): low-velocity missiles (<400 m/s muzzle velocity); medium-velocity missiles (400–500 m/s); high-velocity missiles (>800 m/s). It is clear that high-velocity missile injuries can cause greater internal injuries despite a seemingly small entry wound.

Presentation

The size of a knife and the depth and angle of penetration may predict the likely injury. With gunshot wounds, the location of the entrance and exit wounds together with radiographic location of the bullet identify potential vascular injury. Even when the subclavian or innominate arteries are occluded, the excellent collateral circulation of the scapula anastomoses may maintain a normal distal pulse. Conversely, vascular spasm secondary to adjacent soft tissue/bony injury can cause loss of pulses even in the absence of proximal vessel injury. Auscultation of a systolic bruit should lead one to suspect a false aneurysm while a continuous bruit suggests an AV fistula.

Diagnosis

With injury to mediastinal vessels, radiography of the chest usually demonstrates hemothorax and, if an erect posture is possible, an air-fluid level may be seen in a pneumohemothorax. In a supine patient accumulation of 500–1000 ml of blood may cause only slight opacification of the involved hemithorax. Decubitus films will generally demonstrate layering of blood unless it is loculated or clotted. Pulsation of a foreign body (bullet) caused by its proximity to a major vessel may render its radiographic margins indistinct or 'fuzzy'.

In hemodynamically stable patients, CT scans can identify many injuries that are not apparent on routine radiography. The identification of a constant extravascular 'mass' adjacent to a great vessel generally indicates a contained hematoma.

Arteriography is the gold standard for diagnosing major intrathoracic vascular injuries. A false-negative result may arise if the penetration site is temporarily 'sealed' by hematoma or if the radiographic projection is inappropriate.

A contrast swallow and/or endoscopy should be performed if the patient is hemodynamically stable and if one suspects an associated esophageal or tracheobronchial injury.

Treatment

Although most patients with intrathoracic bleeding can be treated adequately with intravenous fluids and a chest tube, 5–15% of patients require thoracotomy for continuing hemorrhage. This subset includes patients with major vascular injury. If the patient has persistent shock in spite of aggressive fluid resuscitation, an emergency thoracotomy should be performed. Even if the patient's vital signs are stable, thoracotomy is indicated if there is severe, continued bleeding as demonstrated by: (a) more than 1500–2000 ml of blood loss from the chest within the first 4 hours of injury; (b) blood loss from the chest tubes exceeding 200–300 ml/h for 4–5 hours or more; (c) the chest remaining more than half full of blood on radiography in spite of properly positioned chest tubes; and (d) positive arteriography for major vessel injury.

If the patient's condition improves with volume replacement and drainage of the hemothorax, conservative treatment is appropriate. If vital signs deteriorate with drainage of a massive hemothorax, the chest tube should be clamped and the patient expedited to the operating room.

A standard posterolateral thoracotomy provides excellent exposure to almost all parts of the hemithorax. In hypovolemic patients the lateral position can reduce venous return, impair cardiac output and cause a precipitous drop in blood pressure.

A median sternotomy is usually the ideal incision for exploring penetrating wounds of the thoracic inlet or injuries involving the innominate artery, proximal portions of the carotid and right subclavian arteries and pulmonary vessels. Extension of the median sternotomy into the neck along the anterior border of the sternocleidomastoid muscle or along the clavicle (sometimes removing the head of the clavicle) can also provide excellent exposure to the proximal right subclavian and mid-left subclavian arteries, as well as the more distal portions of the right common carotid artery.

An anterolateral thoracotomy is usually the ideal incision for exploring patients with penetrating chest trauma if they are in shock, have moderate to severe hemoptysis, or require internal cardiac massage. Additional exposure can be rapidly obtained by converting this to a bilateral anterior thoracotomy (i.e. a 'clam shell' incision). Once bleeding is controlled, further surgery should be delayed until the patient is adequate resuscitated with fluid/inotropes.

During CPR or management of very severe shock, cross-clamping the descending thoracic aorta may improve coronary and cerebral blood flow. The systolic pressure should be kept below 160 mmHg during this maneuver.

If an adequate repair of the thoracic aorta can be obtained with direct suturing or side-clamping, aortic cross-clamping should be avoided. If the latter is necessary, various methods may be employed: (1) simple cross-clamping of the aorta ('clamp-and-sew') without a shunt or bypass; (2) external heparin-bonded shunt from the proximal aorta to either the distal thoracic aorta or a femoral artery (Gott shunt); (3) partial or complete CPB; and (4) left atrial bypass with a centrifugal pump to the distal thoracic aorta or femoral artery without an oxygenator and with little or no heparinization (heparin bonded circuit). Clamping of the thoracic aorta at the distal arch or isthmus without distal aortic flow for more than 30 min is associated with a high risk of paraplegia.

In most instances, the holes in the great vessels are relatively small (or the patient would have rapidly exsanguinated), and direct repair is often easily accomplished. Whenever possible, sutures in the aorta and large arteries should be tied while the intraluminal pressure is low. Repairs of the proximal common carotid artery in young patients often do not require internal or external shunting unless the occlusion time exceeds 4–5 min. Although gangrene of the upper extremity is unusual with ligation of the subclavian artery, the injured vessel should be repaired whenever possible.

Defects in vena cavae can be repaired by direct venorrhaphy. If the inferior or superior vena cava must be completely clamped in the chest, the sudden, severe reduction in venous return can cause cardiac arrest, particularly in hypovolemic patients. If the descending thoracic or proximal abdominal aorta is clamped or compressed simultaneously, the clamping of an intrathoracic cava is better tolerated.

Further reading

1. Fingleton JG, Gass J, Isoda S, Stephenson LW. Thoracic great vessels. In: *The Textbook of Penetrating Trauma*. Ivaturry RR, Cayten CG (eds). Williams & Wilkins: Baltimore, 1996: pp 512–30.
2. Mattox KL, Wall MJ Jr, Lemaire SA. Injury to the thoracic great vessels. In: *Trauma. 4th Edn*. Mattox KL, Feliciano DV, Moore EE (eds). McGraw-Hill: New York, 2000: pp 559–82.
3. Wilson RF. Trauma to intrathoracic great vessels. In: *Handbook of Trauma: Pitfalls and Pearls*. Wilson RF (ed). Lippincott, Williams & Wilkins: Philadelphia, 1999, pp 266–75.
4. Wilson RF, Stephenson LW. Trauma to intrathoracic great vessels. In: *Management of Trauma: Pitfalls and Practice*. Wilson RF, Walt AJ (eds). Williams & Wilkins: Philadelphia, 1996: pp 361–73.
5. Wilson RF, Tyburski JG. Penetrating trauma to the aortic arch, innominate and subclavian arteries. In: *Current Therapy in Vascular Surgery*. Ernst CB, Stanley JC (eds). Mosby: St. Louis, 1995: pp 608–13.

Related topics of interest

23.3 Blunt cardiac trauma

Robert F Wilson, James G Tyburski

Incidence

Blunt cardiac injury is the most frequent, unsuspected visceral injury responsible for death in accident victims, accounting for about 25% of fatalities. The reported incidence of cardiac injury after blunt chest trauma in patients reaching the hospital alive averages 15–25%, varying from 16% in an autopsy series to 76% in clinical studies.

The most common cause of blunt cardiac trauma is high-speed motor vehicle accidents. Other causes include direct blows to the chest, industrial crush injuries, falls from heights, blast injuries, and athletic trauma.

Types of injuries

Of patients with blunt cardiac injuries, up to 37% have pericardial tears, with left pleuroperi-cardial tears being most common.

Blunt cardiac rupture is usually immediately fatal. In the few who reach hospital alive, the most frequent injury is a tear of the right atrium at its junction with the SVC or IVC.

Patients with a ventricular septal defect (VSD) from blunt trauma are generally critically ill as a result of the shunt and the associated myocardial and pulmonary contusion. Isolated atrial septal defects (ASDs) due to blunt trauma are extremely rare and are rapidly fatal.

Aortic insufficiency is the most common valvular injury caused by blunt trauma. This usually involves rupture of a cusp, at its free border, at its base, or at one of its commissural attachments.

Myocardial contusion

Myocardial contusions constitute over 90% of blunt cardiac injuries. The typical pathologic changes seen at autopsy include subendocardial and interstitial hemorrhage, large surrounding areas of focal myocardial edema, myofibrillar degeneration, myocytolysis and infiltration of polymorphonuclear leukocytes. The anterior right ventricular wall is most frequently involved, followed by the anterior interventricular septum and left ventricular apex.

Myocardial contusions can cause arrhythmias and/or conduction defects, impairing myocardial contractility in 10–20% of patients. Most patients with myocardial contusions have relatively few problems unless:

(a) arrhythmia or conduction defect is present
(b) clinical evidence of heart failure exists
(c) multiple injuries are present
(d) pre-existing cardiac disease is present or
(e) general anesthesia is required.

This is particularly true when surgery is prolonged or involves aortic cross-clamping with significant blood loss. General anesthesia within a month of myocardial contusion carries a significant risk of arrhythmias or hypotension.

Acute dilation of the heart often follows experimental cardiac contusions but this is seldom seen clinically. Chest radiography has its greatest value in the recognition of associated injuries. The major radiographic abnormalities seen with myocardial contusion are fractures of the first two ribs, clavicles, or sternum. In many series, a fractured sternum is most commonly associated with myocardial contusion. However, the reported incidence of myocardial contusion under such circumstances is only 5–6%.

An EKG should be obtained on admission and at 12 and 24 hours post-injury in anyone suspected of a myocardial injury. New EKG changes are unlikely to evolve after 24 hours.

Although many of these patients develop abnormalities on EKG, few require therapy. New atrial fibrillation, multiple ectopics, or conduction disturbances are more important than ST-T segment changes and are virtually diagnostic of direct or indirect (ischemic or hypoxic) myocardial injury. Holter monitoring is more sensitive at detecting arrhythmias although few arrhythmias detected with this technique require therapy.

With acute myocardial contusions, serial troponins should be assessed on admission and at 4–8 hours post-injury. Troponins (I and T), which peak within 4–8 hours, are more sensitive and specific than CK-MB, and have replaced the latter in clinical use.

Transthoracic echocardiography (TTE) has many advantages in the assessment of acute myocardial contusion. Quantitative and qualitative information can be obtained noninvasively on cardiac chamber abnormalities, wall-motion defects, valvular functional integrity, cardiac tamponade, and the presence of intracardiac thrombus or shunts. TTE has been advocated in all suspected cardiac injuries, particularly in the presence of abnormal EKGs or elevated cardiac isoenzymes. Transesophageal echocardiography (TEE) can be used to rapidly and completely evaluate the heart and exclude other injuries, including traumatic aortic rupture. This relatively noninvasive procedure can be performed at the bedside. Unlike TTE, it is unaffected by recent cardiac or abdominal procedures, mechanical ventilation, hemodynamic monitoring lines, chest tubes, or dressings and provides better imaging of the posterior cardiac structures.

First-pass biventricular radionuclide angiography (RNA) can now be performed at the bedside, as well as in the radiology department. This appears to be a very sensitive technique to assess cardiac function, including left and right ventricular ejection fractions, and regional wall-motion abnormalities. However, many patients with an abnormal RNA do not appear to have any clinical cardiac problems. Single-photon emission computed tomography (SPECT) has similar potential for diagnosing myocardial contusions.

Treatment

Patients without identifiable EKG abnormality, myocardial enzyme changes, wall-motion abnormalities on echocardiography or RNA do not require continuous cardiac monitoring, unless indicated for other severe injuries.

Cardiac arrhythmias should be treated promptly with appropriate medication. Prophylactic treatment is generally not indicated. Low-cardiac output or hypotension should be treated with fluids and/or inotropic agents, guided by the response of the PAWP, CVP and cardiac output. If the patient remains hypotensive despite adequate volume replacement, inotropic support, and correction of any mechanical problems (e.g. tamponade), use of an intra-aortic balloon pump (IABP) should be considered.

If intra-mural thrombus is found on echocardiography, it is not clear whether the patients should have prophylactic anticoagulation in the context of recent trauma.

Direct injury to the coronary arteries from blunt chest trauma occurs rarely (<2%). If cardiac tamponade occurs, immediate operation is indicated. Coronary artery thrombosis due to chest trauma is also rare but has been reported.

Hemopericardium or pericardial effusion can occur late (>7 days) even without evidence of associated cardiac injury. Treatment requires drainage and, as with other causes of pericardial effusion, the timing of intervention depends upon the hemodynamic status.

Follow-up

Most patients discharged after blunt cardiac injury will do well. When RNA has been repeated after myocardial contusions, significant improvement is almost uniformly documented by 3–4 weeks. By 1 year, follow-up studies indicate that right and left ventricular ejection fractions, even during maximal workloads, are essentially the same as in control patients.

Further reading

1. Bertinchant J, Polge A, Mohty D et al. Evaluation of incidence, clinical significance, and prognostic value of circulatory cardiac troponin I and T in hemodynamically stable patients with suspected myocardial contusion after blunt chest trauma. *J Trauma* 2000; **48**: 924–31.
2. Ivatury RR. The injured heart. In: *Trauma. 4th Edn.* Mattox KL, Feliciano DV, Moore EE (eds). MacGraw-Hill, New York: 2000: pp 545–58.
3. Wilson RF. Thoracic trauma: heart. In: *Handbook of Trauma: Pitfalls and Pearls.* Wilson RF (ed). Lippincott, Williams & Wilkins: Philadelphia, 1999: pp 255–65.
4. Wilson RF, Stephenson LW. Thoracic trauma: heart. In: *Management of Trauma: Pitfalls and Practice.* Wilson RF, Walt AJ (eds). Williams & Wilkins: Philadelphia, 1996: pp 350–61.

Related topics of interest

23.4 Penetrating cardiac trauma

Robert F Wilson, James G Tyburski

Pathophysiology

All patients who are in shock with a penetrating chest injury anywhere near the heart should be considered to have a cardiac injury requiring an emergency thoracotomy until proven otherwise. With early, aggressive resuscitation and surgery, up to one-third of patients arriving at a trauma center 'in extremis' with penetrating cardiac injuries can be saved. In patients arriving at the operating room with signs of life and a recordable blood pressure, survival rates have exceeded 70% for gunshot wounds and 85% for stab wounds of the heart.

Patients who arrive within 5–10 min of having a penetrating heart injury usually have relatively small cardiac wounds and/or cardiac tamponade. Although cardiac tamponade may prolong life by reducing the severity of the initial hemorrhage, it may be fatal by compromising cardiac diastolic filling.

Diagnosis

Penetrating cardiac injury with isolated tamponade in a normovolemic patient may be diagnosed using the Beck I triad which includes: (1) distended neck veins, (2) hypotension, and (3) muffled heart tones. However, the Beck I triad may be falsely positive or falsely negative in up to a one-third of cases. In addition, the neck veins in patients with shock from cardiac tamponade are not usually distended until any coexistent hypovolemia is at least partially corrected. Cardiac tamponade may also produce the two Kussmaul signs, which are (1) increased neck vein distention during inspiration and (2) pulsus paradoxus with a decrease in systolic blood pressure of 15 mmHg or more during spontaneous inspiration.

If possible, a chest radiograph should be obtained on all trauma victims before they are brought to the operating room. Although chest films are of little help in diagnosing acute cardiac injury, they may reveal a coincident hemopneumothorax that requires chest tube drainage. If the patient is hemodynamically stable, CT scans can be very accurate for diagnosing tamponade or other major injuries. Transthoracic echocardiography may be very helpful, but may be falsely negative in up to 5–10% of cardiac tamponades, especially if a left hemothorax is also present.

If blood is obtained on a paraxiphoid pericardiocentesis and the patient's vital signs improve promptly, a tamponade is almost certainly present. However, the incidence of false-negative pericardiocentesis may be as high as 80%, and the incidence of false positives may be up to 33%. Indeed, if a large amount (>20 ml) of blood is aspirated easily during pericardiocentesis, it is likely that one is aspirating blood from the heart rather than the pericardial cavity.

Another method for diagnosing cardiac injury in a patient who is hemodynamically stable is a subxiphoid pericardial window, usually performed under general anesthesia. If intrapericardial blood is found, as it is in about 14–18% of patients, the incision can be extended up as a median sternotomy to expose and repair the cardiac wound.

Treatment

In patients who are hypotensive and have a low cardiac output, a brief attempt should be made to increase intravascular volume by rapid intravenous infusion of normal (0.9%) saline or Ringer's lactate. If the patient improves and the CVP does not rise as fluid is given rapidly, one can continue to give fluid until systemic pressure and tissue perfusion are adequate. If the CVP rises abruptly with no improvement in tissue perfusion, the patient needs emergency surgery.

In hospitals where adequate facilities, equipment, and trained personnel are present, an emergency department (ED) thoracotomy should be considered in patients who arrive within 10 min of having detectable signs of life. Nevertheless, if the patient can be moved to the operating room with reasonable safety, the results with emergency thoracotomy are much better. This contrasts with blunt cardiac trauma when the outcome of ED thoracotomy for cardiac arrest is uniformly poor.

After the patient is intubated, an anterolateral thoracotomy is performed on the side of the injury, one interspace below the male nipple. If the injury is in the midline, a left anterolateral thoracotomy is performed. If additional exposure to the heart is needed the incision can be extended across the sternum as a bilateral anterior thoracotomy (clam shell incision). This allows wide exposure to both sides of the heart and to the proximal great vessels but requires control of both internal thoracic arteries. If the patient is relatively stable and the cardiac injury is likely to be anterior (as with anterior stab wounds), a median sternotomy can be used to explore the chest.

The pericardial sac is opened in a longitudinal direction 1–2 cm anterior to the phrenic nerve. After the pericardotomy, the surgeon evacuates all blood and clots, begins open cardiac massage as needed, and occludes any bleeding cardiac wounds.

All cardiac wounds are repaired by direct suturing if feasible. Otherwise digital pressure can usually control the bleeding until a repair can be accomplished. A Foley catheter balloon can also be used to occlude the hole until it is repaired. If a posterior cardiac injury cannot be seen, the heart can be swung out laterally and anteriorly out of the pericardial sac to enhance exposure. If it is necessary to lift the apex of the heart in the presence of left-sided or posterior cardiac wounds, this should be undertaken cautiously to minimize the risk of air embolism.

Most atrial wounds can be temporarily controlled by the application of a Satinsky vascular clamp and then sewn with a running polypropylene suture. Wounds of the ventricles can generally be digitally controlled while pledgetted horizontal mattress sutures are passed under the digit and tied by an assistant. When a wound is situated next to a major coronary artery, a pledgetted horizontal mattress suture is placed beneath the artery so as to avoid compression of the vessel. Occasionally, distal bypass grafting may be necessary.

In patients with severe hypotension or cardiac arrest, occluding the descending thoracic aorta will improve coronary and cerebral perfusion. If the patient regains satisfactory cardiac output, the descending thoracic aorta can be gradually unclamped as fluid and blood are infused, aiming for systolic blood pressure around 90–100 mmHg. One should avoid systolic blood pressures greater than 160–180 mmHg when the aorta is clamped because the high pressure may tear open cardiac repairs, excessively dilate the left ventricle (causing irreversible LV failure), or cause intracerebral bleeding.

Ligation of the cut ends is the treatment of choice for lacerations of small coronary vessels. Torn proximal coronary arteries may also be ligated if no evidence of cardiovascular dysfunction exists. If ligation of a proximal coronary artery results in arrhythmias or impaired hemodynamic function, the vessel should be repaired primarily (and usually) on CPB.

Long-term follow-up (months) of these patients is important to detect late complications including valvular dysfunction and septal defects.

Further reading

1. Buckman RF Jr, Buckman PD, Badellino MM. Heart. In: *The Textbook of Penetrating Trauma*. Ivatury RR, Cayten CG (eds). Williams & Wilkins: Baltimore, 1996: pp 499–511.
2. Ivatury RR. The injured heart. In: *Trauma. 4th Edn*. Mattox KL, Felician DV, Moore EE (eds). MacGraw-Hill: New York, 2000: pp 545–58.
3. Tyburski JG, Astra L, Wilson RF, Dente C, Steffes C. Factors affecting prognosis with penetrating wounds of the heart. *J Trauma* 2000; **48**: 587–91.
4. Wilson RF. Thoracic trauma: heart. In: *Handbook of Trauma: Pitfalls and Pearls*. Wilson RF (ed). Lippincott, Williams & Wilkins: Philadelphia, 1999: pp 246–55.
5. Wilson RF, Stephenson LW. Thoracic trauma: heart. In: *Management of Trauma: Pitfalls and Practice*. Wilson RF, Walt AJ (eds). Williams & Wilkins: Philadelphia, 1996: pp 343–50.

Related topics of interest

24 Pulmonary thromboendarterectomy

Stuart W Jamieson

Pulmonary hypertension that results from pulmonary embolism is much more prevalent than recognized, and many patients continue to be misdiagnosed despite the relatively high incidence. It is a progression of acute pulmonary embolism in patients who survive the episode. Over the years, the pathological process that follows in both the affected and the unaffected vessels progresses to a level that is debilitating for the patients. Chronic pulmonary hypertension carries a high mortality rate, with a very poor prognosis. Medical therapy is limited to supportive care, including anticoagulation, diuretics, and vasodilators. The disease, however, is due to a fixed obstructive lesion, making surgery the only curative treatment. Although transplantation for these patients has been suggested and perhaps is still practiced in a few centers, we consider it inappropriate. The mainstay of treatment is surgical removal of obstruction, pulmonary endarterectomy.

Incidence

Although it is impossible to assess accurately the incidence, in 1983 it was estimated that symptomatic pulmonary embolism affected about 630 000 people in the USA with about 500 000 survivors, making it half as common as acute myocardial infarction. The percentage of patients progressing to chronic pulmonary vascular obstruction is also uncertain, but it has been estimated that approximately 100 000 people in the USA have pulmonary hypertension that could be relieved by operation.

Etiology

Even though the majority of patients with chronic pulmonary thromboembolic disease are unaware of a past thromboembolic event, most cases derive from acute embolic episodes. Why some patients are unable to resolve these clots remains uncertain, but it may be a combination of several factors. These include abnormal lytic mechanisms, an overwhelming volume of acute embolic material, repetitive emboli, or embolic substances that cannot be resolved by normal mechanisms (e.g. fat, tumor, or already well-organized fibrous thrombus).

1. Inherited
Ten to twenty percent of patients may possess a higher propensity for thrombosis or a hypercoagulable state. These conditions include inherited deficiencies of antithrombin III, protein C, and protein S, in addition to lupus anticoagulant and dysfibrinogenemias.

2. Acquired
Most patients have a history of embolic disease, and here the etiology is similar to that for deep vein thrombosis, and acute pulmonary embolism. These include malignancy, obesity,

venous stasis, estrogen therapy, and smoking. In some circumstances, chronic indwelling catheters and pacemaker leads are associated with chronic pulmonary emboli.

3. Secondary vasculopathy

After an acute embolic episode, irreversible vascular changes may develop in vessels not affected by the embolus. These changes are not completely explained by simple hemodynamic effects, as a result of redirected blood flow, and other hormonal and neurological factors are probably involved.

Clinical presentation

The clinical presentation of patients with chronic pulmonary hypertension is far from uniform, especially if right-heart failure has not developed. Patients may have a history of progressive dyspnea on exercise. Other symptoms may include chest pain (exertional, or atypical, and often pleuritic), recurrent episodes of thrombophlebitis, hemoptysis, chronic non-productive cough, and perhaps palpitations. Physical findings usually include signs of severe pulmonary hypertension, often combined with evidence of right-heart failure. These may include cyanosis, chronic venous stasis with skin discoloration, and healed varicosities.

Specific investigation

Multiple laboratory, radiographic, and interventional procedure are used as part of the diagnostic work-up. These include blood tests (looking for hypercoagulable states, abnormal liver function, hypoxemia, etc.), chest radiography, EKG, echocardiography, pulmonary function tests, pulmonary ventilation/perfusion (V/Q) scan, chest CT scanning and MRI, pulmonary angiography, and pulmonary angioscopy.

1. V/Q scan

A radionuclide ventilation/perfusion scan is almost always performed. This typically shows multiple punched-out lobar or segmental defects associated with chronic thromboembolic disease, in contrast to a diffuse mottled appearance typical of primary pulmonary hypertension. The perfusion scan has a tendency to underestimate the degree of vascular occlusion, and a moderate probability scan in a patient with other features suggestive of the disease always warrants further investigation.

2. Pulmonary angiography

Selective pulmonary angiography combined with right-heart catheterization remains the gold standard for diagnosis. In addition, with calculation of pulmonary vascular resistance, the study is used to evaluate the severity of the disease, determine the surgical acceptability, and estimate the operative risk. The classical findings are dilated proximal pulmonary arteries, with an irregular lumen, lack of filling out in the periphery often with an abrupt termination of pulmonary vessels, and the appearance of bands or webs. In addition, patients older than 45 years of age undergo coronary angiography so that any significant disease may be dealt with at the time of pulmonary endarterectomy.

3. Angioscopy

When the result of pulmonary angiography is equivocal, and the differentiation between primary pulmonary hypertension and small vessel pulmonary thromboembolic disease difficult, pulmonary angioscopy is employed (about 10–15% of our patients). The angioscope is a fiberoptic scope with a distal balloon, which is inserted through the internal jugular vein. Once in position, the balloon is inflated against the vascular wall, thereby creating a bloodless field for visualization. The characteristic findings in burnt-out embolic disease are intimal thickening and irregularity, pitting, and the presence of pouches, bands, and webs.

Management

Medical management is entirely supportive, and not curative. It consists of chronic anticoagulation, diuretics, vasodilators, and inotropic agents, such as adrenergic agonists, phosphodiesterase inhibitors, and glycosides.

Pulmonary thromboendarterectomy

Pulmonary thromboendarterectomy (PTE) performed by an experienced surgeon is the only curative treatment for thromboembolic pulmonary hypertension. Generally the procedure is offered based on the severity of the disease, and the overall condition of the patient. However, with our increasing experience, we are offering this procedure to all symptomatic patients with angiographic findings suggestive of chronic thromboembolic disease. There are three major reasons to consider pulmonary thromboendarterectomy:

(1) The hemodynamic goal of alleviating right ventricular compromise.
(2) The respiratory goal of improving function by removing the V/Q mismatch.
(3) The prophylactic goal of preventing progression of right ventricular compromise, and preventing secondary vasculopathy in the remainder of the pulmonary circulation.

The procedure is contraindicated in patients with no evidence of pulmonary thromboembolic disease, such as those with primary pulmonary hypertension, severe cardiac failure without thromboembolic disease, or in patients with severe irreversible underlying respiratory disease.

Pulmonary thromboendarterectomy has evolved over the years with certain principles that must be followed. The bilateral nature of the disease, in almost all patients, mandates a median sternotomy to afford access to both sides. Cardiopulmonary bypass is then used to provide hemodynamic stability as well as to allow cooling of the patient, so that circulatory arrest can be achieved. A good surgical outcome can only be accomplished if a complete and effective endarterectomy has been performed – this is only possible in the completely bloodless field provided by complete circulatory arrest. Removal of visible thrombus is only incidental in this operation; the key to success is the recognition and development of the true endarterectomy plane, and a complete endarterectomy to the feathered tail in each branch (Figures 2 and 3).

Over 1000 patients have undergone pulmonary thromboendarterectomy at University of California San Diego since 1990, with a mortality rate of less than 7%. Half of the mortality was related to the patients in whom thromboembolic disease was not the cause of pulmonary hypertension. The differentiation is not always easily made, due to an occasional secondary thrombus that can occur with primary pulmonary hypertension.

The most common complication is reperfusion injury, seen in about 10% of our patients and directly related to this procedure. Other complications include arrhythmias, pericardial effusion, bleeding, volume overload, infection, and persistent pulmonary hypertension. Persistent pulmonary hypertension is usually a diagnostic rather than an operative technical problem.

The only other curative alternative for these patients is transplantation. However, we feel this to be inappropriate. Considering the low morbidity and mortality associated with pulmonary endarterectomy, the long wait for a transplant donor and the mortality during this waiting period, as well as long-term problems associated with rejection and immunosuppression, pulmonary transplantation is not optimal treatment

Further reading

1. Archibald CJ, Auger WR, Fedullo PF et al. Long-term outcome after pulmonary thromboendarterctomy. *Am J Respir Crit Care Med* 1999; **160:** 523–8.
2. Dalen JE, Alpert JS. Natural history of pulmonary embolism. *Prog Cardiovasc Dis* 1975; **17:** 257–70.
3. Jamieson SW, Kapelanski DP. Pulmonary endarterectomy. *Curr Prob Surg* 2000; **37:** 170–252.

25 Surgery for heart failure

25.1 The intra-aortic balloon pump

Alberto Pochettino

History

The concept of diastolic augmentation and systolic unloading was first developed in the 1950s using devices that could remove blood from circulation during systole and replace it during diastole. While physiologic benefits could be demonstrated, severe hemolysis precluded clinical adoption. The use of an intra-aortic balloon was first introduced experimentally in the 1960s. Kantrowitz reported the first successful use of a polyurethane intra-aortic balloon pump (IABP) in humans.

However, direct augmentation of cardiac output (CO) by IABP is limited. Additional benefits are derived from establishing a more favorable balance between myocardial energy supply versus demand, with secondary improvement in cardiac function. The effect is readily lost without IABP support. Early experience suggested that IABP alone may be insufficient to treat cardiogenic shock and often must be combined with inotropic support and arrhythmia management.

Physiology

An intravascular balloon is inflated during diastole soon after aortic valve closure. Depending on the heart rate or the amount of augmentation desired, this inflation can occur at every diastole or at a lower ratio to the native rate (1:2, 1:3). Diastolic inflation displaces blood in all directions. The closer its location to the aortic valve, the greater diastolic pressure augmentation the IABP can generate in the aortic root. The sudden deflation at end diastole creates a vacuum, decreasing afterload in early systole and thereby LV oxygen demand. The net result is a reduction in the tension time index (TTI), which represents myocardial oxygen demand, and an increase in the diastolic pressure time index (DPTI), which represents myocardial oxygen supply (Figure 1).

The flow characteristics that follow these pressure changes depend on vascular resistances. Most vascular beds have significant autoregulation over a wide range of pressures. Therefore in a normal heart, coronary flow measurements during IABP remain stable at all settings. However, during cardiac ischemia or following CPB, autoregulation is often compromised. Under these circumstances, diastolic pressure augmentation can increase flow to myocardium either beyond a critical stenosis or dependent on small collaterals.

Likewise, during cerebral vasoconstriction, when cerebral autoregulation breaks down, IABP can significantly improve cerebral blood flow as the proximity to the balloon favors a re-distribution of flow to the arch vessels. Conversely, a net decrease in blood flow can be

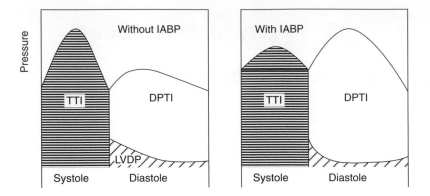

Figure 1 Intra-aortic balloon pump (IABP) augmentation enhances myocardial oxygen supply (DPTI) and reduces myocardial oxygen demand (TTI); LVDP, left venticular diastolic pressure.

demonstrated in organs below the balloon. It has been shown experimentally that renal arterial flow may decrease by 20% during IABP. The further away the balloon is from the renal artery, the lower the negative effect.

The systolic effect of the IABP results in a significant decrease of systolic pressure during cardiac ejection. This decreases myocardial oxygen demand even in states of normal autoregulation. Thus the IABP increases myocardial energy supply during impaired autoregulation, and decreases energy demand at all times. Because the IABP is valveless, blood is displaced in all directions. The net effect is dependent on peripheral vascular resistance, which favors a forward flow by 10–15%. Clinically, CO often increases significantly more than 10–15%. Improved myocardial energy efficiency causes a secondary increase in cardiac output, leading to better organ perfusion.

The cardiac effect of IABP is greater the closer the device is to the heart. However, placement of the balloon near the arch vessels may obstruct flow and cause significant cerebral embolism. The IABP should ideally be deployed immediately distal to the left subclavian artery. To optimize performance, balloon size should match the descending thoracic aorta. Complete balloon obliteration of the descending thoracic aorta may cause intimal damage. Optimal physiologic effect can be achieved when 90% of the aortic cross-sectional area is occupied by the inflated balloon. Distally, a device positioned too low can directly compromise flow and/or occlude the splanchnic arteries. Keeping the balloon well above the diaphragm will minimize the negative flow effect to the mesenteric and renal vessels.

Ideal timing of the IABP is achieved by monitoring the aortic arch and ascending aortic pressures. The IABP is normally triggered by the R wave on the ECG or the arterial pressure trace so that inflation occurs at the dicrotic notch and deflation just prior to the upstroke of the next waveform. This is accomplished by placing the pressure monitor at the tip of the device. With tachycardia and difficulties in obtaining accurate aortic arch pressures, echocardiographic-based timing protocols may generate better diastolic augmentation and systolic unloading, particularly for pediatric patients.

Indications

Today the main indications for IABP are:

- Management of ischemic heart disease where an intervention is planned – IABP may support a catheter-based intervention, e.g. stenting a critical lesion or surgical revascularization in patients with significant LV dysfunction or during OPCAB surgery when cardiac manipulation may cause significant ventricular dysfunction. IABP may also help to control intractable ventricular arrhythmias in patients with ischemic heart disease (IHD).
- Severe ischemic mitral valve insufficiency or post-infarct VSD.
- Post-cardiotomy shock.
- Treatment of conduit vasospasm – support the myocardium and allow vasospasm to respond to vasodilator therapy.
- Management of cardiac disease (IHD, mitral insufficiency and aortic stenosis) in patients undergoing emergent non-cardiac surgery.
- Cerebral vasospasm – cerebral hypoperfusion can be triggered by neurosurgical procedures, sub-arachnoid hemorrhage or even a severe migraine-like syndrome. The IABP has been demonstrated in several small series to increase cerebral flow in these states when standard treatments have failed.

Contraindications and adverse effects

The most common relative contraindications are:

- Aortic valve insufficiency. To obtain effective diastolic augmentation the aortic valve must be competent. Slight regurgitation may decrease effectiveness but does not preclude IABP deployment. Moderate/severe aortic valve insufficiency causes such an increase in regurgitant fraction that it negates the benefit of systolic unloading.
- Small femoral arteries.
- Presence of abdominal or thoracic Dacron graft.
- Severely atheromatous aorto-iliacs with/without mobile plaques.

When the aorto-iliac disease is prohibitive, the IABP can be inserted via a transthoracic route or via the left axillary artery. The presence of large/complex/mobile plaque within the descending thoracic aorta carries prohibitive embolic risk and should be avoided. The presence of an abdominal aortic aneurysm still allows IABP deployment (ideally under fluoroscopic guidance) provided the descending thoracic aorta is relatively normal.

In patients who benefit from increased afterload, e.g. those with hypertrophied ventricles, following aortic valve replacement for critical stenosis with virtual cavity obliteration, or following mitral valve repair with SAM-related mitral regurgitation, IABP should be used cautiously. If diastolic augmentation is desired in these settings, the balloon should be completely deflated well before aortic valve opening to minimize systolic effects.

Recognized complications of IABP (<10%) are:

- limb ischemia, from thromboembolism
- bleeding
- infection
- cerebral embolism and stroke, rarely paraplegia
- mesenteric/renal ischemia.

Future directions

A modification which enhances efficiency is the placement of a distal valve mechanism, such that during deflation all blood displaced would come from the proximal aorta. This would provide maximum afterload reduction and a direct increase in cardiac output of approximately 25%. A variety of designs have been tested. However, as IABP is generally quite effective, there is little driving force behind additional refinements. Furthermore, any modification potentially adds thrombotic complications without proven clinical benefit.

In recent years, efforts have been made to develop a chronic counterpulsation device: Kantrowitz designed an intrathoracic system which consists of a semi-rigid insert sewn to the descending thoracic aorta distal to the left subclavian. A line is then exteriorized and connected to an actuator pump, which controls diastolic inflation of a bladder within the descending thoracic aorta. Because the aortic lumen is enlarged by the device, significantly greater diastolic augmentation is achieved compared to conventional IABP. The intrinsic weak link in the device is the skin connection between the external pump and the intrathoracic device. To decrease infection risk, the skin cuff is infiltrated with autologous skin cells harvested and cultured prior to reimplantation. This device may be particularly useful in patients with end-stage ischemic cardiomyopathy who have exhausted other options.

Further reading

1. Ferguson JJ 3rd, Cohen M, Freedman RJ Jr et al. The current practice of intra-aortic balloon counterpulsation: results from the Benchmark Registry. *J Am Coll Cardiol* 2001; **38**: 1456–62.
2. Pochettino A, Hammond RL, Spanta A. Impaired canine renal blood flow during intra-aortic balloon counterpulsation. *Cardiac Chronicle* 5: 1991; **11**: 1–9.
3. Morewood GH, Weiss SJ. Intra-aortic balloon pump associated with dynamic left ventricular outflow tract obstruction after valve replacement for aortic stenosis. *J Am Soc Echocardiography* 2000: **13**: 229–31.
4. Sirbu H, Busch T, Aleksic I et al. Ischaemic complications with intra-aortic balloon counterpulsation: incidence and management. *Cardiovasc Surg* 2000; **8**: 66–71.

Related topics of interest

25.2 Revascularization for end-stage heart failure

M Pitt, Robert S Bonser

Heart failure or major LV dysfunction (EF <30%) affects 3% of the population and has an incidence of 0.1% per year in those >25 years old. The incidence and prevalence both increase with age. In the developed world, ischemic heart disease (IHD) is the primary cause of heart failure, accounting for more than 50% of cases. While mortality from most cardio-vascular diseases is stable or declining, deaths due to heart failure are increasing.

ACE inhibitors and beta-adrenoreceptor antagonists have been used successfully to atten-uate the detrimental compensatory mechanisms involving the sympathetic nervous system and the renin–angiotensin–aldosterone axis in heart failure. Despite improved medical therapy, both prognosis and quality of life for severe heart failure remain poor with mortality approaching 30% at 1 year. Clearly, alternative techniques are required to improve morbidity and mortality. Recently, attention has focused on the potential benefits of myocardial revas-cularization in ischemic cardiomyopathy. The beneficial effects of revascularization are due to attenuation of ongoing ischemia and improvement in blood flow to chronically underper-fused/repetitively stunned myocardium.

IHD, left ventricular dysfunction, viable and hibernating myocardium

Two concepts – myocardial hibernation and viable myocardium – are important in the evaluation of heart failure due to IHD.

Myocardial hibernation
In recent years reversibility of chronic LV dysfunction has been recognized in a proportion of patients with IHD. This functional recovery can occur in a myocardial region supplied by a stenotic coronary artery following coronary revascularization. These regions are said to be in a functional state of 'hibernation'.

Viable myocardium
Viable myocardium can be defined as:

(1) Resting dysfunctional myocardium (hibernating), displaying improvement in contrac-tile reserve upon stimulation of beta-adrenoreceptors, evidence of sarcolemmal integrity and continued metabolic activity demonstrated by preserved or augmented uptake of exogenous glucose; or
(2) Resting normal myocardial function displaying deterioration with ischemic stress.

Stunned myocardium

Closely associated with hibernation/viability is the phenomenon of myocardial stunning, which is defined as follows: myocardium rendered ischemic, but not irreversibly damaged, which exhibits prolonged depression of regional myocardial function, long after the complete return of blood flow and resumption of a normal EKG. Time to recovery of function is dependent upon the degree and duration of the ischemic insult. The demonstration of myocardial viability distinguishes between myocardium likely to recover function following revascularization and irreversibly damaged myocardium.

Assessment of myocardial viability

The presence of hibernating myocardium can be predicted by several non-invasive imaging techniques, each of which probe different aspects of myocyte function. In brief the techniques used are:

(1) ^{201}Thallium scintigraphy with single-photon emission computed tomography (SPECT).
(2) Technetium-99m (Tc-99m)-tetrofosmin SPECT.
(3) Positron emission tomography (PET) with the glucose analogue [^{18}F]2-fluoro-2-deoxy-D-glucose (FDG).
(4) Dobutamine stress echocardiography (DE).
(5) Dobutamine stress magnetic resonance imaging (MRI).

All of these techniques share similar sensitivity for the detection of myocardial viability, although dobutamine stress echocardiography provides superior specificity.

CABG in LV dysfunction

CABG is well established for the treatment of refractory angina and remains superior to medical therapy and percutaneous coronary intervention (PCI) in terms of functional benefit and survival advantage in certain subgroups. A prospective randomized trial has not yet been conducted to evaluate the role of CABG or PCI compared to medical therapy in ischemic cardiomyopathy.

1. Data from randomized studies

Of the three major trials of coronary artery surgery, only the Coronary Artery Surgery Study (CASS) and Veterans Administration Cooperative Study (VA) enrolled patients with moderate global LV impairment, whereas the European Coronary Surgery Study Group (ECSS) excluded patients with EF <50%. In the VA study, patients with abnormal LV function treated surgically had a survival advantage over the medical group, but this improvement was only detected in those with three-vessel disease. In the CASS study a total of 160 patients with LVEF between 35 and 49% were randomized to medical or surgical therapy. A survival advantage for the surgical group was detected at 7 years in the subgroup of patients with three-vessel disease (88% versus 65%, p = 0.009).

2. Data from non-randomized studies

Several studies suggest superior 3–5-year survival in surgically revascularized patients with

LV dysfunction. The most pronounced survival benefit was seen in the most compromised ventricular function (EF <26%).

CABG for ischemic cardiomyopathy

Initial results for CABG in ischemic heart failure were discouraging, with CASS registry data revealing poor 5-year survival. The survival rate in this series was 23% in both surgically and medically treated patients. Nevertheless, patient numbers were small (72 treated medically and 19 surgically). Subsequently, throughout the 1980s revascularization was not considered the best option. With the recognition that LV dysfunction in patients with IHD may be reversible following revascularization (hibernating myocardium), attention has focused on revascularization for functional and prognostic benefits in patients displaying evidence of myocardial viability but without significant angina.

Except in a few clear-cut cases, e.g. medical therapy in those with prohibitive co-morbidity, in patients with predominant symptoms of ischemic cardiomyopathy, the choice of CABG, heart transplantation or continued medical therapy (including biventricular pacing) is less straightforward. There are no randomized trials comparing these different therapies.

An assessment of myocardial viability should be performed in patients with severe LV dysfunction and IHD amenable to revascularization. Outcome following revascularization may be predicted by a pre-operative viability index. Analysis of data from a number of series reveals that approximately 20% or more of total LV volume must display evidence of viability pre-operatively in order to obtain an improvement in survival. Clearly, the area of viability must correlate with a region of LV dysfunction subtended by stenosed coronary arteries amenable to revascularization. While there is some evidence that CABG may improve prognosis in this patient group, the role of PCI remains undefined.

Risks and benefits of revascularization for heart failure

Improved anesthetic, surgical and myocardial protection techniques have led to decreased risk for CABG in patients with heart failure. Operative mortality has decreased from 11–16% to less than 6%. However, the risk of CABG in patients with severe heart failure remains higher than in patients with moderate LV impairment and is often associated with the need for intensive early postoperative hemodynamic support. Thus the decision to revascularize must balance potential benefits concomitant upon relief of ischemia and subsequent (often delayed) improved LV function against perioperative morbidity and mortality.

The absence of a significant quantum of hibernating myocardium in individual patients is an independent risk factor for increased peri- and postoperative mortality. Application of relatively strict criteria based on extent of viability may allow stratification of patients for revascularization. The potential benefits of CABG in patients with significant hibernating myocardium should perhaps be divided into functional and prognostic, especially in lieu of future long-term data on survival benefit. Recent data from observational studies suggest improvements in quality of life and exercise capacity in patients undergoing CABG in the presence of significant amounts of viable myocardium.

The extent of pre-operative myocardial viability is a determinant of long-term outcome following CABG. Five-year survival rates of 85% have been reported for patients with IHD, heart failure and significant amounts of viable myocardium (>25% of total LV myocardium).

Further reading

1. Braunwald E, Rutherford JD. Reversible ischaemic left ventricular dysfunction: evidence for 'hibernating myocardium'. *J Am Coll Cardiol* 1986; **8**: 1467–70.
2. Fath-Ordoubadi F, Beatt KJ, Spyrou N, Camici PG. Efficacy of coronary angioplasty for the treatment of hibernating myocardium. *Heart* 1999; **82**: 210–16.
3. McDonagh TA, Morrison CE, Lawrence A et al. Symptomatic and asymptomatic left ventricular systolic dysfunction in an urban population. *Lancet* 1997; **350**: 829–33
4. Pagano D, Lewis ME, Townend JN et al. Coronary revascularization for postischaemic heart failure: how myocardial viability affects survival. *Heart* 1999; **82**: 684–8.
5. Rahimtoola SH. The hibernating myocardium. *Am Heart J* 1989; **117**: 211–21.
6. Yusuf S. Effect of coronary artery bypass graft on survival: overview of 10-year results from randomized trials by the Coronary Artery Bypass Graft Surgery Trialist Collaboration. *Lancet* 1994; **344**: 563–70.

Related topics of interest

25.3 Mitral valve surgery for end-stage heart failure

Jennifer A Berry, Vinay Badhwar, Steven F Bolling

Congestive heart failure is one of the world's leading causes of morbidity and mortality. As our population ages and our medical care improves, the number of patients suffering from end-stage heart failure continues to rise. In the USA alone, there are nearly 4.7 million suffering with heart failure. Yet of the 500 000 new patients diagnosed each year, less than 3000 are offered transplantation due to limitations of age, co-morbid conditions, and donor availability. This deficiency has led to new surgical alternatives, such as mitral reconstruction, to treat heart failure effectively. One of the most common and serious problems in cardiomyopathy is the development of mitral regurgitation (MR) which is associated with a significant reduction in long-term survival. The progressive dilatation of the left ventricle initially gives rise to MR that begets more MR and further ventricular dilatation. Mitral reparative surgery for end-stage heart failure thus interrupts this cycle of ventricular deterioration through the restoration of normal cardiac physiology.

Etiology

Effective management of mitral regurgitation begins with a firm understanding of the functional anatomy of the mitral valve. The mitral valve apparatus consists of the annulus, leaflets, chordae tendineae, papillary muscles and the entire left ventricle. Though the pathogenesis of MR in cardiomyopathy is multifactorial, it must be recognized that its etiology is based upon changes in the ventricle. These lead to dilatation of the mitral annulus, resulting in functional MR, or to the distortion of the entire mitral apparatus, resulting in geometric MR.

1. Functional MR

With normal ventricular geometry, the redundant mitral leaflets are responsible for a zone of coaptation that is more than twice the area of the mitral valve orifice. As the failing ventricle dilates, the progressive expansion of the mitral annulus results in incomplete leaflet coaptation and a central regurgitant jet of functional mitral insufficiency. Therefore the most significant determinant of leaflet coaptation in functional MR is the diameter of the mitral valve annulus.

2. Geometric MR

With ischemic cardiomyopathy, a combination of factors contributes to mitral regurgitation. Here, functional MR from annular and ventricular dilatation is compounded by pathologic changes in the subvalvular structures of the ventricle. Ischemic papillary muscle dysfunction is not merely an isolated disorder of the papillary muscle, but actually a disturbance in the coordination of the entire mitral valve apparatus. The resulting distortion of mitral geometry results in an eccentric jet of mitral insufficiency.

Clinical presentation

Symptoms of congestive heart failure are often amplified when MR is present. Clinical signs of decreased cardiac output and pulmonary congestion such as dyspnea and reduced exercise tolerance increase in proportion to the progression of MR. Some of these patients develop myocardial irritability that may manifest in the form of ventricular arrhythmias or sudden death.

Physical examination of MR in cardiomyopathy typically reveals a hyperdynamic cardiac impulse and a characteristic blowing holosystolic murmur that radiates to the axilla, back, or neck. However, with severely depressed ventricular function these clinical findings may be inconspicuous. Radiographically, patients usually have an enlarged cardiac silhouette indicative of left ventricular or atrial enlargement. Typical EKG findings include left atrial enlargement and ventricular hypertrophy.

Diagnostic evaluation

An initial transthoracic echocardiogram (TTE) is helpful to estimate the severity of MR and assess ventricular function. Measurements of left ventricular end-systolic dimension are less dependent on preload than ejection fraction and thus provide a more accurate assessment of ventricular performance. Prior to operation, a TEE must be obtained to evaluate the mitral valve and the coexistence of coronary artery disease should be ruled out by coronary angiography.

1. TEE

Once MR is documented, it is essential to define the mitral pathoanatomy by TEE clearly. Since the surgical approach for functional MR may be different from geometric MR, a detailed understanding of leaflet and chordal excursion including the regurgitant jet characteristics is helpful to plan the correct operation effectively. Though routine color Doppler may provide a semiquantitative analysis of MR, this method is often sensitive to load conditions, ventricular pressure, jet eccentricity and left atrial size and thus may lead to incorrect estimations of the true degree of MR. Proximal flow convergence analysis, which calculates the regurgitant volume by measuring the flow proximal to the mitral valve orifice, may be a preferable method to quantify the extent of MR in heart failure patients more accurately.

2. Angiography

Prior to mitral repair, coronary angiography should be performed to assess the extent of native coronary disease as well as the patency of any prior grafts in patients who have undergone previous revascularization. If occlusions are detected, a study to assess myocardial viability such as dobutamine echocardiography is recommended to determine if concomitant surgical revascularization is warranted.

Management

The successful management of mitral regurgitation in heart failure involves a combined medical and surgical approach. Pre-operatively, the patient is optimized with an aggressive regimen of diuretic and vasodilator therapy to minimize ventricular afterload and normalize the patient's circulating volume. For patients with severe heart failure, a brief period of inotropic therapy for ventricular resuscitation may be necessary. Inability to be weaned from this support is indicative of severe myocardial injury and a poor prognosis with any surgical therapy other than transplantation. Once patients are medically optimized, they are approached surgically based on the etiology and anatomy of their MR.

1. Functional MR

The majority of heart failure patients with MR will have a symmetric central jet from mitral annular dilation. Annular geometry is restored by means of reduction annuloplasty using a circumferential flexible ring. By undersizing the annuloplasty to overcorrect the defect, one can effectively restore the optimal zone of coaptation and function of the mitral apparatus. A size 25 or 26 flexible ring is most commonly used regardless of orifice size, gender or body mass index without resulting in either mitral stenosis or systolic anterior motion.

2. Geometric MR

In cases of anatomic distortion of the valve anatomy, abnormal leaflet or chordal structures often result in the regurgitant jet being eccentrically located. These patients may often require a partial resection and reconstruction to correct leaflet prolapse. Chordal elongation may require shortening and chordal rupture may require reconstruction with an artificial material such as Gore-Tex in order to restore normal leaflet excursion. Each mitral repair is completed with a circumferential annuloplasty.

Mitral reconstruction for end-stage heart failure can be performed with an operative mortality as low as 5%. The 2-year actuarial survival of 80% after successful mitral repair is similar to that of transplantation. With restored ventricular mechanics, the augmented cardiac output of these patients can be seen in their improvements in heart failure symptoms, exercise capacity, and functional status. Intermediate outcome is worse for those with more severe ventricular dilatation associated with pulmonary hypertension or patients with ischemic etiology.

Further reading

1. Bolling SF, Pagani FD, Deeb GM et al. Intermediate-term outcome of mitral reconstruction in cardiomyopathy. *J Thorac Cardiovasc Surg* 1998; **115**: 381–8.
2. Chen FY, Adams DH, Aranki SF et al. Mitral valve repair in cardiomyopathy. *Circulation* 1998; **98**: 124–7.

Related topics of interest

25.4 Ventricular assist devices and artificial hearts

Igor D Gregoric, Wilson J Couto, O Howard Frazier

Chronic, progressive, end-stage heart failure is increasingly prevalent worldwide, causing physical and economic distress for individuals and society. In fact, heart disease kills as many persons as nearly all other causes of death combined.

In 1963, Michael DeBakey implanted a left ventricular assist device (LVAD) into a patient dying of severe heart failure. The LVAD was designed to allow the ventricle to rest and recover. Further clinical breakthroughs were made by Denton Cooley in 1969 with a total artificial heart (TAH); by John Norman in 1976 with an LVAD; and by Cooley and Tetsuzo Akutsu in 1981 with a TAH.

Currently, there are three major indications for mechanical assistance:

- to provide temporary support until myocardial or hemodynamic recovery can occur
- to provide temporary support until cardiac transplantation can be performed
- to provide permanent support for patients who are not transplant candidates (destination therapy).

Each of the available devices addresses at least one of these indications.

Ventricular assist devices

Extracorporeal support

Centrifugal pumps

Except for the intra-aortic balloon pump, centrifugal pumps such as the Bio-Pump® (Medtronic-Biomedicus, Eden Prairie, MN) are probably the most commonly used postcardiotomy cardiac assist devices. These pumps are readily available, cost-effective, and simple to operate. They use high-speed blades, impellers, or concentric cones that rotate at up to 5000 rpm and create a hemodynamic vortex. They yield flows of up to 8 l/min, providing either univentricular or biventricular assistance.

ABIOMED BVS 5000

The ABIOMED BVS 5000 (ABIOMED, Danvers, MA) was the first VAD approved by the United States Food and Drug Administration for supporting postcardiotomy patients. This pulsatile VAD provides short-term uni- or biventricular support. It has three components: (1) dual disposable external pumps, (2) transthoracic cannulas, and (3) a microprocessor-controlled pneumatic device console. Each pump has two chambers, and the atrial bladder, which is vented to the atmosphere and fills passively via a special cannula. The ventricular bladder is connected to the drive console by a pneumatic line. The system provides flows of up to 5 l/min. Although it offers limited mobility, has a limited flow capacity, and necessitates full anticoagulation, it is safe and simple to operate.

Thoratec ventricular assist device

The Thoratec VAD (Thoratec, Pleasanton, CA) is commercially available for providing post-operative support, bridging to cardiac transplantation, and bridging to cardiac recovery. It offers biventricular or univentricular assistance. Its four main components are a blood pump, inflow cannulas, outflow cannulas, and a drive console. Normally, the blood pump is positioned externally on the anterior surface of the abdomen. It provides a stroke volume of 65 ml and flows of up to 6.5 l/min at 100 bpm. The system's chief limitation is restricted patient mobility. As of May 2000, the Thoratec VAD had been implanted in 1376 patients, mainly for bridging to transplantation (828 patients) and postcardiotomy support (195 patients). Sixty percent of the candidates eventually underwent transplantation and their post-transplant survival rate was 86%.

Intracorporeal support

HeartMate left ventricular assist device

The HeartMate LVAD (recently acquired by Thoratec from ThermoCardiosystems) is an implantable pulsatile blood pump that is available as an implantable pneumatic (IP) or a vented electric (VE) model. Both versions feature a titanium alloy pump that consists of a blood chamber, an air chamber, a driveline, and inflow and outflow conduits. The VE-LVAD also contains a motor chamber. It has a maximum stroke capacity of 83 ml and operates at up to 120 bpm, producing peak flows of 10 l/min. Unique blood-contacting surfaces promote development of a continuous cellular lining which ensures a low thromboembolic rate without need for systemic anticoagulation (aspirin used).

The first clinical implant of the HeartMate took place at our hospital in 1986. As of June 1999, 1837 patients worldwide had received a HeartMate (1152 IP; 685 VE), with an approximate success rate of 90% (excluding 30-day perioperative mortality).

Novacor left ventricular assist device

The Novacor LVAD (World Heart Corporation, Ottawa, Canada) was the first electrically powered device designed to be an integrated (and ultimately a totally implantable) system for the definitive treatment of end-stage heart disease. The solenoid-actuated, dual pusher-plate blood pump has a smooth polyurethane sac with polyester valved inflow and outflow conduits. A unique feature of the Novacor LVAD is its complete symmetry. In long-term clinical experiments, the device has proved safe and reliable for extended periods outside the hospital setting.

Jarvik 2000 left ventricular assist device

Recently, our institution has focused on the Jarvik 2000 axial-flow LVAD (Jarvik Heart, Inc., New York, NY). It is a small, lightweight (90 g), valveless continuous-flow pump that is bio-compatible and contains a single moving part (the motor) with blood-immersed bearings. The Jarvik 2000 is powered by either: (1) a percutaneous cable connected to a manually operated controller, or (2) a totally implantable system, with an automatic-rate responsive controller and internal energy coils. At 8000 rpm, against a mean pressure of 60 mmHg, the device produces flows of slightly more than 2 l/min. Our initial clinical experience with the Jarvik 2000 has resulted in physiologic normalization of the cardiac output.

HeartSaver VAD

The HeartSaver (World Heart Corporation, Ottawa, Canada) is a totally implantable intrathoracic VAD that is completely free of external connections. A biotelemetry system allows remote monitoring. Clinical studies of this device are pending.

Total artificial heart

In 1982, the Jarvik 7, a pneumatic TAH, was implanted in Barney Clark, who survived for 112 days before succumbing to infection and thrombosis. As a permanent cardiac substitute, the Jarvik 7 failed, because it required an external pneumatic console and large percutaneous conduits. When later used as a bridge to transplantation, this system (currently known as the CardioWest TAH [CardioWest Technologies, Inc., Tucson, AZ]) permitted 80% survival.

Efforts to develop a more practical heart, which could allow patients to leave the hospital and resume their normal activities resulted in two new models: (1) the Penn State Electric TAH (Penn State University, Hershey, PA), the motor of which receives power from a coil beneath the patient's skin; and (2) the fully implantable ABIOMED AbioCor, in which the electrically driven, dual-chambered, centrifugal pump provides continuous, unidirectional flow via tri-leaflet valves. Alternate right and left systole is produced by a second electric motor that alternately drives the left and right pumping chambers. Studies of the AbioCor in animals began at our institution in 1991. Clinical trials have just begun.

Future perspectives

Because myocardial function can improve with chronic ventricular unloading and because smaller, more effective LVADs and TAHs are becoming available, the future of implantable long-term circulatory support is quite promising. The REMATCH Trial demonstrated conclusively the superior benefits of LVAD over optimal medical therapy in end-stage heart failure. It also highlighted the current shortcomings of this approach as most deaths in the LVAD group were device related. The number of patients who can benefit from these systems will continue to increase, and mechanical circulatory support will eventually become a valid alternative to cardiac transplantation.

Further reading

1. Argenziano M, Oz MC, Rose EA. The continuing evolution of mechanical ventricular assistance. *Curr Prob Surg* 1997; **34**: 322–86.
2. Frazier OH. Mechanical cardiac assistance: historical perspectives. *Semin Thorac Cardiovasc Surg* 2000; **12**: 207–19.
3. Frazier OH, Gregoric ID, Delgado RM et al. Initial experience with the Jarvik 2000 left ventricular assist system as a bridge to transplantation: report of 4 cases. *J Heart Lung Transplant* 2001; **20**: 201.
4. Frazier OH, Macris M, Radovancevic B. *Support and Replacement of the Failing Heart.* Lippincott-Raven: Philadelphia, 1996.
5. Rickenbacher WE. *Mechanical Circulatory Support.* Landes Bioscience: Georgetown, Texas, 1999.

Related topics of interest

25.5 Left ventricular volume reduction

Hisayoshi Suma

Dilated cardiomyopathy (DCM) is a major cause of heart failure and patients are often candidates for heart transplantation. Due to a shortage of donors, heart transplantation is not always available for end-stage heart failure. To treat patients with end-stage DCM, Randas Batista in Brazil introduced partial left ventriculectomy (PLV – the Batista procedure).

This procedure aims to improve the LV function by reducing LV wall tension and LV diameter with wide excision of LV free wall (generally postero-lateral wall between anterior and posterior papillary muscles). This concept was based on Laplace's Law, T = PR/2d (T, wall tension; P, pressure; R, radius; d, wall thickness).

Indication

Patients deemed suitable for the Batista procedure should have been on maximal medical therapy for heart failure and either considered unsuitable or are unlikely to proceed to cardiac transplantation.

- Dilated LV (end-diastolic LV diameter ≥70 mm) and NYHA class III or IV functional status.
- The operation should be performed on an elective basis because emergency operation for cardiogenic shock and multi-organ failure has extremely high operative mortality. For such patients, a left ventricular assist device may be considered as a bridge to PLV.
- Recent investigation has shown that the extent of myocardial fibrosis is not homogeneous in DCM. Consequently, it is important to ensure that the ventricular septum is sufficiently viable and less fibrotic than the LV free wall so that adequate contractile function remains following resection. Otherwise the septal anterior ventricular exclusion procedure should be considered.

Site selection

Because the extent of myocardial fibrosis is not always uniform in DCM, it is dangerous to apply PLV for all dilated left ventricle without knowing left ventricular wall characteristics. Detection of regional myocardial viability is, however, difficult in end-stage DCM. Dobutamine stress echocardiography, MRI, perfusion and metabolic scintiscan and quantitative gated scintigraphy should be used in combination to identify the non-viable parts of the LV.

Intraoperative TEE is useful for detecting changes in LV wall motion and thickness when the LV is decompressed with reduced wall tension during CPB.

Procedure

Through a median sternotomy, the postero-lateral ventricular wall between anterior and posterior papillary muscles is widely excised with CPB. Most patients have concomitant mitral and tricuspid regurgitation due to annular dilation, and therefore valvular reconstruction/replacement may be combined with PLV. TEE may be useful in assessing the extent of ventriculectomy and its effect on LV geometry. The LV should be carefully closed with double-layer sutures to avoid serious bleeding.

Postoperative management

Careful medical treatment should be continued after the operation. Amiodarone is continued unless adverse effects such as pneumonitis or thyroid dysfunction appear. ACE inhibitor and beta-blocker are re-introduced.

Surgical results

- Operative mortality varies between 4 and 30% depending on patient selection and timing of operation, which were not clearly defined.
- One-year and 3-year survival rates are 70–80% and 40–60%, respectively.
- Ejection fraction increases acutely from 10–20% pre-operatively to around 30% after the operation.
- Common causes of late death are heart failure and ventricular arrhythmia.
- Patients with shorter history of heart failure have greater improvement of ventricular function following the operation.
- Outcome for ischemic cardiomyopathy is generally less favorable compared to DCM/Chagas' disease.
- Case selection by intraoperative TEE to detect septal viability improved surgical outcome.

Return of heart failure

Postoperative intractable heart failure is found in about 20% of hospital survivors. Possible causes are:

- residual/recurrent mitral regurgitation
- insufficient left ventricular down-sizing
- too small a left ventricle due to excessive excision
- wrong site excision by removal of the kinetic wall without removal of the weakest area
- extensive fibrosis in retained left ventricle.

Further reading

1. McCarthy PM, Starling RC, Wong J et al. Early results with partial left ventriculectomy. *J Thorac Cardiovasc Surg* 1997; **114:** 755–63.
2. Suma H, Isomura T, Suma H et al. Nontransplant cardiac surgery for end-stage cardiomyopathy. *J Thorac Cardiovasc Surg* 2000; **119:** 1233–45.
3. Frazier OH, Gradinac S, Segura AM et al. Partial left ventriculectomy: which patients can be expected to benefit? *Ann Thorac Surg* 2000; **69:** 1836–41.

Related topics of interest

25.6 Skeletal muscle circulatory support

Augustine TM Tang, Larry W Stephenson

Concept

The ability to harness the biological power of autologous skeletal muscle to provide permanent biomechanical assist to a failing circulation remains an attractive option when compared with other treatments for end-stage heart failure. In particular, it avoids the risks, side effects and costs of chronic immunosuppression; it is not limited by donor availability; and in sharing the workload with the native heart, it also offers potential for myocardial recovery. To ensure long-term success, a large expendible muscle with favorable neurovascular anatomy must be conditioned to perform cardiac-level work, mobilized and connected to circulation so as to maximize assistance in synchrony with cardiac cycle.

Basic principles

Generation of adequate and sustained power

Experimental interest in cardiac assistance from skeletal muscle dates back to 1959 when success was limited by muscle fatigue. Subsequent demonstration of adaptive transformation of a fast-twitch muscle to the slow phenotype, much more fatigue-resistant by appropriate electrical stimulation, revived the concept. This functional transformation is accompanied by biochemical and ultrastructural adjustments, though with some loss of contractile speed and muscle mass. Currently, a regime of postoperative muscle conditioning by progressive electrical stimulation over 8 weeks is used clinically. A 'burst' stimulus generated by an electrical pulse-train at supramaximal voltage induces tetanic contraction in the conditioned muscle to deliver peak power during circulatory assist.

Transfer of power to circulation

Latissimus dorsi muscle (LDM) emerged as the graft of choice because of its large mass, a dominant neurovascular pedicle enabling mobilization and stimulation, its proximity to the heart and aorta and minor functional disability after translocation. The power generated by a conditioned LDM may be transfered to circulation by establishing direct contact with the heart (cardiomyoplasty), aorta (aortomyoplasty), working as an auxillary pumping chamber (skeletal muscle ventricle) or indirectly via a biomechanical device. There is inherent energy loss during coupling but has been particularly unacceptable with biomechanical assist. This indirect approach has been largely abandoned because of failure to establish a reliable and efficient biomechanical interface.

Synchronization with cardiac cycle

Muscle stimulation can be timed to coincide with ventricular contraction (systolic assist) in cardiomyoplasty or occur during diastole (counterpulsation) in aortomyoplasty and skeletal muscle ventricle. In practice, this is achieved by an implantable cardiomyostimulator capable of sensing the R wave on the native ECG via an epicardial electrode and then delivering a burst stimulus to the LDM. Synchronization delay is timed to the closure of mitral valve on echocardiography.

Current applications

Dynamic cardiomyoplasty (DCM)

Currently DCM represents the bulk of our clinical experience with over 700 cases performed globally since its debut in 1985. In this procedure, the left LDM is mobilized on the thoracodorsal pedicle via a flank incision, translocated into the thorax through a window resected in the ribs and wrapped around the ventricles on a beating heart through a sternotomy. Intramuscular electrodes are placed in the proximal LDM and connected to a cardiomyostimulator implanted in the upper rectus sheath which also receives an epicardial sensing wire. After a fortnight of 'vascular delay' believed to promote recovery of muscle blood flow and avoid ischemic damage, a progressive regimen of electrical conditioning of the LDM begins. The transformed muscle provides systolic assist at varying ratios down to 1:4. Operative mortality has steadily declined to 10% in experienced centers largely by excluding patients in NYHA class IV functional status pre-operatively. Currently survival at 1 and 2 years stands around 72% and 60%, respectively. Late postoperative deaths were usually caused by progressive heart failure and ventricular arrhythmia. Incorporation of a cardioverter-defibrillator into the device may partly improve the outcome. Approximately 80% of survivors report subjective benefits including improvements in functional status (NYHA) and quality of life. A survival advantage at 18 months over medically treated controls has also been demonstrated. However, such parameters have not been matched by improvements in objective measures such as hemodynamic and exercise testing.

Dynamic aortomyoplasty (DAM)

In this procedure, the LDM graft is wrapped round the ascending or descending thoracic aorta and functions as a long-term diastolic counterpulsator in a similar fashion to an intra-aortic balloon. However, clinical experience of DAM is currently very limited. Furthermore, some of the problems being addressed experimentally such as the need to sacrifice important aortic branches and for augmentation patches have not yet been resolved.

Skeletal muscle ventricle (SMV)

By wrapping the LDM graft along its length, the resultant SMV can be conditioned and connected to the circulation using artificial conduits in various configurations. A promising approach connects the SMV to the descending thoracic aorta via two separate grafts while ligating the intervening aortic segment. This allows the SMV to function as a diastolic counterpulsator. Early problems of thromboembolism and rupture have largely been resolved. No clinical experience of SMV yet exists, although in-circulation canine SMVs functioning for over 4 years have been reported. This approach may hold the most promise for the future.

Past problems and future trends

Current success in skeletal muscle circulatory support has largely been limited by loss of bio-mechanical performance during muscle transformation, ischemic damage to the distal LDM as a functional graft, the excessive postponement of circulatory assist caused by the vascular delay and conditioning protocol, and the relative inefficient transfer of power from muscle to circulation. Future research directed at such crucial issues may help us to achieve the goal of self-sustained permanent biological circulatory assistance.

Further reading

1. El Oakley RM, Jarvis JC. Cardiomyoplasty: a critical review of experimental and clinical results. *Circulation* 1994; **90**: 2085–90.
2. Magovern GJ Sr, Simpson KA. Clinical cardiomyoplasty: review of the ten-year United States experience. *Ann Thorac Surg* 1996; **61**: 413–19.
3. Niinami H, Greer K, Koyanagi H, Stephenson L. Skeletal muscle ventricles: another alternative for heart failure. *J Card Surg* 1996; **11**: 280–7.
4. Salmons S. Damage in functional grafts of skeletal muscle. In: *Muscle Damage. 1st Edn.* Salmons S. Oxford University Press: Oxford, 1997: pp 215–33.
5. Salmons S, Tang A, Jarvis J et al. Morphological and functional evidence, and clinical importance, of vascular anastomoses in the latissimus dorsi muscle of the sheep. *J Anat* 1998; **193**: 93–104.

Related topics of interest

25.7 Cellular cardiomyoplasty

Sunil K Ohri, Mark Hanson

Current therapies for heart failure

Pharmacology

The mainstay for the majority of patients is drug therapy. This includes the use of vasodilators such as hydralazine and angiotensin-converting enzyme (ACE) inhibitors. More recently angiotensin receptor-1 antagonist, spironolactone and beta-blockers have been shown to incrementally improve mortality when used in combination. Nevertheless, improvements in mortality for patients in severe heart failure have been modest.

Devices

Ischemia also causes conduction abnormalities manifesting as prolonged QT. There is growing evidence that cardiac resynchronization therapy (biventricular pacing) improves cardiac function.

Patients with ischemic LV dysfunction are at increased risk of sudden death from ventricular dysrhythmias. Implantable cardiac defibrillator (ICD) as secondary prevention was found to reduce mortality when compared to optimal medical therapy for acute myocardial infarction (AMI) survivors with ventricular dysrhythmias. Primary prevention in those with inducible ventricular dysrhythmias is also beneficial. The MADIT-2 study recruited patients only on the basis of impaired LV function (30% or less) and found a 31% mortality reduction with the use of an ICD.

Surgery

Current options include:

- orthotopic heart transplantation – limited by supply of human organs and established postoperative complications
- xenotransplantation – remains experimental with concerns surrounding retroviral infection in immunocompromised hosts
- skeletal muscle myoplasty – disappointing outcome related to muscle atrophy
- left ventriculectomy – temporizing procedure for ischemic cardiomyopathy
- ventricular assist devices – further technical improvements in biocompatibility, reliability, prevention of infection, power source, cost and availability are required before they can become accepted therapy.

Cellular cardiomyoplasty

Cellular cardiomyoplasty (CCM) is the transplantation of cells as either autografts or allografts into ischemic fibrosed areas of myocardium, with the anticipated repopulation of these dysfunctional areas with subsequent return of function and/or prevention of ventricular dilatation. A variety of cell types have been investigated in animal models and more recently in the clinical setting. Candidate cells which have been studied include:

- embryonic, fetal and neonatal rodent and porcine cardiomyocytes
- fetal smooth muscle cells
- human adult and fetal cardiomyocytes
- autologous adult atrial cells
- dermal fibroblasts
- skeletal myoblasts
- murine embryonic stem cells
- marrow-derived mesenchymal cells
- hemopoietic stem cells
- endothelial progenitor cells (EPC).

Irrespective of the cell type, improvements in myocardial function have been attributable to:

- ability of some cell types to undertake contractile work
- passive mechanical support, preventing ventricular dilatation
- engrafted cells inducing neoangiogenesis.

Skeletal myoblasts

Skeletal myoblasts are stem cells which are committed to becoming myocytes; they form 3–4% of adult skeletal muscle cells. Their normal function is the restoration of skeletal muscle numbers following injury, disease and apoptosis. These cells both in the rat and humans have been successfully cultured in sufficient quantity (hundreds of millions of cells) to become a potential therapeutic strategy. They may be delivered either by direct myocardial injection or via an intracoronary injection. Survival and subsequent function may be enhanced by genetically modifying myoblasts in vitro by heat shock treatment or transfection with genes encoding for vascular endothelial growth foactor (VEGF) and connexin 43. Although improvements in myocardial function have been documented, which appear to be incremental to the use of ACE inhibitor, at a cellular level these grafts do not form gap junctions. These gap junctions are formed by connexin 43 which are present both at the end and on the lateral aspect of fibers and are necessary for coordinated electromechnical contraction. Furthermore, the dihydropyridine receptors, which act as calcium channels, remain different in the two types of fibers. Cardiac myocytes have fast calcium channels whilst skeletal myocytes have slower calcium channels. These fundamental differences may be overcome by ex-vivo genetic engineering.

Embryonic stem cells

Embryonic stem cells (ESC) are derived from the inner blastocyst of the embryo, whilst embryonic germ cells (EGC) are isolated from primordial germ cells. Both these cells have the ability to differentiate into all three germ cell lines. Thus, within the cardiovascular system, ESC and EGC may differentiate into cardiomyocytes, endothelial cells and vascular smooth muscle cells. Although animal models have demonstrated improvements in cardiac function, ethical, immunological concerns exist, as well as the inability to harvest sufficient numbers of cells to repopulate large infarcts, which will limit their widespread use.

Adult somatic stem cells

Adult stem cells from bone marrow exhibit functional plasticity and, depending on the environment, can differentiate to non-hematopoietic tissue. Conversely, stem cells from non-hematopoietic tissue can differentiate into hematopoietic cells. Three lineages of stem cells from adult bone marrow have been defined:

- mesenchymal stem cells (MSC)
- hematopoietic stem cells (HSC)
- EPC.

Murine stem cells when exposed to 5-azacytidine form microtubules connected by inter-calated disks which beat synchronously and express many of the cardiomyocyte phenotypes. Adult stem cells are found in the bone marrow as stromal cells, which may transform to become cardiac cells either in vitro by modifying culture conditions or in vivo under the influence of local signals. It is uncertain if stem cell transformations result in cells with a phenotype consistent with adult cardiomyocytes. MSC are permissive to the local environment and do not require pre-treatment with azacytidine and when injected into infarcts will differentiate into cardiomyocytes, align themselves with native cells and form intercalated disks. Infarcted/ischemic myocardium may attract MSC from the bone marrow and drive these cells to differentiate into cardiomyocytes, fibroblasts and endothelial cells. EPC have been isolated in the peripheral blood and bone marrow of humans and are responsible for arterio-genesis. HSC in adult male mice have been sufficiently mobilized by stem cell factor and granulocyte colony-stimulating factor to generate de-novo myocardium and vascular structures in the infarcted heart and improve hemodynamics. The advantage of this approach is that immunosuppressive therapy is not required but the functional and electrophysiological properties of MSC- and HSC-derived cardiomyocytes are currently not understood.

Myocardial regeneration

The ability of the human heart to repair damaged muscle after injury is limited after 1–2 years of life. This had been attributed to an irreversible exit from the cell cycle in 'terminally differentiated' cardiac myocytes, although the underlying mechanism(s) limiting further myocyte replication remain unclear. However, recent evidence has cast doubt on this long-held tenet. Cardiac regeneration following injury may be possible using several approaches:

- Angiogenesis induced by cytokines such as isoforms of the VEGF-A gene or members of the fibroblast growth factor (FGF) family: whether given as gene therapy or as recombinant proteins, or transcription factors such as hypoxia-inducible factor-1 (HIF-1), all have potential to induce new blood vessel growth, and clinical trials employing each of these approaches are now underway.
- Formation of large-caliber vessels is dependent upon recruitment of inflammatory cells and bone marrow-derived EPC. There is increasing evidence that recruitment of EPC by cytokines, or ex-vivo expansion of EPC, followed by direct injection into ischemic tissue

or by systemic administration, accelerates new blood vessel formation and enhances cardiac function.

- Recent evidence would suggest that human hearts have a limited ability to regenerate after injury. An autopsy study of adult human hearts of patients who had died following AMI found the expression of the nuclear antigen Ki-67, a marker limited to cells undergoing replication. A number of approaches have been attempted to induce terminally differentiated cardiomyocytes to divide, but most myocytes typically undergo apoptosis when forced into the cell cycle. One approach is the modulation of tumor suppressor cell cycle regulatory genes which participate in the induction of apoptosis following exposure to agents such as simian virus 40. A truncated mutant suppressor protein has been generated (1152stp) that instead of inducing apoptosis enhances myocyte proliferation. Thus, despite the recent demonstration that bone marrow-derived stem cells and/or a reservoir of cells within the myocardium may contribute to cardiac repair following injury, the controlled induction of DNA synthesis, karyokinesis and cytokinesis of adult cardiac myocytes in situ in the adult heart remains a promising therapeutic challenge.

Further reading

1. Menasché P, Hagege AA, Scorsin M et al. Myoblast transplantation for heart failure. *Lancet* 2002; **357**: 279–80.
2. Toma C, Pittenger MF, Cahill KS, Byrne BJ, Kessler PD. Human mesenchymal stem cells differentiate to a cardiomyocyte phenotype in the adult murine heart. *Circulation* 2002; **105**: 93–8.
3. Orlic D, Kajstura J, Chimenti S et al. Bone marrow cells regenerate infarcted myocardium. *Nature* 2001: **410**: 701–5.
4. Assmus B, Schachinger V, Teupe C et al. Transplantation of progenitor cells and regeneration enhancement in acute myocardial injury (TOPCARE-AMI). *Circulation* 2003; **106**: 3009–17.

26 Heart transplantation

26.1 Allografts

Asghar Khaghani, Emma J Birks

Over 57 000 cardiac transplants have now been performed worldwide in 321 centers, although recent activity has declined.

Indications

The main indications for heart transplantation are ischemic heart disease (IHD) and other cardiomyopathies. Other less common indications include valvular heart disease, retransplantation for chronic rejection and congenital heart disease.

Donors

The current supply of organs from brain-dead donors does not meet the continually increasing demand of patients awaiting cardiac transplantation. Unfortunately, >20% of donor hearts offered for transplantation are unusable because of significant myocardial dysfunction. The reasons for the myocardial damage are multifactorial. First, brain death itself has a deleterious effect. Brain death is associated with release of catecholamines, reduction in free thyroxine and free T3, increased reverse T3, reduced cortisol and insulin and increased cytokine production. Secondly, some donors have a sustained cardiac arrest and possibly a period of prolonged hypoperfusion. Thirdly, they are often maintained on large amounts of inotropes that themselves can cause subendocardial necrosis and myocardial damage. Patients need constant intravascular volume replacement (especially as ADH deficiency results in diabetes insipidus), maintaining a CVP around 10–12 mmHg and Hb >10 g/dl, maintenance of acid–base and electrolyte balance, a moderate amount of catecholamine support (usually dopamine first line) and management of other co-morbid conditions such as infection. In an attempt to increase donor numbers, centers have often used older donor hearts (>65 years old), but the results may be less satisfactory.

Survival

Survival is now approximately 80%, 70% and 50% at 1, 5 and 10 years, respectively. After the 20% mortality in the first year there is a constant mortality rate of 4%/year. The most important risk factors known to increase 1-year mortality are recipient age; ventilation prior to transplantation; donor age, especially when combined with long ischemia time; a female donor/male recipient; positive panel reactive antibodies (PRA); and a diagnosis other than IHD or cardiomyopathy.

Post-transplant mortality

Primary graft failure is the most common cause of mortality in the first 30 days after heart transplantation. Acute rejection and infection are the other main causes during this period. These remain the main causes of death in the first year after transplantation. Subsequently transplant coronary disease (TCAD) and malignancy become prime causes of death.

Immunosuppression

Induction therapy using antithymocyte globulin (ATG) is used by most centers, so that in the first 3 days a combination of ATG, corticosteroids and azathioprine or mycophenelate are given. Subsequently the patients are maintained on triple therapy immunosuppression consisting of cyclosporino/tacrolimus, mycophenolate/azathioprine and corticosteroids. Usage of mycophenolate and tacrolimus has increased recently based on evidence of reduced rates of acute rejection and TCAD, and now they are often used as first-line therapy. In about 90% of patients in our institution corticosteroids are weaned off after transplantation.

Post-transplant morbidity

The majority of complications are related to immunosuppression including renal dysfunction, infection, hypertension, diabetes and malignancy (skin tumors and lymphomas). Other important complications are acute rejection and TCAD.

Acute rejection

Following transplantation, patients are monitored by regular EKG, TTE and endomyocardial biopsies for the occurrence of acute rejection. Acute rejection is treated with intravenous methylprednisolone. Severe and repeated rejection or rejection associated with significant hemodynamic compromise is treated in addition with ATG or monoclonal antibodies.

Cytomegalovirus (CMV) infection

CMV remains the most important cause of infective complications. It can cause fever, mononucleosis (including leukopenia and thrombocytopenia), pneumonia, myocarditis, hepatitis and gastrointestinal ulceration. It can also act as a cofactor in the development of both acute and chronic rejection, and post-transplant lymphoproliferative disease. Patients at high risk are those seronegative for CMV who receive a seropositive donor and seropositive individuals who receive ATG or monoclonal antibody therapy. The risk of CMV infection in these groups is 50–75%. Treatment of clinical CMV is with a 10–14 day course of intravenous ganciclovir, which is effective in >90% of patients.

Transplant coronary disease

This is the major cause of death in patients surviving >1 year and affects long-term function of the transplanted heart. It is an accelerated form of coronary disease affecting both intramyocardial and epicardial coronary arteries. Pathological changes range from concentric fibrous intimal thickening to complicated atheromatous plaques. It is likely to be primarily an immune-mediated disease. Although there is partial reinnervation of the cardiac allograft, most patients cannot experience typical angina pain associated with myocardial ischemia, and the first clinical manifestations are often ventricular arrhythmias, heart failure or sudden death. Hence repeated postoperative coronary angiography is performed for diagnostic and surveillance purposes. Intravascular ultrasound is an alternative diagnostic tool as it monitors intimal thickening. Some patients with TCAD are suitable for angioplasty, and very few undergo CABG.

Orthotopic transplantation surgical technique

After a median sternotomy the ascending aorta, SVC and IVC are cannulated, and CPB is established. For conventional orthotopic heart transplantation the native heart is explanted, leaving a small portion of left and right atria behind. The donor heart is prepared for implantation. The anastomosis starts between donor and recipient left atria. This is followed by the pulmonary artery and aortic anastomosis and at this stage the aortic cross-clamp is released, which terminates global myocardial ischemia. The procedure is completed by anastomosing the donor and recipient right atria. Alternatively, separate pulmonary venous and bicaval anastomoses can be performed, which leaves the donor atria intact and is a useful technique for patients with large atria or congenital heart disease.

Domino transplantation

Domino transplantation is a technique originally developed at Harefield Hospital, UK in which the heart from a recipient undergoing heart and lung transplantation for cystic fibrosis or pulmonary hypertension is transplanted into another recipient. This offers the advantage of a heart with a conditioned right ventricle which is advantageous to a recipient with a high transpulmonary gradient, and renders that recipient less likely to develop right-sided failure after transplantation; it has some contribution to the donor pool as well.

Heterotopic transplantation

Background

Heterotopic heart transplantation preserves the recipient heart whilst allowing the donor heart to support the failing native left ventricle. Although earlier reports after heterotopic transplantation showed inferior survival, more recent observations have demonstrated excellent short-term survival after heterotopic transplantation and encouraging medium to long-term results.

Indications and contraindications

Heterotopic transplantation is performed when there is either an undersized donor, pulmonary hypertension in the recipient, or if it is felt that the native heart could contribute significantly to the circulation, especially after concomitant native heart surgery. Contraindications to heterotopic transplantation include patients with significant dysrhythmias, prosthetic valves, presence of LV clot, severe angina or implantable defibrillators.

Surgical technique (Figure 1)

Conventionally, the donor heart is placed in the right pleural cavity and the anastomoses are made between donor and recipient LA, donor and recipient aorta (end to side) and donor pulmonary artery to either recipient pulmonary artery or recipient RA (Harefield's preferred option). Finally, the donor SVC is anastomosed to the recipient SVC to facilitate subsequent endomyocardial biopsy of the transplanted heart.

Outcome

Actuarial survival following heterotopic transplantation is 68% at 1 year, 56% at 5 years and 47% at 10 years. This includes a high-risk group of patients and recipients who have received grossly undersized donor hearts; if these are excluded, survival in the remainder is comparable to orthotopic transplantation. Specific complications that can occur after heterotopic heart transplantation are significant ventricular arrhythmias of the native heart and recurrent angina. Despite the lack of routine anticoagulation, thromboembolic events are uncommon. After an initial improvement in all ventricular parameters, native heart deterioration after heterotopic transplantation is problematic. Following heterotopic transplantation the recipient LV ejects more effectively when it contracts asynchronously with the donor LV. However, this is rarely the situation as the two hearts beat independently of one another and the denervated donor heart tends to beat faster than the recipient. In an effort to improve native heart function a policy of synchronized pacing to coordinate recipient heart systole during donor heart diastole has been introduced in our series.

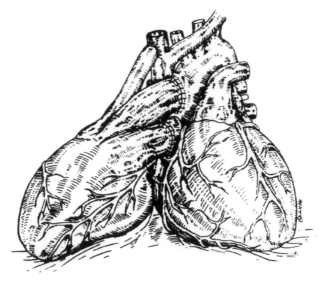

Figure 1 Completed heterotopic heart transplant.

Further reading

1. Del Rizzo DF, Menkis AH, Pflugfelder PW et al. The role of donor age and ischaemic time on survival following orthotopic heart transplantation. *J Heart Lung Transplant* 1999; **18:** 310–19.
2. Heggtveit HA. The donor heart: brain death and pathological changes in the heart. *Laval Med* 1970; **41:** 178–9.
3. Hosenpud JD, Bennett LE, Berkely MK, Boucek MM, Novick RJ. The Registry of the International Society for Heart and Lung Transplantation: Eighteenth Official Report – 2001. *J Heart Lung Transplant* 2001; **20:** 805–15.
4. Khaghani A, Birks EJ, Dyke C, Yacoub MH. Heterotopic heart transplantation. In: *Advanced Therapy in Cardiac Surgery.* Franco KL, Verrier ED, (eds). BC Decker: Ontario, 1999: pp 477–84.
5. Weis M, Von Scheidt W. Cardiac allograft vasculopathy: a review. *Circulation* 1997; **96:** 2069–77.

Related topic of interest

26.2 Xenografts

Shafie Fazel, Heather J Ross, Vivek Rao

Introduction

Although allogenic cardiac transplantation remains the treatment of choice for end-stage heart failure, the majority of transplant-eligible patients die awaiting transplantation because of limited donor availability. The mismatch between organ supply and demand has also driven the very stringent transplant listing criteria. With the aging population, the prevalence of congestive heart failure continues to grow. Xenotransplantation with a theoretically unlimited donor supply is, therefore, very attractive as an alternative treatment for end-stage heart failure patients.

Clinical experience

Ten cases of cardiac xenotransplantation, between 1964 and 1996, have been performed globally with disappointing results.[1] The donor animals included pigs (4), chimpanzees (3), baboons (2), and sheep (1). Three cases have been performed in the cyclosporine era. Most grafts failed within minutes to hours of implantation. The longest graft survival was 20 days when a baboon heart was transplanted into Baby Fae for hypoplastic left-heart syndrome.

Donor animal

The pig is emerging as the donor of choice.

Advantages
- Unlimited availability.
- Good breeding potential with 5–12 per litter.
- Rapid growth to reach adult human heart size in approximately 6 months.
- Right-heart pressures and LV end-diastolic pressures are similar to human.
- Considerable experience with genetically engineered pigs.
- Reduced infective risk compared to primates.
- Domestication of pigs for human use is ethically acceptable.

Disadvantages
- The pig is evolutionarily distant from human (discordant xenograft) and is immunologically subjected to robust hyperacute rejection (described below).
- Significant physiologic differences exist between the pig and the human: the resting heart rate is higher and the mean arterial pressure is lower in pigs.
- Response of the porcine heart to human hormones/soluble factors is largely unknown.

- It is unclear how well the pig heart will function in the upright human.
- The porcine core temperature is nearly 2 degrees higher than the human with potential adverse impact on graft function.
- The growth potential when used in pediatric recipients is unclear.

Immunological barriers

Hyperacute rejection

Hyperacute rejection of the xenograft occurs immediately upon perfusion by recipient blood. Preformed naturally occurring xenoreactive antibodies bind to the porcine endothelium (>90% of xenoreactive antibodies are specific for α1,3 galactose (Gal) expressed on porcine endothelium) and trigger complement activation, resulting in deposition of the membrane attack complex on endothelial cells and release of C3a and C5a anaphylatoxins. The result is extensive endothelial necrosis, platelet thrombi formation and severe interstitial hemorrhage.

Acute vascular rejection (AVR)

This typically begins within 24 hours of reperfusion and may cause graft failure within days to weeks of transplantation. The precise mechanism is unclear although accumulating evidence suggests that it primarily involves xenoreactive antibodies. Temporary depletion of anti-donor antibodies can suppress AVR and permit graft survival, a phenomenon termed accommodation. The specificity of these antibodies has not been fully characterized. It is thought that endothelial damage occurs through antibody-dependent cell-mediated cytotoxicity involving principally the natural killer cells and monocyte/macrophages. Immunosuppression has been shown to blunt AVR.

Acute cellular rejection

Increasing evidence suggests that the T-cell response against xenografts is at least as robust as that against allografts. Human T cells can recognize porcine major histocompatibility complex (MHC) class II antigens through the direct pathway. The xenogenic cellular responses may also be potentially directed at a wider set of protein antigens. The concomitant humoral response also amplifies the cellular response. As such, our traditional immunosuppressive protocols are unlikely to contain acute cellular rejection.

Chronic rejection

Experimental models of xenotransplantation have thus far failed to fully control the aforementioned rejection processes. Long-term data on xenografts are therefore lacking. Chronic antibody production directed against the extracellular matrix and the endothelium of the xenograft has been speculated to mediate late graft failure akin to allograft vasculopathy.

New frontiers

Attempts to control hyperacute rejection have been focused on:

(1) Depletion of xenoreactive antibodies: removal of the anti-Gal antibodies by porcine organ perfusion with recipient blood or immunoadsorption have resulted in a survival of 15 days in pig-to-baboon xenotransplantation.

(2) Inhibition of xenoreactive antibody binding: infusing the recipient with materials that compete for the xenoreactive antibody site resulted in a very limited survival benefit of 18 hours.

(3) Depletion or inhibition of complement: depletion of complement using cobra venom factor or inhibiting the classical and alternative complement cascade with soluble complement receptor 1 (sCR1) have resulted, in combination with immunosuppression and/or splenectomy, in survival of 25 days and 6 weeks, respectively.

(4) Genetic approaches: attempts to create a Gal knockout pig have not been successful, although recently $\alpha 1,3$ galactosyltransferase one-allele-knockout piglets have been cloned. Transgenic pigs, which express other glycosyltransferases that modify Gal on cell surfaces, do not reduce the endothelial-expressed Gal sufficiently to ablate hyperacute rejection. Finally, transgenic pig models with a dominant negative Gal mutation still elicit significant hyperacute rejection. Genetic engineering has also been applied to blunt complement activation. The most successful has been the hDAF pig. Human decay accelerating factor (hDAF) is a protein that inhibits complement activation on the human cell surfaces. The hDAF pig is a transgenic pig whose cells express hDAF. In an orthotopic heart transplant model of hDAF pig into baboon, the recipient survived to 39 days (immunosuppression was achieved with a combination of cyclophosphamide, cyclosporine, mycophenolate mofetil, and corticosteroids).

Infectious disease considerations

Infections transferred with a xenograft are termed xenozoonoses. Considerable media attention has been paid to the risk of infection across different species and subsequent transfer from the recipient to another human. Expert opinion, however, is hopeful that provided the donor animals are bred and housed under very stringent conditions, the risk of xenozoonoses would be less than the risk of infection transfer from a brain-dead human donor. The risk to humans by porcine endogenous retrovirus (PERV) is largely unknown. Recently, PERV has been shown to transfect human cell lines. However, in a study of 160 patients who had been treated with various living pig tissues up to 12 years earlier, no evidence of PERV transmission could be found. Unfortunately, in the absence of clinical trials it is impossible to predict the real risk of xenozoonoses. In January 1999, the European Parliament called for a moratorium on clinical tests involving xenotransplantation in Europe for public health reasons.

Ethical considerations

The major contentious issues are:

(1) Religious and ideological aspects of accepting animal organs.

(2) Psychological and societal impacts of patients with animal organs living in the community.

(3) The view that we will be crossing impermissible natural boundaries.

(4) Genetic modification of living animals for human benefit.

(5) The appropriateness of the intense intellectual and financial focus required to bring xenotransplantation to reality.

The most pressing issue at hand, however, is determining the conditions that should be met before a clinical trial can be conducted. These include the aspects of informed consent and patient selection.

International Society for Heart and Lung Transplantation recommendations

To address these concerns, the International Society for Heart and Lung Transplantation recently published the report of the Xenotransplantation Advisory Committee. A summary of the main recommendations are:

(1) Xenotransplant clinical trials should be undertaken only when experts in microbiology and relevant regulatory bodies consider the risk of xenozoonosis to be minimal.
(2) Government-backed national bodies should control all aspects of the clinical trial, and an international body (e.g. International Society for Heart and Lung Transplantation) should coordinate and maintain a database of trial outcome.
(3) Clinical trials should be undertaken only when >60% survival at 3 months in >10 pig-to-nonhuman primate cardiac xenotransplants is achieved.
(4) The selected patients should be ineligible for allotransplantation but not have such severe co-morbidities that would diminish the potential for benefit in the trial.
(5) The initial trial should only be limited to adults capable of informed consent.

Future

The immunological barriers to xenotransplantation, despite intense research, remain significant. With the increasing success of ventricular assist devices in bridging to allotransplantation/recovery, and as the total artificial heart progresses, the role of xenotransplantation remains undefined for the reasons listed in Table 1.

To paraphrase Dr Norman Shumway, 'xenotransplantation may always be the future of transplantation.'

Table 1 Comparison of xenotransplantation with total artificial heart.

	Xenotransplantation	Total artificial heart
Current clinical trials	No	Yes
Cost	Expensive	Very expensive
Post-discharge care	As per allotransplantation	Very involved
Major barrier	Immunological	Blood–foreign surface incompatibility
Complications	Rejection, cancer, xenozoonosis	Neurological events, bleeding, infection
Projected quality of life	Very good	Good
Patient size limitations	None	Body surface area >1.7 m^2
Pediatric applicability	Yes	No (size limitation)
Ethical considerations	Significant, numerous	Minor, resource allocation
Becoming clinical reality?	No	Yes

Further reading

1. Taniguchi S, Cooper DK. Clinical xenotransplantation: past, present and future. *Ann R Coll Surg Engl* 1997; **79**: 13–19.
2. Platt JL. The immunological hurdles to cardiac xenotransplantation. *J Card Surg* 2001; **16**: 439–47.
3. Vial CM, Ostlie DJ, Bhatti FN et al. Life supporting function for over one month of a transgenic porcine heart in a baboon. *J Heart Lung Transplant* 2000; **19**: 224–9.
4. Michler RE, Chen JM. Cardiac xenotransplantation: ethics and potential application. *J Card Surg* 2001; **16**: 421–8.
5. Cooper DK, Keogh AM, Brink J et al. Report of the Xenotransplantation Advisory Committee of the International Society for Heart and Lung Transplantation: the present status of xenotransplantation and its potential role in the treatment of end-stage cardiac and pulmonary diseases. *J Heart Lung Transplant* 2000; **19**: 1125–65.

Related topics of interest

PART C   PEDIATRIC CARDIAC SURGERY

27 Atrial septal defect

Sunil K Ohri

Etiology

Atrial septal defects (ASDs) form 7% of all congenital heart defects with a female proponderence. In adults, ASDs are the second most common congenital cardiac defect after bicuspid aortic valve. Predispositions to ASDs can be environmental and/or genetic such as trisomy 21 (Down's syndrome) and single gene disorders.

During the 4th to 6th week of gestation the common atrial chamber is divided into two by the growth of endocardial cushions and two septae, the septum primum and the septum secundum. A primum defect constitutes 20% of ASDs and results from failure of fusion of the endocardial cushions with the septum primum. The complex defect involves the inferior aspect of interatrial septum. The mitral valve is often clefted and regurgitant. The postero-medial papillary muscle is more anterior. The abnormal left ventricular cavity has a broad inlet and narrow outlet, producing a characteristic goose-neck appearance on angiography. Other associated anomalies include mitral stenosis, hypoplastic left heart and aortic coarcta-tion. Failure of the septum secundum to fuse with the septum primum results in a patent foramen ovale and if the defect is large a secundum ASD. Seventy percent of ASDs are of the secundum variety. This defect lies at the center of the fossa ovalis but may extend towards the inferior vena cava (IVC) or posteriorly. A multiple defect in the central portion of the fossa ovalis is termed a chiari network. Sinus venosus defects form 10% of ASDs and appear in the interatrial septum above but separate from the fossa ovalis with the right superior pulmonary vein draining into the superior vena cava (SVC). Unroofed coronary sinus defect is a rare anomaly associated with left-sided SVC producing a left-to-right shunt from the left atrium to coronary sinus.

Pathophysiology

Left-to-right shunting results in enlargement of the right atrium, right ventricle and pul-monary vessels. Unlike in ventricular septal defects pulmonary hypertension develops very gradually. Infants very rarely die of surgically uncorrected ASD although they may present with heart failure. Patients may present in and beyond the fourth decade of life with conges-tive heart failure and pulmonary hypertension. This risk does not appear to be different if the patients have a secundum of sinus venosus defect. The main features are reduction in right ventricular function with a posteriorly displaced interventricular septum, impaired left ven-tricular functional reserve and atrioventricular valvular dysfunction. The latter is predomi-nantly tricuspid regurgitation secondary to right ventricular volume overload and annular dilatation. Incidence of supraventricular tachyarrhythmia, including atrial fibrillation, increases with age.

Diagnosis

Clinical features include a pulmonary flow murmur caused by a left-to-right shunt, a diastolic murmur from tricuspid regurgitation and fixed splitting of the second heart sound. Twelve-lead ECG is characterized by right axis deviation and features of right ventricular hypertrophy (prominent R waves in II and III and RSR pattern in V1 with prominent S wave in leads V5 and V6). Primum defects exceptionally produce left axis deviation with overall negative deflection in II and III or prominent S wave in III and AVF. Chest x ray demonstrates cardiomegaly with enlarged right atrium and ventricle. The pulmonary arteries are prominent. Echocardiography may be the only other investigation required for patients who have clinical features, physical examination, chest x ray and ECG all supporting a diagnosis of ASD. Cardiac catheterization is indicated when echocardiography fails to clinch the diagnosis, or when pulmonary hypertension is suspected and also to exclude coronary artery disease in those older than 45 years.

Management

Surgery is indicated in all infants with severe heart failure with or without other associated defects. In asymptomatic children surgery can be delayed until aged 3–4 years. Otherwise ASD repair is indicated when the left-to-right shunt (Qp:Qs) exceeds 1.5:1, when patients have sustained paradoxial embolism or when there is evidence of pulmonary hypertension. Repair is contraindicated when there is shunt reversal and development of Eisenmenger phenomenon which is generally associated with elevated pulmonary vascular resistance (>8 wood units) and/or pulmonary artery pressure of >60 mmHg. The timing of surgical repair may influence long-term prognosis: Murray et al found that the actuarial survival following surgery matched the general population when age of surgical correction ranged between 11 and 24 years; when operation was delayed (after age 41) the 27-year actuarial survival was 40% compared to 59% for the general population.

Surgical closure of an ASD employs either direct suturing or an autologous pericardial patch. Surgery for secumdum defect is low risk with most units reporting mortality approaching 0%. Postoperatively dyspnea may improve but arrhythmia usually persists. Transcatheter closure using the Amplatz™ device, for example, is now increasingly adopted for smaller defects. There is risk of embolization but experience is limited and long-term evaluation awaited. During patch closure of a sinus venosus defect, sutures should be placed to avoid damage to the sinus node or its nutrient artery. Unroofed coronary sinus defect may be treated by patching or closing the coronary sinus ostium while preserving the conduction tissue in triangle of Koch. A primum ASD is closed with autologous pericardial patch either with the coronary sinus to the right or the left side. An existent mitral valve cleft will be repaired unless this results in mitral stenosis. Surgical mortality in uncomplicated primum defects approaches 1% with a re-operation rate of less than 3% and long-term survival approaching that of the general population.

Further reading

1. Murphy JG, Gersch BJ, McGoon MD et al. Long-term outcome after surgical repair of isolated atrial septal defect: follow-up 27 to 32 years. *N Engl J Med* 1990; **323**: 1645.
2. Chan KC, Godman MJ, Walsh K et al. Transcatheter closure of atrial septal defect and interatrial communications with a new self expanding nitinol double disc device (Amplatzer septal occluder): multicentre UK experience. *Heart* 1999; **82**: 300–6.
3. King RM, Puga FJ, Danielson GK et al. Prognostic factors and surgical treatment of partial atrioventricular canal. *Circulation* 1986; **74**: 142–6.
4. Campbell M. Natural history of atrial septal defects. *Br Heart J* 1970; **32**: 820.
5. Shah D, Azhar M, Oakley CM, Cleland JGF, Nihoyannopoulos P. Natural history of secundum atrial septal defect in adults after medical or surgical treatment: a historical prospective study. *Br Heart J* 1990; **71**: 224–8.

Related topic of interest

28 Ventricular septal defect

Henry L Walters III, Ralph E Delius

Introduction

A ventricular septal defect (VSD) is a developmental defect of the interventricular septum (IVS). Isolated VSD is the most common congenital heart defect (2:1000 live births) representing 30–40% of all such malformations. While most commonly single, multiple VSDs can occur. VSDs vary widely in size and location; 50% of patients undergoing surgery for primary VSD have an associated lesion (congenital or acquired). The overall incidence exceeds 50% when the latter group is included.

Morphology

The classification proposed by Anderson is preferred for its accurate anatomical description. Accordingly, VSDs are classified by (1) the boundaries of the defect and (2) the region of the morphological RV into which the defect opens. Variations in the boundaries produce three general classes of VSDs:

Perimembranous defects
Perimembranous defects occupy the membranous IVS adjacent to the anteroseptal commissure of the tricuspid valve. These lesions approximate the aortic valve along the right and noncoronary cusps. Furthermore, the annuli of the tricuspid and aortic valves may form part of the boundary. Perimembranous VSDs can extend into the inlet, outlet, apico-trabecular portions of the RV or a combination of these (confluent). The conduction tissue invariably passes along the posteroinferior rim of the defect.

Muscular defects
Muscular defects have an exclusively muscular boundary. Purely muscular VSDs are termed inlet, outlet and apical-trabecular when they open into the respective portions of the RV. Multiple apico-trabecular defects produce a 'Swiss cheese' septum. When a muscular VSD does not extend into the perimembranous IVS, the conduction tissue follows a normal course. Therefore, the relation of the conduction tissue to the VSD depends upon where the defect opens into the RV.

Doubly committed/juxta-arterial defects
These defects are subarterial defects and exist beneath both the aortic and pulmonary valves. The superior border is formed by fibrous tissue between the leaflets of the aortic and pulmonary valves (not muscle). These VSDs are particularly associated with aortic valve leaflet prolapse causing progressive aortic regurgitation.

Associated lesions

- Pulmonary stenosis (20%).
- ASD (17%).
- Coarctation of the aorta (17%).
- Persistent left SVC (9%).
- PDA (6%).
- Aortic valve (right coronary) leaflet prolapse and progressive valvular regurgitation.
- Fibromuscular subvalvular aortic stenosis and/or RVOT obstruction.

Pathophysiology

A large VSD (≥ aortic annulus) causes systemic (=LV) RV systolic pressure. Infants with large VSDs may remain asymptomatic until after 6 weeks when reduction in pulmonary vascular resistance maximizes left-to-right shunting of blood and markedly increase the ratio of pulmonary to systemic blood flow (Qp:Qs). Moderate-sized VSDs are 'restrictive' allowing for moderate elevation of Qp:Qs and RV systolic pressure at approximately 50% systemic values. These patients may develop relatively mild symptoms or remain asymptomatic. Those with small VSDs associated with near-normal right-heart pressures and minimally increased Qp:Qs usually have little or no symptoms.

In some infants, the VSD becomes restrictive as the heart grows so that severe pulmonary vascular disease (PVD) does not develop. Spontaneous complete closure of VSDs, even large ones, may occur in 25–50% of patients during childhood. These children develop normally.

In infants with untreated and persistently large VSDs, severe PVD and a significant increase in PVR emerge by 6–12 months. As the PVD progresses, left-to-right shunting diminishes and may become predominantly right-to-left (patient becomes cyanotic) when fixed pulmonary hypertension occurs (Eisenmenger's syndrome).

Clinical presentation

- Symptoms: tachypnea, poor feeding, failure to thrive, exercise intolerance, frequent respiratory infections.
- Signs: subcostal retractions, sweating with feeds, malnourishment, hyperdynamic precordium with palpable thrill (3rd to 5th left intercostal space), loud split second heart sound, loud pansystolic murmur, diastolic mitral flow rumble when Qp:Qs is large, hepatosplenomegaly.
- Chest x ray: usually normal with small VSDs; otherwise, enlarged central pulmonary arteries, pulmonary vascular congestion and cardiomegaly.
- EKG: with significantly raised Qp:Qs tall R waves in the right precordial leads and tall R waves with tall peaked T waves in the left precordial leads.

Specific investigation

(1) **Echocardiogram** is the gold standard test in the overwhelming majority. It provides detailed information on the location, size, number and direction of shunt through the VSD(s).

(2) **Cardiac catheterization/angiography** adds information when there are rare anatomical ± physiological questions unanswered by echocardiography. Cardiac catheterization is certainly justified in older patients who may have fixed pulmonary hypertension. These patients should have PVR assessed on room air and following pulmonary vasodilation with 100% oxygen or nitric oxide.

Management

1. Expectant

Patients with small VSDs may never require surgical repair. They should be observed closely for the development of symptoms, pulmonary hypertension or acquired complications including aortic regurgitation, subaortic fibromuscular stenosis and/or RVOT obstruction.

2. Medical

Patients with large VSDs and/or symptoms of congestive heart failure may require nutritional supplementation and treatment with diuretic ± systemic vasodilator.

3. Surgical

Important considerations include the presence of congestive heart failure or growth failure, the likelihood of severe pulmonary vascular disease and the possibility of spontaneous closure. Indications include:

- persistent congestive heart failure ± failure to thrive despite medical therapy
- persistent pulmonary hypertension
- failure of spontaneous VSD closure
- progressive LV dilatation
- associated progressive aortic incompetence, subaortic obstruction or RVOT obstruction.

Operative risk increases and long-term effectiveness declines with pre-operative pulmonary hypertension, particularly if it remains fixed. Surgery is clearly contraindicated in Eisenmenger's syndrome.

Surgical techniques

- Median sternotomy.
- CPB with bicaval cannulation.
- Cardioplegic arrest.
- Transatrial approach to VSD through the tricuspid valve.
- Synthetic patch defect closure using interrupted or running suturing.
- Avoid suturing close to the conduction tissue with consequent complete heart block.
- If transatrial approach gives inadequate exposure, VSD closure can be performed through a right ventriculotomy.
- Doubly committed/juxta-arterial defects are best repaired through a transpulmonary approach.
- Any associated lesions are repaired simultaneously along with the VSD closure.
- Total circulatory arrest, using a solitary venous cannula, is recommended in neonates weighing less than 3 kg.

- PA banding is recommended only when there are serious coexisting medical conditions (prematurity, weight below 2 kg, serious non-cardiac disorders) or compelling anatomical situations ('Swiss cheese septum') that preclude VSD closure. Every effort should be made to remove the band and perform a definitive repair within 6 months.

Outcome

Repair of isolated VSDs, even in very small infants, can be safely accomplished in experienced centers with <1% mortality. The most significant risk factor for death after repair of isolated VSD is poor pre-operative condition of the patient from serious coexisting non-cardiac medical problem(s). Major associated cardiac lesions are also an incremental risk factor for postoperative mortality.

Further reading

1. Anderson RH, Wilcox BR. The surgical anatomy of ventricular septal defect. *J Cardiac Surg* 1992; 7: 17–36.
2. Walters HL, Pacifico AD, Kirklin JK. Ventricular septal defects. In: *Textbook of Surgery. The Biological Basis of Modern Surgical Practice*. Sabiston DC (ed). WB Saunders: Philadelphia, 1997: pp 2005–18.

Related topics of interest

1.1   Heart valves
1.3   Conduction system
27   Atrial septal defect
43   Palliation versus correction of congenital heart defects

29 Atrioventricular septal defect

William Brawn

Introduction

Atrioventricular septal defects (AVSDs) are characterized by maldevelopment of the atrio-ventricular septum producing a common atrioventricular junction. The prevalence of AVSD is 0.2 per 1000 live births. Eighty percent of AVSD patients have Down's syndrome, whilst 35% of Down's syndrome patients have AVSD.

This complex mixing defect may cause cyanosis, congestive cardiac failure, recurrent chest infections and failure to thrive. Survivors may develop pulmonary hypertension and pulmonary vascular disease. Surgery is indicated early in infancy for the complete form of AVSD, to facilitate normal development and growth and avoid pulmonary vascular complications. Antenatal diagnosis of Down's syndrome has dramatically reduced the occurrence of AVSD, since many families choose to terminate pregnancy.

Morphology

In AVSD there is a contiguous ASD and VSD, resulting in a common atrioventricular junction, i.e. there are no separate mitral and tricuspid valves. In the complete form of AVSD, a common five-leaflet atrioventricular valve guards the atrioventricular junction. In partial AVSD the common atrioventricular valve is divided into morphologically abnormal mitral and tricuspid valves. Furthermore, the VSD is usually wholly or partially closed and not hemodynamically significant.

Rastelli's classification of atrioventricular septal valve morphology based on the anatomy of the superior bridging leaflet is helpful (Table 1).

The majority of common atrioventricular valves are Rastelli type A, a few are Rastelli type C and the minority Rastelli type B.

Table 1 Rastelli's classification of atrioventricular septal valve morphology.

Type	Description of anatomy
Type A	Superior leaflet may be attached to the ventricular septum and variably divided
Type B	Rarely there may be a cleft in the superior leaflet, but the attachments to the chordal apparatus are to the right side of the ventricular septum
Type C	Superior leaflet may be completely free floating and not attached to the ventricular septum

Complete AVSD can also occur in the setting of Fallot's tetralogy, double outlet RV and various forms of heterotaxy. However, the general principles of valve repair used in uncomplicated AVSD can be applied to this more complex group.

Repair of complete AVSD

To achieve a normally functioning left atrioventricular valve, both the ventricular and atrial septal defects are closed prior to reconstruction of a left and right atrioventricular valve. A two-patch repair technique has been successfully utilized. Initially CPB with hypothermic circulatory arrest was utilized for almost all small patients, but latterly bi-caval cannulation with continuous hypothermic CPB and only short periods of circulatory arrest has been utilized uniformly with cardioplegic arrest. The surgical technique involves assessing the atrioventricular valve and placing marking sutures on the functional zones of apposition or the 'created cleft' of the superior and inferior components of the common atrioventricular valve. This assessment is facilitated by insufflating the ventricular cavity with cold crystalloid solution to close the leaflets under pressure. The zones of apposition are then inspected to determine the correct placement of a marking suture. The marking suture is placed at a point of leaflet apposition and where the VSD patch will be attached to the valve tissue. The VSD patch, usually Dacron, is then sutured with multiple interrupted mattress Prolene sutures pledgeted with Teflon to the rightward side of the ventricular septum. This avoids the bundle of His which passes from the inferiorly displaced atrioventricular node, along the crest of the ventricular septum to its midpoint, before passing to the left side of the ventricular septum and into the LV. Simple mattress sutures are then placed through the free edge of the Dacron patch out through the atrioventricular valve tissue of the superior and inferior components of the atrioventricular valve. These sutures are then passed through either native or bovine pericardial patch and individually tied down to sandwich the superior and inferior components of the atrioventricular valve between the upper border of the VSD patch and the ASD patch. Thus the VSD is closed, and the common atrioventricular valve is divided into left and right components. In general, the tricuspid valve working at lower pulmonary pressures does not create problems with competency or stenosis; this valve is not repaired unless postoperative pulmonary hypertension is anticipated.

The left atrioventricular valve is then insufflated with crystalloid solution to test its competency. Whether it is competent or not, it is our routine to close the zone of apposition or 'cleft' between the superior and inferior leaflets with interrupted simple Prolene sutures. Closure of this 'cleft' is important to achieve a competent left atrioventricular valve. In general, the cleft is closed along its length to the insertion of chordae tendonae into the leaflet tissue. Having achieved a competent left atrioventricular valve, the ASD is closed by suturing the native or bovine pericardial patch with a continuous Prolene suture so that the coronary sinus is closed to the pulmonary venous atrium. Where there is a left SVC it is possible to sew inside the orifice of the coronary sinus to avoid the atrioventricular node and to allow the left SVC to continue to drain to the RA. In order to avoid postoperative pulmonary hypertension, surgical repair below 4 months of age is advocated.

Other methods of AVSD repair have been described and applied successfully, including division of the superior leaflet of the atrioventricular valve and placement of a single patch to close both the ventricular and atrial septal defects. More recently, a few centers have described a technique whereby the superior and inferior components of the common atrioventricular valve are directly sandwiched or sutured on to the ventricular septum. The ASD is then closed with a single patch of pericardium. This technique has been reported as being widely applicable to the repair of AVSD with any size of VSD. However, the longer-term function of the left atrioventricular valve utilizing this technique is undetermined.

Following repair of the left atrioventricular valve and separation from CPB, on-table echocardiographic assessment of the repair is undertaken. If the atrioventricular valves are competent with good ventricular function, then with monitoring of LA pressure and possibly PAP if pulmonary hypertension is anticipated, the postoperative course is usually straight-forward. However, these children may have quite flimsy atrioventricular valve tissues and recurrent left atrioventricular valve regurgitation occurs in 5–10%. Our experience suggests that disruption of the repair can occur in the sutures at the 'cleft' and that the attachment of the superior component of the atrioventricular valve can tear away from the intracardiac patches. Whilst re-repair can be difficult, it is possible to achieve a competent valve by patching these areas with pericardial tissue and reinforcing the sutures lines with pericardial pledgets. Whilst a completely competent valve may not be achieved, mild or even mild-to-moderate atrioventricular regurgitation may be quite well tolerated.

The repair of the atrioventricular valve in partial AVSD is simpler, in that the ventricular septum is intact and the left atrioventricular valve is already formed as a separate entity. To achieve a competent left atrioventricular valve the 'cleft' is directly sutured with interrupted sutures. It is important, even if the left atrioventricular valve seems to be competent when tested by LV crystalloid insufflation, that the cleft is closed. Recurrence of the left atrioventricular valve regurgitation during follow-up is always through the zone of apposition where sutures have torn through or the 'cleft' has not been closed. Other unusual complications of AVSD repair include complete heart block requiring a pacemaker insertion and significant residual VSD requiring re-operation.

Rarely AVSD is associated with Fallot's tetralogy where there is malalignment of the ventricular septum superiorly with deficiency in the ventricular septum at this point. This is associated with marked fibromuscular subpulmonary stenosis. Repair of this condition requires placement of an enlarged VSD patch superiorly and resection of the muscular outflow tract obstruction to the pulmonary artery with patching of the RV outflow tract.

Outcome

Surgical repair should be performed in the first few months of life and, in uncomplicated cases, can be achieved with an early mortality of 5% or less. Early re-operation may be necessary in a small percentage of cases because of disruption of the repair and again this re-operation is usually successful. In the longer term, operations may be necessary for residual atrioventricular valve regurgitation, either to re-repair or to replace that valve, or because of the development of LV outflow tract obstruction. In those patients where there is sound repair, which is maintained in the early postoperative period, the longer-term outlook seems very satisfactory.

Further reading

1. Anderson RH, Ebels T, Yen Ho S. The surgical anatomy of atrioventricular septal defect. In: *Annual of Cardiac Surgery. 7th Edn.* Yacoub M, Pepper J (eds). Current Science: London, 1994: pp 71–9.
2. Rastelli GC, Kirklin JW, Titus JC. Anatomic observations in complete form of persistent common atrio-ventricular canal with special reference to atrioventricular valves. *Mayo Clinic Proc* 1966; **41**: 296.
3. Weintraub RG, Brawn WJ, Venable AW, Mee RBB. Two-patch repair of complete atrioventricular septal defect in the first year of life. *J Thorac Cardiovasc Surg* 1990; **99**: 320–6.
4. Redmond JM, Silove ED, DeGiovanni JV et al. Complete atrioventricular septal defect: the influence of associated cardiac anomalies on surgical management and outcome. *Eur J Cardiothorac Surg* 1996; **10**: 991–5.
5. Nicholson IA, Nunn GR, Sholler GF et al. Simplified single patch technique for the repair of atrio-ventricular septal defect. *J Thorac Cardiovasc Surg* 1999; **118**: 642–7.

Related topics of interest

30 Patent ductus arteriosus

Constantine Mavroudis, Carl L Backer

Anatomy and physiology

The ductus arteriosus (DA) of Botalli is a normal fetal structure arising from the left sixth aortic arch. In utero the DA connects the main pulmonary artery to the upper descending thoracic aorta just distal to and opposite the origin of the left subclavian artery. The origin and insertion of the ductus can be highly variable; the ductus may be bilateral (right and left ductus) or absent (tetralogy of Fallot with absent pulmonary valve). In infancy the length of the ductus varies from 2 to 8 mm with a diameter of 4–12 mm, averaging 7 mm. Histologically, the media of the DA is deficient in elastic fibers and the smooth muscle is especially sensitive to prostaglandin-mediated relaxation and oxygen-induced vasoconstriction.

Circulating prostaglandins maintain ductal patency during the fetal period. At birth an elevated arterial pO_2 inhibits prostaglandin synthetase, resulting in ductal constriction. Permanent DA closure requires loss of cells from the muscular media and neointimal proliferation. The fibrosed DA becomes the ligamentum arteriosum. Functional closure of the DA occurs within a few hours of birth in term infants and is usually irreversible within 6 weeks.

Natural history

Patent DA (PDA) accounts for 5–10% of all congenital heart defects. Twice as common among females, PDA occurs in approximately 1 in 1600 term live births. Maternal rubella virus during the first trimester is associated with an increased incidence of PDA. The incidence of PDA in preterm infants is increased in comparison to full-term infants; the overall incidence in preterm infants is 20–30%. With earlier gestational age and lower birth weight, the incidence rises sharply: 21% at gestational age 34–36 weeks, 44% at 31–33 weeks and 77% at 28–30 weeks. Immature ductal tissue is less sensitive in preterm infants to oxygen-mediated constriction and more sensitive to prostaglandin vasodilation. In preterm infants, a PDA may contribute to morbidity from necrotizing enterocolitis, abnormal cerebral blood flow, respiratory distress syndrome, and chronic lung disease. Retrograde blood flow in the descending aorta in diastole leads to decreased systemic flow and predisposition to end-organ ischemia (renal failure, necrotizing enterocolitis). In term infants and older children, a small PDA may be hemodynamically insignificant and detected only by echocardiography ('silent' ductus). A large nonrestrictive ductus with no other congenital cardiac defects produces a large left-to-right shunt with LA dilation, left ventricular volume overload, and progressive congestive heart failure. Left untreated, a large PDA may lead to pulmonary arteriolar hypertension with the eventual shunt reversal (Eisenmenger syndrome). Significant elevation in PVR may develop by as early as 6 months of life and result in supra-systemic PAP. Other complications include endarteritis, ductal aneurysm, aortic aneurysm, pulmonary artery aneurysm, and aortic dissection. During the pre-antibiotic era the average life span of a patient with PDA was 36 years and endarteritis was the most common cause of death (45% of mortality). The risk of endarteritis in the antibiotic era is clearly much lower than the historical studies mentioned.

At present, the risk of developing congestive heart failure and/or pulmonary hypertension with a moderate or large ductus along with the (low) risk of endarteritis for even a small ductus are indications for intervention in nearly all patients with an isolated (clinically audible) PDA. The management of the 'silent' ductus detected only by echocardiogram remains controversial and one that may be best addressed individually.

Clinical features and diagnosis

Symptoms and physical findings depend on the size of the ductus as well as the PVR and associated intracardiac defects. With a small ductus, the degree of left-to-right shunting is restricted by the narrow lumen, and the child may be asymptomatic. A typical continuous 'machinery' murmur is heard in the left second intercostal space. With a moderate-sized PDA, the shunt increases significantly over the first few months of life as the PVR falls. These children tend to have failure to thrive, recurrent upper respiratory tract infections, and fatigue with exertion. The pulse may be bounding along with an overactive cardiac impulse and continuous murmur. With a large PDA, an infant develops heart failure in the first weeks of life with tachypnea, tachycardia, and poor feeding. Physical findings include an overactive precordium, wide pulse pressure, and an enlarged liver. Preterm infants with a large ductus will frequently have respiratory distress and require intubation and ventilation.

Abnormalities on the chest x ray are proportional to the degree of left-to-right shunting; a large ductus results in enlargement of the LA and LV, increased pulmonary vascular markings, and interstitial pulmonary edema. Electrocardiographic changes indicative of LVH and LA enlargement are present. TTE can accurately identify ductal anatomy and characterize shunt flow. A LA-to-aortic diameter ratio of greater than 1.2:1 is present in the majority of premature infants with a significant PDA. Most infants and children with physical findings and an echocardiogram indicating isolated PDA do not require cardiac catheterization, unless catheter occlusion is to be the treatment strategy. However, if the TTE findings suggest severe pulmonary hypertension, pre-intervention cardiac catheterization should be performed. With elevated PAP, pulmonary reactivity is assessed using oxygen and pulmonary vasodilators. Patients with fixed pulmonary hypertension will have systemic desaturation and exhibit differential cyanosis, with pink face and right hand, and cyanosis of the feet. Patients with fixed elevated PVR are not candidates for ductal closure because of the high risk of RV failure, and must be considered for lung transplantation and simultaneous ductal closure. MRI can also identify ductal anatomy and characterize ductal flow and pressure gradients.

Management

Since the first successful ligation of a PDA by Gross in 1938, in a 7-year-old girl through the left chest, subsequent experience has proven the efficacy of PDA closure with low morbidity, mortality and excellent clinical results. The introduction of new surgical techniques and improvements in anesthetic management and intensive care have resulted in minimized risks, shorter hospital stays, and safer operations, particularly on low birth weight infants.

Technological advances in recent years have made possible percutaneous trans-catheter ductal closure and thoracoscopic ligation.

Pharmacologic advances have also focused on medical management of PDA. For infants with ductal-dependent congenital heart disease (e.g. hypoplastic left heart syndrome), prostaglandin E1 infusion maintains ductal patency. Recently ibuprofen, which significantly reduces plasma levels of prostaglandins, has been used for ductal closure in premature infants because of fewer side effects, compared to indomethacin, on mesenteric, renal, and cerebral perfusion. For those infants who fail to respond to pharmacologic management, thoracoscopic clipping of the PDA has been used in premature infants (<1200 g). In these infants, trans-catheter closure is difficult as the vessels encountered are extremely small, and positioning of the occluders requires fluoroscopic control necessitating removal of infants from incubators.

The safe and efficacious surgical interruption of the PDA in the older child remains the gold standard to which alternative interventions compare (Figure 1). Video-assisted thoracoscopic surgery (VATS) can be applied to a wide range of patients requiring ductal closure and has a lower incidence of residual or recurrent shunting than coil occlusion. This technique obviates the need for intravascular foreign bodies, and addresses patient/parent esthetic concerns. With increased use of critical pathways management of surgical/hospital stays, perceivable differences in hospital length of stay and costs have narrowed. On the other hand, continued transcatheter device development has led to improved outcomes with multiple coil placements, and it is likely that in the future improved devices will address outstanding concerns of embolization and residual or recurrent shunting. Recently, intravascular ultrasound guidance has been used during trans-catheter coil closure of PDA, with excellent agreement between the ultrasound guidance and angiography.

The adult with a PDA presents unique challenges, e.g. calcification of the ductal tissue, relatively old age with associated heart failure, pulmonary hypertension, and other systemic health concerns. Recent reports have described coil embolization of PDA in adults. While residual shunting occurred, the reduction in shunt size and resultant improvement of heart

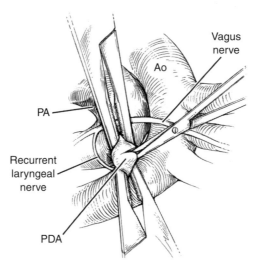

Figure 1 Division and oversewing of a patent ductus (Ao = aorta). (Reproduced with permission from Hillman N, Backer CL, Mavroudis C. PDA. In: *Pediatric Cardiac Surgery. 3rd Edn.* Mavroudis C, Backer CL (eds). McGraw-Hill: New York, 2002.)

failure were deemed acceptable in view of overall status improvement. Controversy surrounds the surgical approach to PDA in the adult. Some advocate the use of CPB to allow balloon occlusion of the ductus and patch or direct closure of the ductal orifice via a transpulmonary approach. Others recommend the transaortic closure of the patent ductus, using temporary heparin-coated aortic shunts for safe temporary aortic occlusion without the need for heparinization or CPB. This procedure may be contraindicated in patients in whom there is a severe degree of aortic atherosclerosis.

Further reading

1. Burke RP, Jacobs JP, Cheng W, Trento A, Fontana GP. Video-assisted thoracoscopic surgery for patent ductus arteriosus in low birth weight neonates and infants. *Pediatrics* 1999; **104:** 227–30.
2. Campbell M. Natural history of persistent ductus arteriosus. *Br Heart J* 1968; **30:** 4–13.
3. Mavroudis C, Backer CL, Gevitz M. Forty-six years of patent ductus arteriosus division at Children's Memorial Hospital of Chicago. Standards for comparison. *Ann Surg* 1994; **220:** 402–9.
4. Radtke WA. Current therapy of the patent ductus arteriosus. *Curr Opin in Cardiol* 1998; **13:** 59–65.
5. Toda R, Moriyama Y, Yamashita M et al. Operation for adult PDA using cardiopulmonary bypass. *Ann Thorac Surg* 2000; **70:** 1935–7.

Related topics of interest

31 Tricuspid atresia

Gordon A Cohen, Martin J Elliott

Anatomy

Tricuspid atresia is a condition that is characterized by the absence of the tricuspid valve with varying degrees of RV hypoplasia. The morphological RA is usually muscular and blind-ending with no vestigial tricuspid valve in its floor. The RV is usually rudimentary and completely lacks an inlet component because of this absent connection. The apical trabecular part of the incomplete ventricle is separated from the LV by the apical trabecular septum. With atresia or absence of the tricuspid valve, the only exit from the right atrium is either through a patent foramen ovale or through an ASD.

Tricuspid atresia is relatively uncommon and occurs in about 2% of all cases of congenital heart disease. This condition is almost always associated with a VSD but may also be associated with pulmonary stenosis, transposition of the great vessels and aortic coarctation.

Pathophysiology

The absence of a communication between the RA and RV results in blood being shunted right-to-left across the intra-atrial communication to produce complete mixing of systemic and pulmonary venous blood in the LA. This shunting results in cyanosis with left-heart volume overload.

Natural history

The survival of a neonate with tricuspid atresia is dependent on the degree of shunting present. In children with a restrictive atrial level communication, pulmonary oligemia and severe cyanosis will be present and death may ensue if no intervention is taken to permit mixing. Neonates with either severe pulmonary stenosis or coarctation of the aorta may be dependent on a patent ductus artenosus (PDA) and may collapse if the duct closes. In new-borns with no pulmonary stenosis and an unrestrictive VSD, heart failure with high pulmonary blood flow can occur when the pulmonary vascular resistance falls shortly after birth. Irrespective of the precise anatomy, survival beyond infancy is rare without intervention.

Clinical presentation

Neonates with tricuspid atresia are always cyanotic, even in those with high pulmonary blood flow. Cardiac auscultation usually reveals a single, loud second heart sound. If the VSD is restrictive, a harsh holosystolic murmur may be heard at the lower left sternal border. Associated pulmonary stenosis often causes a mid-systolic murmur in the left upper sternal border. Physical examination may demonstrate unequal pulses or blood pressures between the upper and lower extremities if aortic coarctation is present. CXR will demonstrate cardiomegaly and LV hypertrophy with either increased or decreased pulmonary vascular markings depending on the underlying associated anatomy of the defect. EKG will demonstrate RA enlargement, left axis deviation and LV hypertrophy. Two-dimensional TTE almost always gives definitive anatomical information about the defect. With the effectiveness of echocardiography, cardiac catheterization is usually not necessary to obtain a diagnosis but is required later in life for hemodynamic assessment of suitability for a total cavopulmonary connection.

Management

1. Newborn/neonatal period

Immediately after birth, the circulation may be dependent on the presence of a PDA and thus a prostaglandin infusion may be necessary to maintain ductal patency. If the anatomical defect is such that there is a reduction in pulmonary blood flow, then the use of a neonatal shunt (modified BT shunt) is necessary and must be performed shortly after birth. If the anatomical defect results in a high pulmonary blood flow state, then pulmonary artery banding is indicated to protect against pulmonary vascular disease. In patients where there is a restrictive atrial communication, a balloon atrial septostomy (Rashkind's procedure) should be performed. In some cases a surgical atrial septectomy may be necessary.

In patients with significant subaortic obstruction, which may occur when transposition is present, a Damus–Kaye–Stansel procedure may be performed at the time of systemic–pulmonary arterial shunting. The basic principle of this operation is to allow all blood leaving the heart through either the aortic valve or pulmonary valve to be directed in a common fashion into the aorta for systemic blood flow.

2. Long term

The definitive treatment for patients with tricuspid atresia is a total cavopulmonary artery connection (Fontan-type operation). The basic principle of the Fontan operation is to divert systemic venous return back to the pulmonary artery without the use of a functional ventricle. The total cavopulmonary connection directs, rather than pumps, systemic venous return into the pulmonary arteries. This then allows the functional ventricle of the heart to be used for providing systemic blood flow. In the modern era, this operation is usually performed in a staged manner. The first step is a bi-directional Glenn shunt (superior cavopulmonary anastamosis) which is commonly performed on children at approximately 6 months of age. Patients usually live with this surgical configuration until 2–5 years of age when they then undergo a completion total cavopulmonary anastamosis (completion Fontan procedure).

Outcome

Data from the Pediatric Cardiac Care Consortium collected between 1984 and 1993 demonstrated that for all patients undergoing a Fontan operation for a functional single ventricle, patients who have a primary diagnosis of tricuspid atresia and undergo this type of surgical correction seem to have an overall lower mortality and a better long-term survival. In addition, patients with tricuspid atresia also have the best long-term quality of life. The reason that these patients do better than other patients with a functional single ventricle is, presumably, because in most cases the left ventricle serves as the systemic ventricle.

Further reading

1. Wilcox BR, Anderson RH. *Surgical Anatomy of the Heart. 2nd Edn.* Gower Medical Publishing: London, 1992.
2. Archer N, Burch M. *Paediatric Cardiology, An Introduction.* Chapman & Hall Medical: London, 1998.
3. de Leval M. Right heart bypass operations. In: Surgery for Congenital Heart Defects. *2nd Edn..* Stark J, de Leval (eds) WB Saunders: Philadelphia, 1994: pp 569–87.
4. Hagler DJ. Fontan. Surgery of congenital heart disease: Pediatric Cardiac Care Consortium 1984–1995. In: *Perspectives in Pediatric Cardiology.* Moller JH (ed). Armonk, NY: Futura Publishing, 1998: **6:** 345–52.

Related topics

32 Pulmonary atresia with intact ventricular septum

Victor T Tsang, Vibeke E Hjortdal

Pulmonary atresia with intact ventricular septum (PA/IVS) is difficult to manage. The prognosis for this rare malformation (approximately 1:22 000 live births) has improved, partly related to the use of prostaglandin (PGE1) infusion to maintain the duct-dependent pulmonary circulation. Another important contribution is a better understanding of right ventricle (RV) morphology and its use in the management strategy. The ideal approach is to restore continuity between RV and pulmonary artery (PA), when the RV is adequate for supporting the pulmonary circulation. This also decompresses the hypertensive RV and may promote growth of the hypoplastic cavity. Precise management in an individual patient will be governed by the varying degrees of RV hypertrophy/cavity hypoplasia, tricuspid valve (TV) dysplasia and RV-dependent coronary circulation.

Anatomical consideration

The RV morphology varies from severe cavity hypoplasia to gross enlargement, with different extents of hypertrophy and TV anomalies. Most newborns have RV cavity hypoplasia and hypertrophy, both of which may be severe. Classifying the RV on the basis of a tripartite concept (outlet, trabecular, and inlet portions) may assist management strategy. It has also been shown that TV dimension relates to the degree of RV cavity hypoplasia. An atrial septal defect (ASD) is constant. Occasionally the communication may be restrictive. The pulmonary arteries are usually good-sized vessels.

Two main forms are generally recognized. Those with mild-to-moderate RV cavity hypoplasia tend to have a reasonably well-developed infundibulum, and the pulmonary valve may be a fibrous membrane. Severe RV hypoplasia is usually associated with severe infundibular stenosis/atresia. In some patients, fistulae develop between the diminutive hypertensive RV cavity and the coronary arteries, resulting in myocardial ischemia. The proximal coronary arteries may be stenosed or occluded; the involved regions depend on a collateral supply of deoxygenated blood from the hypertensive RV.

These morphological features dictate whether patients are suitable for biventricular repair, or if the 'Fontan' route should be the preferred surgical option.

Assessment of RV size

The degree of RV cavity hypoplasia is the main determinant of the appropriate surgical option. However, assessment of RV size can be difficult because of its unusual geometry.

Methods hitherto incorporated the tripartite concept, or a complex score of RV size, or measurement of TV annulus diameter or 'eyeballing' the RV. Sometimes the simple approach is probably sufficient for clinical decision-making.

The relationship between RV size and TV dimension has been described for PA/IVS. de Leval suggested that an RV with TV diameter within 3 standard deviations (SD) of normal can support adequate pulmonary blood flow in a biventricular circulation. However, it would be unsafe to consider biventricular repair in a small RV without the trabecular portion and with a TV diameter of <3 SD of normal. There is evidence that LV function can be compromised by a hypertensive and hypertrophied RV, thus raising the question of whether RV decompression should be performed even if it is unsuitable for biventricular repair.

Hanley suggested using the z value (standard deviation units) of the TV diameters to guide the management of neonates with PA/IVS:

- z value ≥−1.5 (normal or mildly hypoplastic): an early pulmonary valvotomy or right ventricular outflow tract (RVOT) procedure without a concomitant shunt. A transannular patch may be necessary if infundibular stenosis coexists, thus creating unobstructed forward flow from the RV. A patent foramen ovale (PFO) can be left open.
- z value between −1.5 and −4: a transannular RVOT patch without closing the PFO and a concomitant systemic to pulmonary shunt.
- z value ≤−4, patients without an infundibulum or with significant coronary fistulae: only a systemic-to-pulmonary shunt should be performed. In the presence of an RV-dependent coronary circulation, the hypertensive RV perfuses portions of the ventricular myocardium with desaturated blood during systole. During diastole reversed blood flow may cause 'coronary steal' into a relaxed RV. In this instance RV decompression would exacerbate myocardial ischemia.

Neonatal management

PA/IVS is often diagnosed prenatally. The progression of critical pulmonary valvar stenosis towards PA/IVS has also been observed prenatally. Cyanosis is present at birth and becomes severe with ductal closure. Following diagnosis, the most important aspect of immediate treatment is to maintain ductal patency with PGE1. The next stage is to provide reliable, adequate pulmonary blood flow to ensure survival beyond the newborn period. Ideally, treatment should establish the RV as the pulmonary pump, and, if not possible, to decompress a hypertensive RV.

In practice, echocardiography should reveal the size and geometry of RV cavity, the level of atresia (valvar or valvar and infundibular), TV size and competence, size and confluence of the pulmonary arteries, size of the ASD, size of the patent duct, and LV function. Angiography is not routinely necessary but is useful for demonstrating RV-to-coronary artery fistulae which may influence surgical management.

Surgical relief of the RVOT obstruction to increase pulmonary blood flow and to stimulate RV growth can be accomplished using various procedures. The RV may be decompressed by closed valvotomy without CPB or a transannular patch of the RVOT. It may be difficult to predict postoperative RV performance. Subsequent pulmonary regurgitation may interfere with the diastolic function. It is advisable to leave the ASD open for right-to-left shunting. Advances in interventional cardiology have reduced the number of patients needing urgent RVOT surgery. Balloon valvotomy is likely to succeed with isolated valvar atresia with a patent infundibulum. The prostaglandin infusion is slowly weaned off over a few days postoperatively.

The presence of severe TV hypoplasia and a diminutive RV offer little potential for subsequent growth. An early systemic-to-pulmonary shunt aiming towards eventual Fontan conversion remains the palliation of choice in the majority. This group of patients with the smallest RV is most prone to develop RV-to-coronary fistulae. This may partly explain a significant incidence of sudden, presumably dysrhythmic deaths from myocardial ischemia.

Survivors of neonatal palliation

Patients who fulfill the aforementioned morphological criteria, either since birth or as a result of a satisfactory decompression, can undergo radical repair leading to a biventricular circulation. This consists of relieving any residual RVOT obstruction, restoring RV-to-PA continuity, closing the ASD and the extracardiac shunt if present and TV repair for regurgitation. Some or all of these procedures can be performed by percutaneous intervention.

However, it is sometimes difficult to predict RV intrinsic growth. Despite RV-to-PA continuity, there may be a subset of patients with near-normal RV cavity size and good RV systolic function, but impaired diastolic function. In this situation, the RV may be unable to sustain adequate pulmonary blood flow. There may be excessive RA and systemic venous pressure if the ASD is restrictive, or marked right-to-left shunting with a large ASD.

Patients whose decompressed RV has not grown sufficiently to fully support the pulmonary circulation can benefit from different operations. If the RV can handle a proportion of systemic venous return, the superior vena cava (SVC) can be connected to the right PA. Inferior vena cava (IVC) return is directed to the left PA via the RV following relief of RVOT obstruction. The ASD should ideally be closed to separate the pulmonary and systemic circulations. This 'partial biventricular repair' would harness RV capability. The ASD can also be left partially open, fenestrated or adjustable if the RA pressure is excessive. The theoretical concern of this operation is that during ventricular systole, peak PA pressure can exceed SVC pressure, resulting in retrograde caval blood flow.

Incorporating a non-functional RV in a biventricular circulation can be detrimental and the Fontan route may be preferable. In patents with coronary fistulae, a total cavopulmonary artery connection is preferred to an atriopulmonary connection as the former allows saturated blood from the LA to reach the RV and then the coronary circulation. Desaturated systemic venous blood is isolated from the RV by this approach.

Further reading

1. Daubeney PE, Sharland GK, Cook AC et al. Pulmonary atresia with intact ventricular septum: impact of fetal echocardiography on incidence at birth and postnatal outcome. UK and Eire collaborative study of pulmonary atresia with intact ventricular septum. *Circulation* 1998; **98**: 562–6.
2. de Leval M, Bull C, Hopkins R et al. Decision making in the definitive repair of the heart with a small right ventricle. *Circulation* 1985; **72**: II52–II60.
3. Gibbs JL, Blackburn ME, Uzun O et al. Laser valvotomy and balloon valvuloplasty for pulmonary atresia with intact ventricular septum: five years' experience. *Heart* 1997; **77**: 225–8.
4. Hanley FL, Sade RM, Blackstone EH et al. Outcomes in neonatal pulmonary atresia with intact ventricular septum. A multiinstitutional study. *J Thorac Cardiovasc Surg* 1993; **105**: 406–27.
5. Mair DD, Julsrud PR, Puga FJ, Danielson GK. The Fontan procedure for pulmonary atresia with intact ventricular septum: operative and late results. *J Am Coll Cardiol* 1997; **29**: 1359–64.

Related topics of Interest

33 Tetralogy of Fallot

James L Monro

Anatomy

In 1888, Fallot described the association of overriding aorta, VSD, pulmonary stenosis and RV hypertrophy. This situation arises due to the cephalad and anterior deviation of the infundibular septum. This septal displacement narrows the RV outflow tract (RVOT), with failure of the main body of the interventricular septum to meet the infundibular septum, thus creating a VSD. RV hypertrophy results because of pressure equalization across a large VSD. The pulmonary stenosis may be valvular (a bicuspid valve is frequently present). More rarely, this may be supravalvular and usually subvalvular, where bands of infundibular muscle cause RVOT obstruction (RVOTO). Furthermore, there may be obstruction at all three levels, resulting in considerable hypoplasia of the RVOT. Further narrowing of the RVOT leads to pulmonary atresia and thus pulmonary atresia and VSD in the extreme form of tetralogy of Fallot (TOF). Other variants include TOF with absent pulmonary valve syndrome, where the valve is narrow, regurgitant and represented just by a ridge. The resulting turbulence of blood flowing through into the PAs can cause huge PA dilatation, with resulting bronchial compression. Other associated abnormalities include complete AVSD, multiple VSDs and anomalous coronary artery patterns.

Clinical presentation

Pathophysiologically, TOF results in much of the desaturated blood coming into the RV preferentially channeling through the VSD into the LV, rather than through the stenosed RVOT. The EKG typically shows patterns of RV hypertrophy and strain. Chest x ray reveals a classical 'boot-shaped' heart due to RA and RV enlargement with pulmonary oligemia. The subvalvular muscle of the RVOT can constrict as when the child gets upset, causing more right-to-left shunting, increasing cyanosis and thus causing a 'blue spell'. Many children with TOF remain acyanotic beyond the first year of life, but then become progressively more cyanosed, whilst others with more severe early cyanosis may die prematurely.

Palliation

The first successful operation on a child with TOF was performed by Alfred Blalock in 1945, before the era of open heart surgery. Using the idea from his cardiology colleague Helen Taussig, he divided the right subclavian artery distally and turned it down and anastomosed it to the right PA (the Blalock–Taussig shunt). The increased pulmonary blood flow resulted in more saturated blood returning to the heart and therefore reduced cyanosis. In 1948,

Brock described an operation to improve pulmonary blood flow by punching out infundibular muscle from below, and Holmes-Sellors performed a closed pulmonary valvotomy with a similar result. In 1962, Waterston described a further palliative procedure with a direct anastomosis of the right PA to the back of the ascending aorta. It was difficult to achieve exactly the correct size shunt, and this operation was superseded, in the 1970s, by the introduction of the modified Blalock–Taussig shunt. This involved a Gore-Tex conduit interposed between the right subclavian artery and the right PA. This has been the preferred palliative procedure for TOF for the last two decades but can lead to distortion of the PA.

Repair

Lillehei, in 1956, was the first surgeon to successfully repair TOF. Although some pioneering operations using CPB had been performed, the results were disappointing and Lillehei used a cross bypass circulation-technique from the father while he performed the repair by closing the VSD and relieved the RVOTO. This technique, although used successfully on many occasions, was rather cumbersome and in the latter half of the 1950s several surgeons, notably Kirklin, began to get better results in children using CPB. However, the results in infants (<1 year) were poor and most surgeons continued to use a palliative procedure with staged correction. This two-stage approach continued, but in the early 1970s some surgeons began to get good results with correction in infancy and gradually over the last 30 years, many more children with TOF are being repaired in infancy. Initially this was in cyanosed infants who required surgery, but gradually the indication expanded to those who were asymptomatic. Provided this can be achieved with an acceptable mortality, this results in preservation of RV function, reduced late arrhythmia and improved oxygenation and childhood development. If repair is to be performed, it is important that the PAs are of adequate size as they will have to accommodate the cardiac output. Generally palliation is preferred to repair in the presence of (a) very small pulmonary arteries or (b) an anomalous LAD from the RCA.

Repair is undertaken with CPB. The surgical technique requires VSD patch closure (pericardium, Gore-Tex or Dacron) and relief of the RVOTO. Traditionally the VSD was approached through a right ventriculotomy, but over the last decade or so, the right atrial approach has gained popularity. The relief of the RVOTO depends on its extent. Virtually all patients require removal of obstructing muscle bundles in the infundibulum and usually this can be done through the RA. When the pulmonary annulus is small, it may be necessary to insert a patch across the valve up into the main PA. Transannular patching relieves the stenosis but inevitably results in pulmonary regurgitation (PR), which is tolerated very well for many years. However, some patients may develop severe PR and RV dilatation even after 20 years, requiring insertion of a homograft conduit in the RVOT. It requires a fine sense of judgement to know when a transannular patch is necessary and the recommendations of Pacifico are very helpful: they provide the minimally acceptable pulmonary annulus diameter indexed to weight/surface area based on anatomical studies of the normal pulmonary annulus diameter. If the diameter of the annulus is less than this, a transannular patch is needed..

Surgical efficacy (relief of RVOTO) can be assessed by measuring left and right ventricular pressures when CPB is discontinued. If the RV pressure is <80% of LV pressure it is likely that adequate relief has been achieved. Even higher ratios may be acceptable as the obstruction normally regresses further during the next 24 hours.

Results

The early mortality (within 30 days) is <5%, and even in infants approaches 0% in some units. Early complications such as bleeding, residual VSD and heart block are now rare. However, late complications are associated with the correction of RVOTO, particularly in those with a narrow pulmonary valve annulus. With a transannular patch, late regurgitation is inevitable and this may require conduit replacement, usually many years later. Persistent residual RVOTO (gradient >60 mmHg) usually requires re-operation within 1–3 years. Rare late complications requiring re-operation include residual VSD (Qp:Qs >2.0) and aneurysm of the RVOT patch. There is therefore a significant incidence of re-operation, but otherwise most children who have had repair of TOF have normal life expectancy.

Further reading

1. Alexiou C, Mahmoud H, Al-Khaddour A et al. Outcome after repair of tetralogy of Fallot in the first year of life. *Ann Thorac Surg* 2001; **71**: 494–500.
2. Kirklin JW, Barratt-Boyes BG. Tetralogy of Fallot with pulmonary stenosis. In: *Cardiac Surgery. 2nd Edn.* Churchill Livingstone: New York, 1993; **2**: 861–1012.
3. Monro JL, Shore G. Correction of Fallot's tetralogy. In: *A Colour Atlas of Cardiac Surgery: Congenital Heart Disease.* Walker WF (Ed). Wolfe: London, 1984: pp 109–28.
4. Pacifico AD, Kirklin JW, Blackstone EH. Surgical management of pulmonary stenosis in tetralogy of Fallot. *J Thorac Cardiovasc Surg* 1977; **74**: 382–95.

Related topics of interest

34 The Fontan circulation

Constantine Mavroudis, Carl L Backer

Introduction

A physiologic repair separating the systemic and pulmonary circulations for the successful treatment of tricuspid atresia was reported by Fontan in 1971. Modifications of anatomical configurations, connections, and anastomotic techniques (see Table 1) were successively reported, but the basic principle of diverting systemic venous return to the pulmonary circulation, thus bypassing the right heart, remained unchanged. Perioperative mortality after the Fontan procedure declined steadily against a backdrop of higher-risk patients being referred for surgery (younger age, more complex univentricular heart defects).

Complications

With improved perioperative and long-term survival following Fontan surgery, late complications have become evident. Most of these occur in Fontan patients with atriopulmonary (AP) connections as opposed to the newer total cavopulmonary artery connections (TCPC) using lateral tunnel or extracardiac techniques. The TCPC, in particular, by excluding most of the right atrium from the systemic venous circulation, is believed to reduce postoperative development of debilitating atrial arrhythmias because of reduced atrial distention and avoidance of a right atriotomy and extensive atrial suture lines. However, long-term outcome is awaited.

Thromboembolism

The incidence of thromboembolism is variable (0–19%) and depends upon the diagnostic test used. Risk factors have not yet been identified because of the small numbers in each series. Several Australian and Canadian centers are currently enrolling patients in a randomized controlled trial comparing prophylactic antiplatelet with anticoagulation therapies in order to develop antithrombotic guidelines.

Protein-losing enteropathy (PLE)

Excessive protein loss within the gastrointestinal tract is poorly understood. An international multicenter study reported a 3.7% incidence of PLE. Medical treatment only resulted in complete resolution of symptoms in 25%, no improvement in 29%, and death in 46%. Surgical treatment was associated with relief in 19%, no improvement in 19%, and death in 62%. The etiology of PLE is multifactorial. Two major factors are decreased cardiac output and compensatory flow redistribution with elevated mesenteric vascular resistance. Despite the many treatments currently used (heparin, prednisolone, elemental diet, atrial septostomy, atrial pacing) the outlook is uniformly poor with transplantation being considered for many end-stage sufferers.

Pulmonary arteriovenous fistula formation

Patients with polysplenia syndrome and single ventricle anatomy may have interrupted inferior vena cava (IVC) with azygos or hemiazygos continuation to the superior vena cava (SVC). AP Fontan with a classic Glenn shunt predisposes to pulmonary arteriovenous fistulas when the hepatic venous return is excluded from part of the pulmonary circulation. This can be reversed with subsequent pathway revision (reconnecting divided pulmonary arteries and TCPC) to include hepatic venous drainage.

Arrhythmia

Recurrent atrial arrhythmia in single ventricle physiology causes unfavorable hemodynamic consequences that are less well tolerated than in patients with two functioning ventricles. Three factors are considered important: injury to the sinoatrial node or its blood supply, extensive atrial incisions and sutures lines, and chronic atrial hypertension. Uncommonly, in the presence of atrioventricular discordance or heterotaxy with intrinsic abnormalities of the conduction system, the underlying anatomic substrate and hemodynamic disturbance predispose to tachyarrhythmias. The type of Fontan connection, however, is not strongly predictive. Atrial flutter (incidence 16%) developed sooner and was more likely to occur in patients who were older at the time of the initial Fontan operation.

Technical modifications that minimize sinus node injury and atrial suture lines, together with early interventions for AV valve regurgitation, have reduced the risk of arrhythmias. Management options for recurrent or persistent postoperative arrhythmias after Fontan procedures include drug therapy, pacemaker implantation, catheter ablation or in some cases surgical conversion to TCPC (lateral tunnel or extracardiac conduit).

Pathway obstruction

This most commonly involves obstruction in a calcified homograft conduit used for the AP connection. Alternatively, extrinsic compression of the native pulmonary artery by a greatly distended right atrium can also cause significant reduction in pulmonary blood flow. Patients present with increasing dyspnea, cyanosis and 'spelling'. Its presence and extent is best assessed by cardiac catheterization and angiography.

Fontan conversion

Complications following AP Fontan connections are often amenable to reconstruction and arrhythmia ablation. Fontan conversion with arrhythmia surgery is safe and efficacious. Indications for conversion include development of significant late complications such as pathway obstruction, significant arrhythmias, and valvular dysfunction. A significant number of patients who meet these selection criteria have ventricular dysfunction. If the ventricular function can be improved by arrhythmia cessation or valve repair, conversion to TCPC is recommended; otherwise, transplantation is indicated. Surgical intervention prior to the development of atrial fibrillation results in less surgical morbidity. Other beneficial effects of early operation include preservation of myocardial function, avoidance of toxic antiarrhythmic agents and improved functional class. Cardiac transplantation may, however, be required following Fontan conversion.

A current approach combines conversion to TCPC, atrial reduction, a modified maze procedure, and permanent pacing. Arrhythmia ablative techniques used at conversion

Table 1 Historical evolution of the Fontan procedure.

Author	Technique	Advantages	Disadvantages
1971 Fontan et al.	• Classic Glenn anastomosis • Atrial septal defect closure • Direct connection RA to proximal end LPA using aortic homograft • Main pulmonary artery ligated • Homograft valve inserted in orifice of IVC	• Incorporate RA as pump	• Valve dysfunction • Atrial suture lines • Anterior anastomosis • RA dilates
1973 Kreutzer et al.	• Mobilized and anastomosed MPA and valve to RA appendage using rigid Teflon ring around pulmonary valve annulus to prevent its collapse • Partial closure of patent foramen ovale	• Incorporate RA as pump	• Prosthetic material • Atrial suture lines • Anterior anastomosis • RA dilates
1973–74 Multiple authors	• RA–RV connection using valved conduit	• Incorporate RV to augment PA flow	• Conduit obstruction • Atrial suture lines • Anterior anastomosis
1978 Bowman et al.	• RA–RV connection using valved conduit with distal portion of conduit sutured to splayed RV	• Incorporate RV to augment PA flow • Enlarge RV chamber	• Conduit obstruction • Long vertical RV incision
1979 Björk et al.	• Patch closure of septal defect(s) • Direct anastomosis of posterior wall of RA appendage to everted edge of RV incision, anterior roofing of communication with pericardium	• Incorporate RV to augment PA flow	• Atrial suture lines • Anterior anastomosis

Year / Author	Procedure	Advantages	Disadvantages
1982 Kreutzer et al.	• Direct roof of RA (or appendage) – RPA anastomosis	• Incorporate RA as pump	• Atrial suture lines
1988 de Leval et al.	• Cephalad end of transected SVC anastomosed to right PA, enlarged cardiac end of SVC anastomosed to main PA • Intracardiac cavocaval channel, either prosthetic or composite	• Technically simple • Applicable to multiple chamber vessel arrangements • Excludes RA from circuit	
1990 Marcelletti et al.	• Extracardiac conduit IVC–PA	• Intraatrial prosthetic materials avoided • Obstruction to pulmonary venous return reduced	• Potential thrombosis of conduit • Need for anticoagulation
1992 Bridges et al.	• Baffle fenestration	• Maintains cardiac output • Limits RA pressure	• Reinterventions sometimes necessary • Potential for cerebrovascular accident
1994 Kao et al.	• Conversion of AP to TCPC Fontan	• Reduces RA distention • Excludes RA from circuit • Improves hemodynamics	• Need for anticoagulation • Major reoperation
1999 Mavroudis et al.	• Conversion of AP to TCPC Fontan • Concomitant arrhythmia surgery	• Reduces RA distention • Addresses arrhythmia foci • Improves hemodynamics	• Need for anticoagulation • Major reoperation

include standard right-sided and biatrial procedures to treat atrial re-entry tachycardia and atrial fibrillation, respectively. Reports of Fontan conversion performed without arrhythmia surgery demonstrated improved hemodynamics but with a 76% postoperative arrhythmia recurrence. The hazards of resternotomy due to previous surgery and a giant right atrium can be reduced by using vacuum-assisted venous drainage and femoral cannulation. Unwanted cavitary entry in a Fontan patient causes more hemodynamic compromise than in the patient with two functioning ventricles. In addition, conduit placement, chamber enlargement, and chamber/vessel malposition present unique challenges in entry. The Fontan circuit can be reconstructed using extracardiac techniques that connect the IVC to the pulmonary artery using a large (20–24 mm) Gore-Tex tube and direct SVC anastomosis to the pulmonary artery. In patients with divided pulmonary arteries (unilateral cavopulmonary artery anastomosis and right atrial-to-contralateral pulmonary artery connection), they may be reconnected with an interposition graft (Gore-Tex tube or a nonvalved homograft) to restore hepatic venous flow to both lungs and prevent pulmonary arteriovenous fistulas.

Concomitant epicardial pacemaker implantation may be performed for therapeutic or prophylactic reasons. Atrial antitachycardia, atrial rate-responsive, or dual-chamber pacemakers may be implanted. Single-agent therapy (beta-blocker for re-entry tachycardia and amiodarone for AF) may be necessary following surgery.

Outcome following Fontan conversion

In the Chicago experience of 73 patients, overall arrhythmia recurrence after conversion to TCPC with concurrent arrhythmia surgery and pacemaker placement was 17% with less than 10% receiving chronic antiarrhythmic medications. Since introducing the more extensive modified right-sided maze procedure for atrial re-entry tachycardia, no recurrence of atrial tachycardia has been observed. AF is managed with a Cox-maze III procedure. Although a right-sided procedure alone is considered effective by some, isthmus cryoablation with lesions limited to the right atrium was ineffective. This has been eliminated with the use of the Cox maze III procedure which combines the right-sided maze procedure, appropriate for anatomic substrate, with a left-sided series of incisions, excisions, and cryoablations. Intraoperative radiofrequency and microwave energy ablation are less effective.

The Chicago series included patients with severe ventricular dysfunction, cyanosis-causing pulmonary AV fistulas, significant associated cardiac lesions, and PLE. Perioperative mortality (no early and one late death) and re-operation for bleeding rates were low. However, acute renal failure has been observed more than other complications, probably due to underlying chronic renal insufficiency, prolonged CPB time, excessive cardiotomy suction and resultant hemoglobinuria. Cardiac transplantation after Fontan conversion was performed in three patients in the Chicago series, which compares well with other series.

Further reading

1. Balaji S, Gewillig M, Bull C, de Leval MR, Deanfield JE. Arrhythmias after the Fontan procedure. Comparison of total cavopulmonary connection and atriopulmonary connection. *Circulation* 1991; **84**: III–162–7.
2. Burke RP, Jacobs JP, Ashraf MH, Aldousany A, Chang AC. Extracardiac Fontan operation without cardiopulmonary bypass. *Ann Thorac Surg* 1997; **63**: 1175–7.
3. de Leval MR, Kilner P, Gewillig M, Bull C. Total cavopulmonary connection: a logical alternative to atriopulmonary connection for complex Fontan operations. Experimental studies and early clinical experience. *J Thorac Cardiovasc Surg* 1988; **96**: 682–95.
4. Gandhi SK, Bromberg BI, Rodefeld MD et al. Lateral tunnel suture line variation reduces atrial flutter after the modified Fontan operation. *Ann Thorac Surg* 1996; **61**: 1299–309.
5. Marcelletti CF, Hanley FL, Mavroudis C et al. Revision of previous Fontan connections to total extracardiac cavopulmonary anastomosis. A multicenter experience. *J Thorac Cardiovasc Surg* 2000; **119**: 340–6.
6. Mavroudis C, Backer CL, Deal BJ, Johnsrude C, Strasburger J. Total cavopulmonary conversion and maze procedure for patients with failure of the Fontan operation. *J Thorac Cardiovasc Surg* 2001; **122**: 863–71.

Related topics of interest

35 Hypoplastic left heart syndrome

Marcus M Haw

Hypoplastic left heart syndrome (HLHS) is a spectrum of congenital heart anomalies involving hypoplasia of the left heart. The diagnosis ranges from critical neonatal aortic valve stenosis to complete absence of the LV. Nearly all patients with HLHS have coarctation but the condition is categorized by four subtypes:

- aortic stenosis and mitral stenosis
- aortic atresia and mitral atresia
- aortic atresia and mitral stenosis
- aortic stenosis and mitral atresia.

Aortic atresia is associated with the most severe hypoplasia of the ascending aorta, which may be <2 mm in diameter. The aortic arch diameter is normally between 3 and 5 mm. Perfusion to head and neck vessels and coronary arteries is normally retrograde from the ductus arteriosus. Coarctation is present at the junction of the ductus in most patients. The PA is often the only visible outflow from the heart and appears continuous with the massive ductus arteriosus. The right PA has its origin very close to the commissures of the pulmonary valve and the left PA a little more distally. The left PA is often smaller than the right PA. The LA is small with an enlarged RA and normally a mildly restrictive stretched PFO. However, there may be a large atrial septal defect (ASD) or an intact atrial septum. The latter leads to collapse at birth with the need for an emergency intervention.

Associated cardiac anomalies

- Tricuspid valve (particularly the septal leaflet).
- Bicuspid pulmonary valve.
- VSD/AVSD.
- Interrupted aortic arch.
- Rarely total anomalous pulmonary venous connection.

Associated extracardiac anomalies

In an autopsy study performed in the Children's Hospital, Philadelphia an overall genetic abnormality rate of 28% was found, including Turner's syndrome, diaphragmatic hernia, hypospadias and omphalocele. In our experience the extracardiac anomaly rate in patients undergoing surgical repair is much lower.

Pathophysiology

Antenatally, there is obstruction of blood from the pulmonary circulation and the RV outflow is directed across the ductus arteriosus. Blood passes retrogradely to the head and neck and down the miniscule ascending aorta to the coronary arteries. At birth there is immediate reduction in PVR, which reduces the proportion of cardiac output passing to the systemic circulation. If the duct remains patent, viability is dependent on the balance between PVR and SVR. If the duct begins to close, severe cardiovascular collapse is immediate and a common form of death. In cases of a PDA there is excessive pulmonary blood flow which increases with the reduction in PVR over the first few days of life.

Management of antenatal HLHS

Following antenatal diagnosis (by fetal ultrasound) advice should be sought from a unit experienced in the management of HLHS. Parents should be counseled and given the opportunity to discuss the treatment options with the pediatric cardiologist and surgeon involved. Many parents choose termination. If they choose to continue with the pregnancy, then the mother should be admitted to the maternity unit attached to the cardiac surgical center for obstetric management.

Pre-operative presentation

Often the undiagnosed neonate presents within the first 24–48 hours of life with mild cyanosis. If the duct closes then cardiovascular collapse is experienced, as a greater proportion of the systemic flow is pushed by the closing duct into the lungs. Often the situation is exacerbated by the administration of supplemental oxygen, further reducing the PVR. Once a diagnosis is made or suspected from the clinical presentation, a prostaglandin E1 (PGE1) infusion should be commenced and supplemental oxygen should be avoided. The neonate should be transported to a cardiac unit. If intubated, oxygen should be avoided, using air for ventilation.

Pre-surgical management of the stable neonate

Many neonates remain stable, self-ventilating on air with a prostaglandin infusion and SaO_2 monitoring. This is the ideal pre-surgical state. However, excess pulmonary blood flow may necessitate the use of head box N_2 to reduce the FiO_2 to <20%. Monitoring capillary blood gases for serum lactate is a useful guide to cardiac output in this stage.

Management of the pre-operative neonate requiring resuscitation

The medical management by the obstetric and the transport team is essential to the outcome. Early infusion of PGE1 and the avoidance of supplemental oxygen are key points. Reliable pulse oximetry is essential in monitoring treatment progress. Arterial blood gas analysis is nearly always required in unstable patients. In severe cardiorespiratory collapse, sodium bicarbonate or THAM (tromethamine) buffer may be indicated. Tracheal intubation may be necessary and umbilical venous line offers the safest venous access. If an adequate cardiac output is not obtained with PGE1, inotropic support should be considered. After arrival at the tertiary cardiac unit, the neonate should not undergo surgery until all organs are functioning normally and a period of time (4–5 days) is allowed for reduction in PVR.

Surgical techniques

We normally perform a Norwood Stage I procedure for this condition using a pulmonary homograft for the ascending aortic and arch reconstruction. Profound hypothermia (16°C) and circulatory arrest is routinely employed. Occasionally, circulatory arrest is used later in the operation if the ascending aorta is large enough to take the arterial cannula.

Goals of the Stage I procedure are to:

- avoid any outflow obstruction
- restrict pulmonary blood flow
- remove any pulmonary venous obstruction
- preserve PA growth
- preserve tricuspid valve function.

This will optimize the heart for future Fontan surgery. Our technique is modified from that described by Norwood (1983). In the first stage of the operation (Figure 1), the PA is transected below the bifurcation and closed either with a direct suture or with a circular patch to avoid stenosis. The PDA is ligated and divided and the aortic coarctation tissue is excised and an incision from the descending thoracic aorta around to the proximal ascending aorta is made (Figure 1). The patch of PA homograft using its right PA branch is fashioned. The patch is sutured to the underside of the aortic arch and around the orifice of the main PA (Figure 1). The main PA itself is fixed to the end of the incision in the ascending aorta with three interrupted everting sutures. This is particularly critical in the very small ascending aorta as coronary supply finds its way to the aortic root via this tiny orifice. The reconstructed outflow is without obstruction and a Gore-Tex shunt is placed between the innominate artery and the right PA (Figure 1). Following completion of surgery the hematocrit is increased using modified ultrafiltration whilst correcting the acid–base status and biochemistry as required. Milrinone is given during the rewarming period in order to improve diastolic function before weaning from CPB. The shunt size is critically important to the control of pulmonary blood flow, and we generally use thin-walled Gore-Tex shunts of 3–4 mm diameter. On occasions when the pulmonary venous return has been obstructed antenatally, a larger shunt may be necessary. A period of stability is established following discontinuation of CPB indicated by a falling serum lactate and good systemic blood pressure. When both systolic arterial pressure and SaO_2 are in the 70s, the sternum is stented open and the neonate transferred to the intensive care unit (ICU).

Postoperative management

Cardiopulmonary stability is the chief goal. It allows an assessment of myocardial function and pulmonary blood flow to be undertaken. If pulmonary blood flow is excessive, our

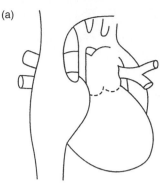

Hypoplastic left heart
Single right ventricle
Diminutive ascending aorta
Large pulmonary artery
Duct-dependent circulation

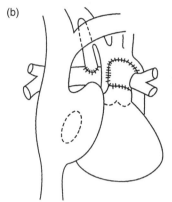

After surgery
PA-aortic anastomosis using homograft patch
Disconnected branch pulmonary arteries
Modified BT shunt: innominate-RPA
Atrial septectomy

Figure 1 (a) Hypoplastic left heart. (b) After surgery.

approach is to place Liga clips to the Blalock–Taussig (BT) shunt to reduce blood flow guided by serial blood gas analysis often at the cotside in the ICU. Inotrope is used for myocardial dysfunction. When cardiorespiratory stability has been achieved, the sternum is closed (usually 24–48 hours postoperatively). We aim for early extubation facilitated by maintenance of good cardiac output, urine output and fluid balance.

Second-stage procedure

We electively bring children forward for the bi-directional Glenn procedure 3–9 months following the Norwood Stage I procedure. Timing varies with cyanosis and clinical condition. Pre-operative angiography will confirm anatomic abnormalities of the PA or the arch reconstruction. Hemodynamically significant lesions should be addressed concomitantly. The bi-directional Glenn procedure is performed without CPB using SVC to right PA anastomosis after excising the BT shunt.

Stage III Norwood procedure

The third stage involves completion of the Fontan circulation. Our preferred approach is extracardiac total cavopulmonary artery connection with TCPC and fenestration performed using CPB but on a beating heart. Additional palliative surgery such as tricuspid valve annuloplasty or arch reconstruction may be required. We normally perform all corrective surgery before the final Stage III procedure.

Surgical outcomes

The greatest risk is at the Stage I Norwood procedure where published mortality is 20–50%. Our overall early mortality for the Stage I Norwood procedure is 25% (10% in the last 2 years). However, we have observed occasional sudden death in the community in children who were otherwise well. There are patients with pre-operative poor RV function who survive the Norwood procedure and possibly the Stage II procedure but who have inadequate cardiac function to sustain them. There is undoubtedly a significant attrition rate between Stage I procedure and final palliation. In those patients who are suitable for continuing palliation, the mortality at Stage II and Stage III procedures should be acceptable. It is likely that in most programs only 50% of the children who start along the surgical protocol will survive to have an effective TCPC procedure. Despite early reports of adverse neurological outcomes, recent experience suggests that children who have undergone this treatment are not significantly different from others with major cardiac anomalies. Recent reports suggest improved early outcome for the Stage I procedure using RV-PA conduits as a source of pulmonary blood flow. We have not changed our practice as the reported outcomes are not superior to our current results.

Further reading

1. Pigott JD, Murphy JD, Barber G, Norwood WI. Palliative reconstructive surgery for hypoplastic left heart syndrome. *Ann Thorac Surg* 1988; **45**: 122–8.
2. Iannettoni MD, Bove EL, Mosca RS et al. Improving results with first-stage palliation for hypoplastic left heart syndrome. *J Thorac Cardiovasc Surg* 1994; **107**: 934–40.
3. Pizarro C, Malec E, Maher KO et al. Right ventricle to pulmonary artery conduit improves outcome after stage I Norwood for hypoplastic left heart syndrome. *Circulation* 2003; **108**: 155–60.

Related topics of interest

36 Transposition of the great arteries

Mark D Rodefeld, V Mohan Reddy, Frank L Hanley

Introduction

Transposition of the great arteries (TGA) is incompatible with life without intervention. Infants typically present early in the neonatal period with profound cyanosis. Current survival is greater than 90% with the arterial switch operation. This chapter focuses on the most common form of TGA: that defined as atrial situs solitus, atrioventricular concordance, and ventriculoarterial discordance (SDD), also called D-TGA.

Incidence and natural history

TGA accounts for 5–10% of all cardiac malformations.

Mortality rates if untreated:
- 30%: 1 week
- 50%: 1 month
- 90%: 1 year.

Anatomy

In TGA, the aorta arises from the anatomic right ventricle, while the pulmonary artery arises from the anatomic left ventricle (ventriculoarterial discordant connection) (Figure 1). As a result, systemic venous blood is ejected into the systemic arterial circulation without passing through the lungs. Pulmonary venous blood returning to the left atrium is ejected back through the pulmonary arterial circuit. Survival depends upon the degree of mixing of oxygenated and deoxygenated blood at any of three levels: a patent ductus arteriosus, an atrial septal defect, or ventricular septal defect. Most commonly, the ventricles are normally positioned and the aorta is malposed anteriorly and rightward in relation to the pulmonary artery. A well-developed subaortic conus is present and there is typically fibrous continuity between the mitral and pulmonic valves without subpulmonary conus.

Anatomic variation

Approximately 50% of cases of D-TGA have an intact ventricular septum (TGA-IVS). In other cases, the most typical associated findings are:
- 25%: isolated ventricular septal defect (TGA-VSD)
- 25%: VSD with left ventricular outflow tract obstruction (pulmonic or subpulmonic stenosis)
- 10%: coarctation of the aorta
- 40%: coronary artery abnormalities.

Ventricular septal defect

When present, the morphology of the ventricular septal defect is variable. It may be anteriorly malaligned, resulting in varying degrees of overriding of the pulmonary annulus onto the right ventricle. In the most severe form, this culminates as double outlet right ventricle with subpulmonic ventricular septal defect, also known as the Taussig–Bing anomaly. Subaortic stenosis caused by anterior malalignment of the infundibular septum is associated with coarctation, aortic arch hypoplasia, or interrupted aortic arch depending on the severity of the lesion.

Coronary artery anomalies

Coronary arteries take the 'shortest route' to an aortic sinus. The two aortic sinuses of Valsalva which 'face' the pulmonary artery contain the ostia of the coronary arteries in more than 99% of cases. The aortic commissure, which separates the two facing sinuses, is typically directly aligned with the pulmonary commissure which separates the two facing sinuses. These anatomic features permit transfer of the coronary arteries in the arterial switch operation. The most common or 'normal' coronary pattern in TGA (60–70% of cases) is similar to that seen with normal cardiac anatomy in which the left main arises from the left anterior facing sinus, branching to give off the circumflex and LAD, and the right coronary artery arises from rightward posterior facing sinus. Coronary abnormalities are frequently encountered in TGA (30–40% of cases). The most common abnormal pattern is when the circumflex arises from the right coronary artery off the right posterior facing sinus, and passes behind the great vessels. Other variations of coronary patterns are common, including intramural course of the coronaries, and single origin coronary arteries.

Pathophysiology

The systemic and pulmonic circuits are in parallel rather than in series (Figure 2). As a result, output from each ventricle is recirculated through that ventricle. This results in hypoxemia and excessive right and left ventricular workload. Oxygenation is dependent on mixing between the two circuits either through an intracardiac shunt (PFO, ASD, VSD) or extracardiac shunt (PDA, bronchopulmonary collaterals). The extent of shunting is determined by local pressure gradients dependent upon respiratory cycle phase, compliance of the ventricles, heart rate, and the volume of blood flow and vascular resistance in each of the circulations. Poor mixing is marked clinically by decreased pO_2, increased pCO_2, and metabolic acidosis.

Specific investigation

Echocardiographic evaluation is typically sufficient for most patients. Cardiac catheterization is rarely needed unless confounding variables are present which need further clarification. Echocardiography should specifically address the following issues: ventricular function; presence or absence of ASD and VSD; anatomy and function of the tricuspid and mitral valves; status of the left ventricular outflow tract and pulmonic valve – this will become the systemic outflow tract after the arterial switch operation; coronary artery anatomy; caliber of the distal aortic arch and presence of coarctation.

Management

Initial management goals are to stabilize the patient medically by reversing profound hypoxemia and acidosis.

1. Maximize mixed venous oxygen saturation
(a) Improve O_2 delivery:
  • inotropic agents
  • optimize hematocrit.
(b) Decrease O_2 consumption:
  • paralysis and sedation
  • mechanical ventilation.

2. Ensure adequate mixing
(a) Rapid institution of prostaglandin E1 (PGE1) infusion to maintain ductal patency.
(b) Emergent balloon atrial septostomy (Rashkind). Under echo guidance, a balloon catheter which has been introduced through a peripheral vein is placed across the ASD, the balloon is inflated, and then is forcefully pulled back, tearing open the atrial septum and resulting in an unrestricted atrial septal defect. This may be a lifesaving maneuver if PGE1 fails or if there is inadequate atrial level shunting in the setting of clinical instability.

Surgical repair

Goal

The goal is to re-route systemic venous blood to the pulmonary arterial circulation and pulmonary venous blood to the systemic arterial circulation. Historically, this was accomplished at the atrial level by atrial baffles (Mustard, Senning), but atrial repair is disadvantageous, in that it is physiologic, not anatomic. The morphologic right ventricle functions as the systemic ventricle. Late deterioration in systemic right ventricular function remains a problem. In some cases, dynamic left ventricular outflow tract obstruction may develop from systemic right ventricular pressure loading. Atrial baffle repair is also associated with a high incidence of late sinus node dysfunction, atrial dysrhythmias, and systemic venous obstruction.

Repair at the arterial level (arterial switch) results in the morphologic left ventricle as the systemic ventricle, providing an anatomic as well as physiologic repair. Although the operation is technically challenging, the long-term results appear to be more promising than those seen with other types of corrective surgery.

Timing of surgical repair

The left ventricle must be able to eject against systemic afterload after the arterial switch is performed. The left ventricle remains adequately 'prepared' for systemic pressure loads for only 2–4 weeks after closure of ductus arteriosus, after which it adjusts to the lower pressure work required for the pulmonary arterial circulation. Although pulmonary arterial pressure (left ventricular pressure) can be maintained in the presence of a non-restrictive PDA or a large VSD, providing the option for surgery to be electively delayed for several weeks if needed, the ideal time for corrective repair is within the first days to first week of life after initial medical stabilization of hypoxemia and acidosis.

Arterial switch operation

Technical features

(1) Full mobilization of the great vessels, pulmonary arteries beyond the lobar branches.

(2) Great vessels are transected above the semilunar valves. The aorta is transected just above the commissures, and the pulmonary artery is transected closer to the pulmonary artery bifurcation.

(3) Coronary orifices are inspected and gently probed if necessary to ensure complete understanding of the coronary arterial anatomy.

(4) Coronaries are dissected, along with a cuff of sinus tissue, and translocated posteriorly to sites on the neo-aorta (Figure 1a).

(5) Coronary reimplantation on the neo-aorta (Figure 1b), preferably at sites higher on the pulmonary artery than the deep portions of the valve sinuses to avoid kinking.

(6) The posteriorly positioned branch pulmonary arteries are brought anterior to aorta. This is known as the Lecompte maneuver (Figure 1c).

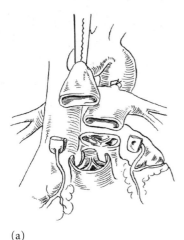

(a)

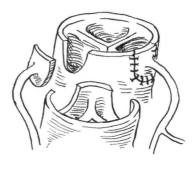

(b)

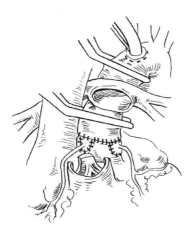

(c)

Figure 1 (a) Preparation for transfer of coronary buttons. (b) Coronary button transfer. (c) Lecompte maneuver.

(7) The proximal neo-aorta (above the coronary anastomoses) is connected end-to-end to the ascending aorta.

(8) Right atrium opened and ASD and/or VSD repaired.

(9) Coronary donor sites repaired with patches of autologous pericardium (Figure 2a).

(10) The proximal neo-pulmonary artery is connected to the transverse pulmonary artery confluence (Figure 2b).

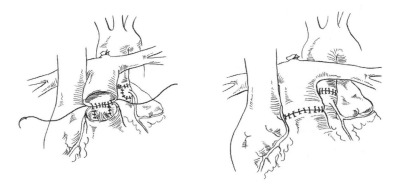

(a)   (b)

Figure 2 (a) Formation of neopulmonary artery. (b) Completed arterial switch procedure.

Surgical results

Arterial switch operation

The overall surgical mortality is approximately 5%. By 6–12 months post-operation, the survival after arterial switch is the same as that for an age-, race-, and sex-matched population.

Arterial switch: postoperative issues

1. Risk factors for death:
   - very low birth weight
   - long circulatory arrest duration
   - abnormal coronary artery pattern
        intramural course of left coronary artery
        retropulmonary course of left coronary
   - complex arch abnormalities
   - right ventricular hypoplasia
   - multiple ventricular septal defects
   - dextrocardia (<5%).
2. Coronary arteries are generally the most technically challenging aspect of the operation. Coronary insufficiency is detected early after weaning from cardiopulmonary bypass, and, if not corrected, long-term survival is jeopardized.

3. Perioperative left ventricular dysfunction:
   - diastolic dysfunction is common due to poorly compliant ventricles
   - gentle volume administration is critical
   - afterload reduction may be helpful.
4. Arrhythmia complications <2–4%.
5. Late complications: amongst the most common late complications is supravalvar pulmonary stenosis, with a 5% re-intervention rate.
6. Long-term issues not yet determined:
   - coronary arterial stenosis, especially at the origins
   - long-term function of the neo-aortic valve under systemic pressure.

Further reading

1. Casteneda AR, Trusler GA, Paul MH et al. Congenital Heart Surgeons Society: the early results of treatment of simple transposition in the current era. *J Thorac Cardiovasc Surg* 1988; **95**: 14.
2. Colan SD, Boutin C, Casteneda AR, Wernovsky G. Status of the left ventricle after arterial switch operation for transposition of the great arteries: hemodynamic and echocardiographic evaluation. *J Thorac Cardiovasc Surg* 1995; **109**: 311.
3. Wernovsky G, Mayer JE, Jonas RA et al. Factors influencing early and late outcome of the arterial switch operation for transposition of the great arteries. *J Thorac Cardiovasc Surg* 1995; **109**: 289.

Related topics of interest

37 Double outlet right ventricle

Marcus M Haw

Anatomic classification

Double outlet right ventricle (DORV) is the term given to all morphological variations in which both great arteries arise wholly, or in their greater part, from the RV. There are some variations including heterotaxy syndromes, or mitral atresia where the LV is inadequate to support the systemic circulation. These univentricular forms will not be considered here. Biventricular forms of DORV display a spectrum of anatomy from tetralogy of Fallot (TOF) at one end to transposition of the great arteries (TGA) at the other. This variation is both anatomic and physiological, with completely different surgical solutions. Many authors differentiate DORV from TOF by the presence or absence of aortic to mitral fibrous continuity as assessed by 2-D-echocardiography. This is not always precise, but it is equally difficult to define the subaortic fibrosa at surgery. Although the differentiation is not always essential to the surgeon, awareness of the possibility is important, as the length of the intraventricular patch will in general be significantly larger in DORV than in TOF.

Position of the VSD

The VSD in DORV may be subaortic, sub-pulmonary, doubly committed or non-committed. The anatomy and physiology of DORV with subaortic VSD is usually similar to that of TOF. Patients with a sub-pulmonary VSD behave more like TGA. In these circumstances the surgical treatment is fairly clear. There is a spectrum between these two extremes where the ability to perform an intraventricular repair depends on the distance between the pulmonary valve annulus and the tricuspid annulus. A special type of DORV is the Taussig–Bing defect. Here the aortic and pulmonary valves are supported on separate and individual conus. The VSD is sub-pulmonary but separate from the pulmonary valve. The aorta and pulmonary valve arise entirely from the RV, and the aortic and pulmonary valves are at the same level and side by side.

Pathophysiology

The tetralogy type of DORV is generally cyanotic depending on the degree of RVOT obstruction. With muscular obstruction the likelihood of cyanotic spells increases with age. When the VSD is sub-pulmonary, presentation depends on the degree of intraventricular mixing. There is often streaming of blood within the ventricular cavities leading to cyanosis despite high pulmonary blood flow. Sometimes there is additional muscular subaortic obstruction, which may exacerbate this effect.

Investigation

Chest x ray appearance will depend on the type of DORV, and the degree of pulmonary blood flow, and may present as a spectrum from a tetralogy-like appearance with a boot-shaped heart and oligemic lung fields, to cardiomegaly and pulmonary plethora in patients with transposition plus VSD physiology. In nearly all of these infants, the 2-D-echocardiography is diagnostic and all that is required prior to operation.

Key surgical features include the separation of the pulmonary valve from the tricuspid valve in relation to the diameter of the aortic valve, the development of the conal septum, and the attachment of chords to the conal septum, all of which will influence the surgical approach. Coronary artery anatomy is determined and aortic arch abnormalities excluded. When sub-pulmonary stenosis is observed, a cardiac catheter may be useful to visualize the branch pulmonary arteries in tetralogy, and to assess pulmonary artery pressure in transposition. In transposition DORV cyanosis may be profound and a balloon atrial septostomy may be required to improve mixing at an atrial level.

Surgical management

There is little place for medical management in these defects.

Transposition variants (sub-pulmonary VSD, Figure 1)

In the current author's practice the procedure of choice is the arterial switch procedure and closure of the VSD in the majority of situations. This choice has not been influenced by variations of coronary anatomy, which are common in DORV. If pulmonary or sub-pulmonary stenosis is so severe that an arterial switch procedure is not possible, then a modified Blalock–Taussig shunt is performed to support pulmonary blood flow as a neonate. A

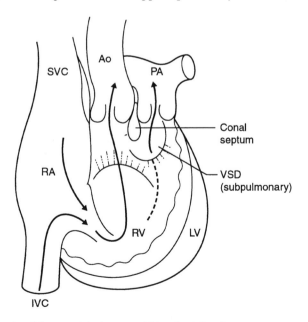

Figure 1 Double outlet right ventricle (transposition physiology).

Rastelli-type procedure is then performed at a later date with a conduit from the RVOT to pulmonary artery and closure of VSD at approximately 1 year of age. Positioning the conduit may be particularly difficult in this condition, especially if the LAD arises from the right coronary artery. The great vessels are to a greater or lesser degree side by side; thus, reconstruction of the RVOT is obliquely across the anterior or left coronary artery. The author has used interposition grafts or incision into the right pulmonary artery in order to avoid the neopulmonary artery compressing this area.

Tetralogy and intermediate variants (subaortic VSD, Figure 2)

In patients presenting like TOF with cyanosis, and or spells, early and sometime neonatal repair is preferred. Primary repair includes pulmonary valvotomy and possible resection/division of obstructing muscle bundles from the RVOT. The VSD is generally very large and has a somewhat distant medial border. Although transatrial closure is preferred, a ventriculotomy may be necessary for adequate exposure. The VSD may be some distance from the aortic valve and this should have been predicted by the pre-operative assessment. If so then a Gore-Tex tube is used to fashion the VSD patch, thus creating an intraventricular tunnel for the left ventricular outflow tract (LVOT). The length and diameter of the patch are critical to the outcome. If too short or too narrow then there will be LVOT obstruction; if too generous then the patch will obstruct the RVOT. The space between the pulmonary valve and the tricuspid annulus must be large enough to contain the full width of the LVOT. There must be enough septum to allow for future growth. Chords of the tricuspid valve inserted into the sub-pulmonary conus may be divided and re-inserted into the patch after its insertion. Generally the VSD is large and does not need to be enlarged. Additional maneuvers may be necessary such as transannular patch and or pulmonary artery augmentation as in standard tetralogy repairs.

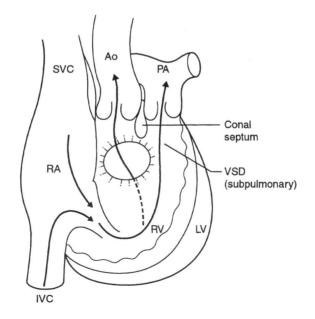

Figure 2 Double outlet right ventricle (tetralogy physiology).

Expected results of surgery

This is a heterogeneous group of patients with variable complexity. In the author's practice there have been 17 DORV repairs. Six patients underwent intraventricular tunnel repair with no deaths. Eleven patients underwent arterial switch procedure and closure of VSD. Three patients also had subaortic resection for sub PS; one of these patients died in the postoperative period. It is expected that during the next 20 years a number of patients will present for redo surgery with pulmonary and or aortic insufficiency, as seen in patients following tetralogy repair or arterial switch. Pulmonary stenosis is a problem of the reconstructed pulmonary outflow after arterial switch, particularly in the side-by-side anatomy of the great vessels.

The functional result of uncomplicated cases is generally excellent.

Further reading

1. Lev M, Bharati S, Meng CCL et al. A concept of double outlet right ventricle. *J Thorac Cardiovasc Surg* 1972; **64**: 271.
2. Anderson RH. Double outlet right ventricle. *Eur J Cardiothorac Surg* 2002; **22**: 853.
3. Lacour-Gayet F, Haun C, Ntalakoura K et al. Biventricular repair of double outlet right ventricle with non-committed ventricular septal defect (VSD) by VSD rerouting to the pulmonary artery and arterial switch. *Eur J Cardiothorac Surg* 2002; **21**: 1042–8.
4. Castenada AR, Jonas RA, Mayer JE, Hanley FL (eds). Double outlet right ventricle. In: *Cardiac Surgery of the Neonate and Infant.* WB Saunders: Philadelphia, 1994.

Related topics of interest

38 Truncus arteriosus

Ralph E Delius, Henry L Walters III

Introduction

Truncus arteriosus (TA) is a comparatively rare (2–3% of all defects) congenital lesion consisting of a single great vessel arising from the heart. A single semilunar valve is present. This single great vessel (truncus) gives rise to the coronary arteries, aorta and pulmonary arteries (PAs). Almost invariably a ventricular septal defect (VSD) is present. One-third of patients with TA have DiGeorge syndrome characterized by thymic aplasia/hypoplasia, hypoparathyroidism, hypocalcemia, dysmorphism and chromosome deletion (22p11).

Embryology

TA belongs to the conotruncal family of defects. During the third week of fetal development a common arterial trunk arises from the heart which soon divides into the PA and aorta by means of a caudally progressive spiral conotruncal ridge. This structure also participates in the final closure of the ventricular septum. Failure of this complex process results in TA and almost invariably an associated VSD.

Morphology

The truncus is typically larger than a corresponding aorta. The truncal semilunar valve is usually abnormal (thickened/deformed leaflets). The number of leaflets varies from 1 to 5 cusps. Valvar regurgitation is more common than stenosis. Coronary artery distribution is usually normal although the site of the coronary ostia can vary greatly (caudal, above sinotubular junction, from PA, etc.).

PA anatomy varies considerably in TA and forms the basis for the most commonly used classification schemes (Collett and Edwards, Van Praagh). However, in clinical practice these schemes have limited value as distinction between types is often not easily seen, e.g. the most common PA anatomy is often termed Type I–II as it fits into neither type accurately. Collett–Edwards Type IV, with PAs arising from the descending aorta, is now considered to represent tetralogy of Fallot with pulmonary atresia. The PAs are occasionally discontinuous with one artery (L>R) arising from a posterior descending coronary artery (PDA).

The aortic arch is usually of normal caliber but often right-sided. The PDA is usually absent or small except in cases of discontinuous PAs or interrupted aortic arch (IAA). IAA coexists in 15–20% of TA (Type B most common).

The VSD is typically immediately below the truncal valve and represents absence of the infundibular septum. It is approximately triangular, made up of:

- superior border – truncal valve
- anterior border – anterior limb of the trabecula septomarginalis
- posterior border – ventriculoinfundibular fold.

In approximately one-third of patients the ventriculoinfundibular fold is absent and the posterior border abuts the tricuspid annulus and the conduction pathway.

Clinical presentation

Mixing of unsaturated and saturated blood occurs at VSD and truncal artery levels with relatively mild cyanosis. There is unrestricted pulmonary blood flow contributing to congestive heart failure once pulmonary vascular resistance (PVR) falls after birth. Any truncal valve dysfunction will further complicate the hemodynamics. Coexisting IAA may further alter pathophysiology with ductal closure leading to lower torso hypoperfusion and shock.

Uncorrected TA is lethal, with a 1-year survival of 10%; approximately half the deaths occur during the first month of life, typically from severe congestive heart failure. Pulmonary vascular disease can develop after 6 months and is the leading cause of death in late survivors.

TA with IAA is almost uniformly fatal by 1 month of age without prostaglandin infusion to maintain ductal patency.

Specific investigation

Echocardiography is central to the diagnosis. Cardiac catheterization may be valuable in selected cases if there are concerns with coronary artery anatomy, PA continuity, PVR and in older patients (>6 months).

Due to the frequent association of DiGeorge syndrome, all TA sufferers should be genetically evaluated for this disease.

Management

Since medical therapy is usually unsuccessful in controlling heart failure, surgery is performed early (usually within 2 weeks of life). Through a median sternotomy, venous drainage can be accomplished by either right atrial (RA) or bicaval cannulation. Immediately prior to commencing cardiopulmonary bypass (CPB) the right and left PAs are snared and then occluded once CPB is initiated. This prevents flooding of the pulmonary vascular bed at the expense of the systemic circulation. The patient is usually cooled to 18°C. After aortic cross-clamping and cardioplegic arrest, both PAs are carefully dissected from the truncal root with every effort made to preserve their continuity. Care must be exercised during this maneuver as the left coronary artery ostium may abut the PA origin from the truncus. The resulting defect in the truncal root can be closed primarily or with a patch. The VSD is exposed through a vertical right ventriculotomy which should be large enough to allow VSD closure and provide unobstructed blood flow from the right ventricle (RV). The VSD is closed with standard techniques, with the superior edge of the VSD patch attached to the margin of the ventriculotomy. Right ventricular outflow tract (RVOT) is reconstructed usually with a pulmonary homograft although some surgeons prefer other conduits. The proximal anastomosis of the homograft to the ventriculotomy is usually augmented by means of a pericardial patch (glutaraldehyde-treated autologous/bovine). An associated atrial septal defect (ASD) is usually partially closed, but a patent foramen ovule (PFO) is typically left alone to allow for right-to-left shunting during the early postoperative period.

Reactive pulmonary hypertension is a primary concern immediately post-operation although this has become less common with early neonatal repair. Preventive measures include adequate sedation, mild hyperventilation with respiratory alkalosis and hyperoxygenation (PaO_2 >100 mmHg). Another early postoperative complication is junctional ectopic tachycardia, which invariably leads to diminished cardiac output and impaired perfusion. This arrhythmia results from increased automaticity, typically of the bundle of His, which exceeds the sinus rate. Treatment includes digoxin (controversial), topical cooling (approximately 35°C) and intravenous amiodarone.

Outcome

Surgical outcome of TA took a remarkable step forward with publication of a surgical series by Dr Paul Ebert in 1984. He described 106 patients undergoing TA repair with overall mortality of 11%. Subsequent improvements in operative mortality have been comparatively modest, current reports demonstrating 5–10%. Late survival is approximately 85% at 10 years, with truncal valve regurgitation being the primary determinant of longevity. Patients invariably undergo re-operations for RVOT conduit replacements. Approximately 15–20% of patients ultimately require truncal valve replacements although recent reports of truncal valve repair have been encouraging.

Further reading

1. Ebert PA, Turle K, Stanger P et al. Surgical treatment of truncus arteriosus in the first 6 Months of Life. *Ann Surg* 1984; **200**: 451–6.
2. Mavroudis C, Backer CL. Surgical management of severe truncal insufficiency: experience with truncal valve remodeling techniques. *Ann Thorac Surg* 2001; **72**: 396–400.
3. Thompson LD, McElhinney DB, Reddy M et al. Neonatal repair of truncus arteriosus: continuing improvement in outcomes. *Ann Thorac Surg* 2001; **72**: 391–5.

Related topics of interest

39 Interrupted aortic arch

Constantine Mavroudis, Carl L Backer

Interrupted aortic arch (IAA) is rare (0.5–1.3% of congenital heart disease) with loss of luminal continuity between the ascending and descending aorta. Blood flow into the descending aorta is through a large PDA. If untreated, median survival is 4 days with death precipitated by ductal closure. The vast majority have associated anomalies including VSD (90%), bicuspid aortic valve (30–50%), LV outflow tract obstruction (LVOTO) (25–40%), DiGeorge syndrome (15–30%), truncus arteriosus (10%), single ventricle (5%), aortopulmonary window (4%), and transposition of the great arteries (TGA) (3%).

Anatomy and embryology

First described in 1778, IAA was later classified into three types by Celoria and Patton (Figure 1).

- Type A (25–35%) occurs distal to the left subclavian artery. The innominate, left carotid, and left subclavian arteries all originate from the ascending aorta. The descending aorta is supplied with blood from the PDA (Figure 1a).
- Type B (60–70%) occurs between the left common carotid artery and the left subclavian artery, and is frequently associated with aberrant origin of the right subclavian artery from the descending aorta and LVOTO from subaortic stenosis (Figure 1b).
- Type C (<5%) occurs between the innominate artery takeoff and the left common carotid (Figure 1c).

The embryology of IAA is multifactorial. The large VSD causes preferential shunting of blood into the PA and PDA in utero, leading to diminished flow in the ascending aorta. Failure of embryonic development of the various components of the aortic arch (3rd and 4th branchial arches) has been postulated as cause of the three IAA subtypes. Neonatal hypocalcemia and defective thymic-dependent cellular immunity (DiGeorge syndrome) are related to abnormal development of the thymus and parathyroid glands, which are derived from the 3rd and 4th pharyngeal pouches, and many of these patients have IAA.

Pathophysiology and clinical evaluation

Ductal closure reduces systemic blood flow to the lower extremities causing acidosis, anuria, necrotizing enterocolitis, and hepatic ischemia. Additionally, the pulmonary circulation is flooded as the PVR drops, causing severe congestive heart failure and death if untreated.

Resuscitation with prostaglandin E1 restores a PDA and systemic perfusion. It is important to maintain elevated PVR and divert blood flow from pulmonary to the systemic circulation.

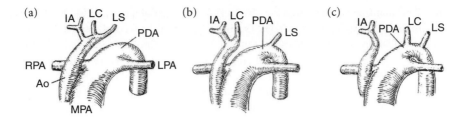

Figure 1 Classification of IAA. (a) Type A, (b) Type B, (c) Type C. (A, aorta; IA, innominate artery; LC, left carotid artery; LPA, MPA, RPA, left, main, and right pulmonary arteries; LS, left subclavian artery; PDA, patent ductus arteriosus.) (Reproduced with permission from Jonas RA. Interrupted aortic arch. In: *Pediatric Cardiac Surgery. 2nd Edn.* Mavroudis C, Backer CL (eds). Mosby-YearBook: St. Louis, 1994: p 184.)

This can be achieved by avoiding high FiO_2 and respiratory alkalosis from hyperventilation (pCO_2 around 40–50 mmHg). Metabolic acidosis should be corrected. Dopamine is used in ischemic renal insult. Most infants recover following resuscitation and intubation and may be operated on an elective basis. Neonates with DiGeorge syndrome require treatment for hypocalcemia and should receive only irradiated blood.

Historically, angiography has been used to assess the hemodynamics, intracardiac morphology, and precise arch anatomy of IAA. The ascending aorta is usually about half the normal diameter; it has no arch curvature but ascends straight towards the head, generally with two branches of equal size – the angiographic 'V' sign. The main PA is very large, with the descending aorta a direct continuation of the PDA. More recently, TTE has been used alone for diagnosis. This should localize the site and extent of interruption, demonstrate the narrowest dimension of the LVOT as related to the posterior displacement of the conal septum, and assess the diameter of the aortic annulus and ascending aorta. Echocardiographic measurements of aortic valve diameter and subaortic diameter index may predict subsequent LVOTO after primary repair of IAA.

Surgical management

The first successful correction of isolated IAA was performed by Chamberlin in 1954, using an aortic homograft via left thoracotomy. Samson described a successful staged repair in 1955 in a short-segment Type A IAA in which the VSD was closed 4 years later.

IAA repair originally involved staged correction. Initial palliation was by PA banding followed by subsequent intracardiac repair and debanding. Single-stage complete repair in infancy using a Dacron graft was first reported in 1972 by Barratt-Boyes. Trusler in 1975 performed single-stage repair without the use of prosthetic material. Single-stage complete repair is now preferred at most centers but some aspects remain controversial.

Staged correction

Prior to the widespread use of CPB in neonates, staged correction was the only safe approach. The first operation is through a left posterolateral thoracotomy. Following PDA ligation the operation must progress swiftly because of lower extremity ischemia. The aortic arch may be reconstructed directly using endogenous vessels or a prosthetic interposition graft. A PA band is tightened until distal PA pressure is <40% systemic systolic blood pressure. The banding should increase the peripheral arterial pressure by 10–15 mmHg whilst maintaining peripheral SaO$_2$ >85%. Optimal timing of the second stage is 2–3 months after initial palliation. Using median sternotomy and CPB, the VSD is closed and the PA debanded. If a prosthetic graft was used in the initial repair the child will outgrow the conduit and develop an anastomotic gradient. Often a second conduit (16–20 mm) can be added between the ascending and descending aorta to augment neonatal graft flow. Although the survival in some series is quite good, others have reported poor outcomes using a staged approach.

Single-stage repair

Single-stage repair is preferable to a staged approach. Early reports of primary repair utilized an interposition graft with VSD closure while more recent series have emphasized direct arch anastomosis. This approach avoids the potential problems of a prosthetic graft that cannot grow and the complications associated with PA banding. The one-stage repair is more complex and has unique complications including compression of the right PA or the left main bronchus.

Through a median sternotomy the head vessels, right and left PA and PDA are encircled with vessel loops. Double cannulation of the ascending and descending aorta (via the PA and PDA) may be employed to facilitate cooling to 18°C. During CPB the right and left PAs are occluded with tourniquets to prevent flooding of the lungs and to maintain systemic pressure. Circulatory arrest is used for resection of all ductal tissue followed by end-to-side anastomosis of the descending and ascending aorta. The VSD is closed through the pulmonary trunk or the RA.

The largest multi-institutional series of IAA (n = 183, from 1987 to 1992) is from the Congenital Heart Surgeons' Society. Of these, 116 underwent single-stage repair with 44 deaths (38%). Forty underwent staged repair of IAA with 14 deaths (35%). Risk factors for death were low birth weight, younger age at repair, IAA Type B, outlet and trabecular VSD, smaller size of the VSD, and subaortic stenosis.

Associated defects

IAA with severe subaortic stenosis

Complete single-stage repair of this lesion with resection of the infundibular septum and VSD closure via either a transpulmonary artery or transatrial approach has been successful. Others advocate preservation of the conal septum and placement of the VSD patch on the left side of the septum to deflect the conal septum anteriorly and away from the subaortic area. This approach has improved survival.

IAA with TGA

This occurs in 3% of IAA. The current approach is complete primary neonatal repair with arterial switch, simultaneous aortic arch reconstruction and VSD closure. A comparison between single- and two-stage repair reported improved early mortality and reduced re-operation rate with a single-staged approach.

IAA with truncus arteriosus

In truncus arteriosus with IAA (usually Type B), the truncus gives rise to an ascending aorta with brachiocephalic vessels and a PA that gives rise to the branch PAs and a PDA connected to the descending aorta. In a series of seven infants who underwent repair with circulatory arrest, the aortic arch was reconstructed by direct anastomosis with total excision of ductal tissue. RV-to-PA continuity was established with a valved conduit. There was no reported mortality.

Re-interventions

LVOTO development and recurrent or persistent aortic arch obstruction are the most common indications for re-operation. Modifications to the operative technique, e.g. placement of the VSD patch on the left side and direct anastomosis instead of patch aortoplasty, have reduced complications. When direct anastomosis is used, recurrent aortic arch obstruction is often successfully treated with percutaneous balloon aortoplasty. Patients with associated truncus arteriosus may need re-operation for progressive RVOT conduit stenosis/ insufficiency.

Further reading

1. Haas F, Goldberg CS, Ohye RG, Mosca RS, Bove EL. Primary repair of aortic arch obstruction with ventricular septal defect in preterm and low birth weight infants. *Eur J Cardiothorac Surg* 2000; **17**: 643–7.
2. Jonas RA, Quaegebeur JM, Kirklin JW, Blackstone EH, Daicoff G. Outcomes in patients with interrupted aortic arch and ventricular septal defect. A multiinstitutional study. Congenital Heart Surgeons Society. *J Thorac Cardiovasc Surg* 1994; **107**: 1099–113.
3. Salem MM, Starnes VA, Wells WJ et al. Predictors of left ventricular outflow obstruction following single-stage repair of interrupted aortic arch and ventricular septal defect. *Am J Cardiol* 2000; **86**: 1044–7.
4. Sano S, Brawn WJ, Mee RBB. Repair of truncus arteriosus and interrupted aortic arch. *J Cardiac Surg* 1990; **5**: 157–62.
5. Van Mierop LHS, Kutsche LM. Development of the aortic arch system and pathogenesis of coarctation of the aorta and interrupted aortic arch. In: *Coarctation and Interrupted Aortic Arch*. Mavroudis C, Backer CL (eds). *Cardiac Surgery: State of the Art Reviews*. Hanley & Belfus, Philadelphia: 1993; **7**: 1–22.

Related topics of interest

40 Coarctation of the aorta

Frank L Hanley

Epidemiology

Aortic coarctation is a congenital luminal narrowing anywhere from the arch to the aortic bifurcation which obstructs blood flow (98% centered around the origin of the left subclavian artery). Coarctation represents 5–8% of congenital heart disease (incidence is 1:1200 live births). Males are affected 2–5 times more frequently, with a reduced incidence in the black population. Of those patients with Turner's syndrome, 15–36% have coarctation. Coarctation is strongly associated with other cardiac malformations (PDA, VSD, bicuspid aortic valve, mitral valve abnormalities).

Anatomy

Coarctation is usually diagnosed in infancy with 50% becoming symptomatic within 1 month of life. The lesion may be a discrete isolated obstruction or a diffusely narrow segment. When diffusely narrowed, the aortic isthmus is most frequently involved (tubular hypoplasia). In 1903, Bonnet divided the patients with coarctation into two groups: infantile and adult. In the infantile group, there is preductal coarctation of the aorta associated with isthmic tubular hypoplasia. In the adult group, the narrowed segment is isolated and located at (juxtaductal) or just below the ductus (postductal). The critical factors that determine the hemodynamic burden are the size of the transverse arch and the severity of the coarctation.

In surgical series, to evaluate outcomes, a classification into three groups has been described:

- group 1: patients with isolated coarctation
- group 2: patients with coarctation and VSD
- group 3: patients with coarctation and complex cardiac anomaly.

Coarctation causes progressive development of collateral blood flow predominantly derived from the subclavian artery and its branches (internal thoracic, intercostal, musculophrenic, transverse cervical, scapular, lateral thoracic, superior epigastric, and spinal arteries). Coarctation is associated with cerebral aneurysms which remain undetected until rupture.

Pseudocoarctation is defined as kinking of the aorta, which radiographically mimics coarctation, but without functional obstruction.

Embryology

- Flow theory – blood flow through cardiovascular structures during fetal growth determines their size at birth (diminished flow = diminished growth).

- Ductal sling theory – abnormal extension of contractile ductal tissue sling into the aorta with subsequent contraction and fibrosis during ductal closure.

The flow theory does not explain isolated coarctation. Both theories may apply in the same patient. There are other less convincing ideas including neural crest maldevelopment.

Natural history

Coarctation tends to present in one of two distinct modes:
(1) Infants with associated cardiac anomalies and severe coarctation with ductal-dependent blood flow to the lower extremities present at ductus closure with cardiovascular collapse, acidosis and renal failure. The sudden increase in LV afterload precipitates congestive cardiac failure.
(2) Older patients remain essentially asymptomatic and present with hypertension and its complications such as cerebral artery aneurysm rupture.

Morphology

- Hypoplasia of the proximal aortic arch (between innominate artery and left common carotid artery) = cross-sectional diameter ≤60% of the descending aorta.
- Hypoplasia of the distal arch (between left common carotid artery and left subclavian artery) = cross-sectional diameter ≤50% of the ascending aorta.
- Isthmic hypoplasia (between left subclavian artery and ductus insertion) = cross-sectional diameter ≤40% of the ascending aorta.

Associated defects

More frequent with infantile coarctation, 85% of neonates and 50% of infants have associated left-sided obstructed lesions (aortic stenosis/atresia, bicuspid aortic valve, subaortic stenosis, Shone's syndrome), and lesions with abnormal interventricular or great vessels communication (VSD, VSD+TGA, or VSD+DORV, AP Window). Coarctation is rarely associated with the right-sided obstruction.

Pathophysiology

Following birth, the pathophysiology depends on three factors:

- the degree of obstruction
- the status of the ductus arteriosus
- associated intracardiac lesion.

Diagnosis

Infants with critical coarctation and ductus closure present in shock. The infant may be tachypneic, tachycardic, and pale. Upper extremity pulses may be thready and lower extremity pulses absent. The patient may be hypotensive with hepatomegaly. Chest radiograph will demonstrate cardiomegaly and congestive cardiac failure. The TTE will confirm the diagnosis showing a lack of pulsatile flow in the descending aorta, the coarctation site, the size of the transverse arch, and any other associated intracardiac anomaly.

Physical examination of an asymptomatic older child may reveal upper extremity hypertension with absent or faint femoral pulses. Chest radiograph will demonstrate rib 'notching' in those >4 years old. The classic '3 sign' is caused by dilatation of the subclavian artery, narrowing at the coarctation site, and poststenotic dilatation of the descending aorta. Accurate diagnosis can be established using echocardiogram, cardiac catheterization, CT, and MRI.

Management principles

Prognosis is related to:

(1) age (risk increased in younger patients)
(2) the number and extent of associated defects
(3) the anatomy of the coarctation (greater risk with arch hypoplasia).

- PGE1 infusion for neonates in extremis restores ductal patency and improves distal perfusion.
- ICU monitoring and ventilatory support to avoid apnea (15–20%) with PGE1.
- Muscle paralysis, inotropic support, sodium bicarbonate supplementation, and diuretic therapy.
- The patient is placed in right lateral decubitus position.
- A right radial artery line and a lower extremity arterial line together are used to assess post-repair pressure gradient.
- The core temperature is carefully maintained at 35°C. Spinal cord ischemia is rare in neonates and infants, but has been reported with higher core temperatures during aortic cross-clamping.

Surgical options

Gross undertook experimental repair in 1938, the first successful resection and end-to-end anastomosis was performed by Craaford in 1944. Subsequently, different techniques were developed. Current surgical options are:

Subclavian flap aortoplasty
Advantages
(1) All-natural tissue.
(2) Avoidance of tension on the suture line.
(3) Less overall dissection.
(4) No circumferential scar.
(5) Option to retain a PDA.

Disadvantages
(1) Interruption of left arm blood flow and potential growth retardation.
(2) Retention of abnormal ductal tissue.
(3) Inability to correct arch hypoplasia.
(4) Potential for late aneurysm formation.

Resection and primary anastomosis

Advantages
(1) Complete removal of ductal tissue.
(2) Ability to correct arch hypoplasia.

Disadvantages
(1) Potential for tension on the suture line.
(2) Greater technical difficulty.
(3) Requires extensive dissection.
(4) Cannot retain a PDA.

Synthetic patch aortoplasty

Advantages
(1) Minimal dissection.
(2) Left arm perfusion preserved.
(3) Short clamp time (5–8 min).
(4) Option to retain a PDA.

Disadvantages
(1) Aneurysm formation (opposite to the patch).
(2) Retention of abnormal ductal tissue.
(3) Inability to correct arch hypoplasia.

Interposition graft

Advantage
Less suture line and clamp time when coarctation segment is extremely long.

Disadvantage
No growth potential.

Currently mortality is low using all techniques. However, the incidence of recurrent coarctation in neonates remains significant (7–25%) with each method. Other potential complications are listed in Table 1.

Table 1 Potential complications after surgery

Early complications	Late complications
(a) Hemorrhage	(a) Re-stenosis
(b) Recurrent laryngeal nerve injury	(b) Aneurysm
(c) Phrenic nerve injury	(c) Left arm ischemia
(d) Horner's syndrome	
(e) Chylothorax	
(f) Hypertension	
(g) Paraplegia/stroke	
(h) Aneurysm	
(i) Re-coarctation	
(j) Left arm ischemia	

Results

Hospital mortality in neonates with coarctation associated with cardiac defect is 2–9%. In older patients, hospital mortality should approach zero. Influenced by the age at operation (inversely proportional), technique used, quality of the initial repair, and growth at the repair site, recurrent coarctation (gradient >20 mmHg) develops in 5–20% of the patients. In most cases, these can be resolved with balloon angioplasty. Otherwise a variety of redo surgical techniques may be utilized, including patch aortoplasty (discrete re-coarctation), subclavian flap aortoplasty (in infants who require preservation of a PDA), and extended end-to-end repair. Alternatively, an extra-anatomic bypass should be considered (tube graft from ascending to descending aorta) to avoid dissection around the previous repair and risk of paraplegia.

Further reading

1. Bouchart F, Dubar A, Tabley A. Coarctation of the aorta in adults: surgical result and long-term follow-up. *Ann Thorac Surg* 2000; **70**: 1481–9.
2. Castaneda AR, Jonas RA, Mayer JE Jr, Hanley FL. Aortic coarctation. In: *Cardiac Surgery of the Neonate and Infant*. WB Saunders: Philadelphia, 1994: pp 333–52.
3. Magee AG, Blauth CI, Quereshi SA. Interventional and surgical management of aortic stenosis and coarctation. *Ann Thorac Surg* 2001; **71**: 713–15.
4. Vouhé PR, Trinquet F, Lecompte Y et al. Aortic coarctation with hypoplastic aortic arch: results of extended end-to-end aortic arch anastomosis. *J Thorac Cardiovacs Surg* 1988; **96**: 557–63.
5. Quaegebeur GM, Jonas RA, Weinberg AD, Blackstone EH, Kirklin JW. Outcomes in seriously ill neonates with coarctation of the aorta. A multi-institutional study. *J Thorac Cardiovasc Surg* 1994: **108**: 841–54.

Related topics of interest

41 Valvular disease in children

James L Monro

Valvular disease in children is mostly congenital, although rheumatic fever accounts for mitral stenosis in many children in developing countries. Valves may be regurgitant, stenosed or atretic. Complete atresia interrupting normal blood flow is life threatening in contrast to some stenoses which can be quite mild and where operation can be safely postponed for years. Although mild regurgitation may take years to become severe, timely intervention may avoid cardiac enlargement and failure.

Aortic valve

Stenosis (valve area < 0.5 cm^2/m^2)

1. Valvular

Valvular stenosis is the most common and may present at any age. Critical neonatal aortic stenosis is life threatening and requires urgent operation. Many children do not require surgery until after the first year of life. Typically, there is a bicuspid valve with fusion of the cusps anteriorly. This can be treated successfully by open valvotomy with CPB. Even a small split may result in significant improvement of the valve orifice area and cardiac output. As long as there are no complicating features, such as a small or even hypoplastic left ventricle, the results are very good. Although, re-operation is inevitable later, even infants can usually grow to a size where an adult size prosthesis can be inserted at re-operation with or without aortic root enlargement.

The outcome of blind valvotomy with a dilator passed through the apex of the ventricle is poor and has been largely abandoned. Percutaneous balloon valvuloplasty is usually successful but carries a significant risk of vascular complications, cusp avulsion and severe regurgitation. Despite this, balloon valvuloplasty is the treatment of choice in most units.

2. Supravalvular

Stenosis is rare and is frequently associated with Williams syndrome. It is repaired by patch aortoplasty.

3. Subvalvular

Stenosis is probably acquired and of uncertain etiology. A circumscribed fibrous ridge develops just below the aortic valve and this can usually be enucleated with blunt dissection. Some subvalvular stenoses with a tunnel-like outflow tract are more difficult to repair.

Regurgitation

This may be associated with a VSD (juxta-arterial), in which case the VSD should be closed and it may be possible to repair the valve by plicating the prolapsing right coronary cusp. Regurgitation may be present with a bicuspid valve when a cusp prolapses. It may be iatrogenic, or even follow what was initially a satisfactory valvotomy. Rheumatic fever, Marfan's syndrome and endocarditis are also recognized causes.

Except when associated with a VSD, repair is usually not successful and valve replacement is required with severe regurgitation. There is an increasing trend towards pulmonary valve autograft replacement (Ross procedure). This has the advantage that the patient does not need anticoagulants, but the disadvantage that the pulmonary valve needs to be replaced with a homograft, which will require multiple replacements. Homografts can also be used in larger children but are in short supply. Heterografts have been shown to calcify early in children and should not be used.

Mechanical valve replacement is very satisfactory, particularly with modern carbon bi-leaflet valves. However lifelong anticoagulation is essential. It is usually possible to implant an adult-size prosthesis, although root enlargement may be necessary. Mechanical valve replacement is recommended for Marfan's syndrome.

Aortic atresia

Aortic atresia is part of the hypoplastic left heart syndrome and is not amenable to direct repair. Most infants die in the first week of life, but with the Norwood repair, subsequent cavopulmonary anastomosis and a Fontan procedure around 4 years of age, approximately 50% of these children survive into teenage.

Mitral valve

Stenosis

A variety of mitral valve abnormalities cause congenital stenosis such as a 'parachute valve'. This has a single papillary muscle and short chordae, and may be amenable to repair by splitting the papillary muscle along its length. Other valvular pathologies may be amenable to repair and each has to be assessed and treated accordingly. However, many repaired valves will subsequently develop increasing recurrent stenosis and require re-operation.

Regurgitation

If secondary to annular dilatation, competence can be achieved by annular reduction with an annuloplasty suture running along the posterior annulus over Teflon pledgets (De Vega type). Following repair of partial AVSD, if the 'cleft' between the anterior and posterior bridging leaflets was not sutured, late regurgitation may develop which can be adequately repaired by suturing the cleft. Following repair of complete AVSD, where leaflet tissue may be inadequate, severe regurgitation may develop which is usually not repairable and replacement is required. The use of TEE is very helpful in defining the regurgitation pre-operatively and assessing the adequacy of repair.

If repair is not possible, replacement will be necessary and a mechanical valve should be used. It is unlikely that an adult-size prosthesis can be inserted in small children and therefore a further operation will be necessary as the child grows. Despite the need for anticoagulation, late results are surprisingly good, even in small children.

Pulmonary valve

Stenosis

Stenosis, which may present in early infancy, is now usually dealt with by the cardiologist using balloon dilatation. However, it may occasionally be necessary to perform a surgical valvotomy and sometimes to excise a very dysplastic valve with or without a transannular patch.

Obstruction of the right ventricular outflow tract may be caused by tetralogy of Fallot, a stenosing and calcifying homograft inserted in the repair of truncus arteriosus, pulmonary atresia or the Ross procedure. When the obstruction is severe (usually when RV pressure is 2/3 systemic) the homograft needs to be replaced.

Regurgitation
Regurgitation most frequently follows repair of Fallot's tetralogy when a transannular patch has been used. Regurgitation is inevitable, but usually well tolerated for years. However the RV enlarges and it is prudent to insert a homograft into the outflow tract before irreversible RV damage ensues.

Pulmonary atresia
Pulmonary atresia can occur with or without a VSD. The former is like an extreme form of Fallot's tetralogy. With an intact septum, the RV is usually very small, and all the blood returning to the RA must go through an ASD to the left side. An initial shunt and later Fontan type of procedure usually results in reasonable long-term results.

Tricuspid valve

Stenosis
Stenosis is rare, and may be congenital or rheumatic. If the annular size is reasonable, a valvotomy is usually adequate. If the annulus is small, it may be possible to insert an RA-to-RV valved conduit (e.g. homograft) in parallel, but this can be a very difficult situation to treat satisfactorily.

Regurgitation
Regurgitation may be due to dilatation of the RV stretching the annulus, in which case treatment of the underlying cause with or without a tricuspid annuloplasty is appropriate.

Ebstein's malformation is an important, although rare, cause of often severe tricuspid regurgitation. The valve is displaced down into the RV, leaving above it an atrialized RV wall. Repairs have been described, and that by Carpentier seems the most satisfactory. However it may occasionally be necessary to replace the valve, and a stented tissue valve is suitable in older children.

Further reading

1. Alexiou C, McDonald A, Langley SM et al. Aortic valve replacement in children: are mechanical prostheses a good option? *Eur J Cardiothorac Surg* 2000; **17**: 125–33.
2. Carpentier A, Chauvaud S, Mace L et al. A new reconstructive operation for Ebstein's anomaly of the tricuspid valve. *J Thorac Cardiovasc Surg* 1988; **96**: 92–101.
3. Elkins RC, Knott-Craig CJ, Ward KE, Lane MM. The Ross operation in children: 10-year experience. *Ann Thorac Surg* 1988; **65**: 496–502.
4. Kirklin JW, Barratt-Boyes BG. Congenital aortic stenosis. In: *Cardiac Surgery. 2nd Edn.* Churchill Livingstone: New York, 1993, **2**: 1195–237.
5. Kirklin JW, Barratt-Boyes BG. Congenital mitral valve disease. In: *Cardiac Surgery. 2nd Edn.* Churchill Livingstone: New York, 1993; **2**: 1343–59.

Related topics of interest

42 Total anomalous pulmonary venous connection

Stephen M Langley

The pulmonary veins (PVs) are disconnected from the LA in total anomalous pulmonary venous connection (TAPVC). Blood enters the systemic circulation by passing through an atrial communication (ASD/PFO) from the RA into the LA. Consequently, the pulmonary and systemic venous return mix within the RA.

TAPVC is relatively uncommon, accounting for 1.5–3% of congenital heart disease. About one-third of cases coexist with other major cardiac abnormalities including truncus arteriosus, transposition of the great arteries, pulmonary atresia, aortic coarctation, tetralogy of Fallot and a functional single ventricle including hypoplastic left heart syndrome. In young patients a PDA is common.

Embryology

The lung buds develop as an outpouching from the primitive foregut, taking with them a plexus of veins derived from the splanchnic venous plexus which drain to the heart through paired common cardinal, umbilical and vitelline veins, i.e. systemic venous drainage. Subsequently, the common PV evaginates from the LA and fuses with the pulmonary venous plexus surrounding the lung buds. TAPVC results from failed fusion with persistent connection of the pulmonary plexus to the splanchnic plexus. The PVs therefore drain to the heart via a systemic vein.

Anatomy

There are three main types of TAPVC.

1. Supracardiac (45%)

In the most common form, the PVs drain into a common retrocardiac venous confluence which, via an ascending vein in the mediastinum, joins the innominate vein or the SVC ultimately. Occasionally, the confluence drains via a vein coursing beneath the heart before ascending in the right paravertebral gutter to join the azygous vein. The connecting vein between the PV confluence and the systemic vein can obstruct as it passes between the left PA and the left main bronchus (broncho-pulmonary vice).

2. Cardiac (25%)

The common PV drains directly into the coronary sinus or very rarely the left and right pulmonary veins join the posterior RA wall separately. PV obstruction is relatively uncommon.

3. Infracardiac/infradiaphragmatic (25%)

The common PV drains via a descending vein which invariably accompanies the esophagus through the diaphragmatic esophageal hiatus to reach the portal venous system, or rarely the IVC. Obstruction is very common either at the diaphragm, or typically following closure of the ductus venosus when blood must then pass through the hepatic sinusoids before returning to the RA via the hepatic veins and IVC.

In approximately 5% of cases mixed drainage occurs with different veins connecting to separate anomalous sites.

Pathophysiology

As both the systemic and all the pulmonary venous blood returns to the RA, survival depends on blood shunting into the LA across the ASD. Mixing of the systemic and pulmonary venous blood causes variable cyanosis, the extent of which is related to the size of the ASD and to any PV obstruction. A restrictive ASD is rare but limits systemic perfusion and promotes pulmonary hyperemia and edema. A larger non-restrictive ASD allows greater systemic perfusion and more balanced Qp:Qs. PV obstruction may cause secondary PA and RV hypertension, which when severe produces right-to-left shunting at atrial and ductal levels. Combined with severe pulmonary edema, this results in severe hypoxemia in the neonate.

Clinical features

Presentations depend on:

- size of the ASD
- extent of pulmonary venous obstruction
- associated cardiac malformation.

Unobstructed TAPVC is usually asymptomatic at birth. Subsequently, increased pulmonary blood flow causes tachypnea in the first weeks of life, progressing to respiratory infections, failure to thrive and cardiac failure by 6 months. Cyanosis may be absent. Gross PV obstruction presents within hours of birth with severe cyanosis, respiratory distress and hypoperfusion.

Diagnostic imaging

Chest x ray (CXR)

- Pulmonary hyperemia or oligemia (PV obstruction), dilated RA and RV.
- In older children with TAPVC to the innominate vein the 'figure-eight' or 'snowman' appearance.
- Normal heart size and diffusely hazy lung fields with Kerley B lines obscuring the cardiac silhouette with PV obstruction.

Echocardiography
- Confirms diagnosis, determines site of connection of the PV confluence, evaluates obstruction and coexisting cardiac abnormalities.
- RV volume overload, RA enlargement and leftwards bowing of the atrial septum.
- Color-flow mapping quantifies flow through the anomalous connections.
- Doppler echocardiography quantifies PV obstruction.

Cardiac catheterization
- Contraindicated in critically ill neonates with obstructed TAPVC, as the osmotic load can exacerbate pulmonary edema.
- Indicated for older children to determine RV and PA pressures plus PV obstruction.
- Step-up in oxygen saturation in the systemic veins localizes the site of PV connection.
- Balloon septostomy of a restrictive ASD may temporarily palliate, although many centers prefer early surgical correction.

Medical management

In obstructed TAPVC, alprostadil (prostaglandin E1) to delay PDA closure is not effective. Intubation, ventilation with 100% oxygen and correction of metabolic acidosis are necessary prior to emergency surgery. In unobstructed TAPVC, as PVR decreases after birth volume, loading of the right heart gradually increases. Medical treatment for congestive heart failure is required.

Surgical management

Obstructed TAPVC represents a true surgical emergency as no effective medical palliation exists. Surgical repair should immediately follow echocardiographic diagnosis. In unobstructed TAPVC, surgery should be undertaken in early infancy before the sequelae of cyanosis and volume overloading of the heart and lungs ensue.

Surgical technique

The supra- and infracardiac types are repaired by anastomosing the PV confluence to the posterior LA wall and ligating the systemic venous connection. The ASD is usually closed unless pulmonary hypertension is a serious concern. Indwelling PA and LA monitoring lines are sited.

The cardiac type is repaired by incising the tissue between the foramen ovale and the coronary sinus ostium and placing a pericardial baffle over the two orifices to close the ASD and redirect coronary sinus return into the LA.

Postoperative management

In obstructed TAPVC, the muscularized pulmonary arterioles remain labile postoperatively. Fentanyl infusion is used to maintain anesthesia and minimize reactive pulmonary vasoconstriction. Hypocapnia ($PaCO_2$ approximately 4 kPa), hyperoxygenation and inhaled nitric oxide keep PA pressure ≤ systemic pressure. Sedation is gradually weaned after 24–48 hours of hemodynamic stability.

Outcome

Before 1970, TAPVC repair carried >50% mortality. This has subsequently fallen to <10% in modern series. PV obstruction is a significant postoperative problem in 10% of cases manifesting in the first few months after correction. It is usually remote from the anastomotic site and affects the PVs close to their junction with the confluence. Obstruction is caused by intimal fibrous hyperplasia and is unresponsive to balloon dilatation and difficult to repair surgically. In this respect, the pre-operative diameter of the individual PV may influence long-term outcome. Anastomotic stenosis may occur and can usually be surgically corrected. Late death is often related to PV obstruction.

Further reading

1. Kirshbom PM, Myung RJ, Gaynor JW et al. Preoperative pulmonary venous obstruction affects long-term outcome for survivors of total anomalous pulmonary venous connection repair. *Ann Thorac Surg* 2002; 74: 1616–20.
2. Caspi J, Pettitt TW, Fontenot EE et al. The beneficial hemodynamic effects of selective patent vertical vein following repair of obstructed total anomalous pulmonary venous drainage in infants. *Eur J Cardiothorac Surg* 2001; 20: 830–4.
3. Hyde JA, Stumper O, Barth MJ et al. Total anomalous pulmonary venous connection: outcome of surgical correction and management of recurrent venous obstruction. *Eur J Cardiothorac Surg* 1999; 15: 735–40; discussion 740–1.
4. Bando K, Turrentine MW, Ensing GJ et al. Surgical management of total anomalous pulmonary venous connection. Thirty-year trends. *Circulation* 1996; 94: II12–16.

Related topics of interest

43 Palliation versus correction of congenital heart defects

Stephen M Langley

Introduction

Surgical management of congenital heart defects (CHDs) strives to create a heart which is fully septated into two atria and two ventricles with the morphologic LV supplying the systemic circulation and the morphologic RV supplying the pulmonary circulation. In certain conditions, one or a number of palliative procedures are required before this optimum situation can be achieved. In other conditions, full correction is not possible and the palliation will be permanent.

Temporary palliation

Prostaglandin E1 (PGE1) is used in neonates with severe cyanosis resulting from CHD causing reduced PA blood flow (PBF) such as tetralogy of Fallot (TOF), pulmonary atresia or tricuspid atresia. PGE1 therapy is a temporizing measure which stabilizes the critically ill neonate prior to surgery. It maintains patency of the ductus arteriosus (PDA), and thereby increases PBF, preventing arterial desaturation and acidosis. Therefore PGE1 is ineffective treatment where cyanosis is due to reasons other than a reduced PBF, e.g. total anomalous pulmonary venous connection in which cyanosis results from pulmonary venous obstruction. An intravenous infusion of PGE1 is also essential to maintain right-to-left shunting through the PDA in neonatal coarctation or interrupted aortic arch. In these patients, congestive heart failure and shock may occur suddenly if the duct closes. Maintaining ductal patency with PGE1 allows perfusion to the lower half of the body prior to surgical correction.

Palliation to improve pulmonary blood flow

A systemic to PA shunt is created to improve PBF in patients with right-to-left shunts with reduced PBF, such as tricuspid atresia, pulmonary atresia or those with TOF not suitable for early complete correction. The classical Blalock–Taussig shunt involves an end-to-side anastomosis of the subclavian artery to the ipsilateral PA. A modified Blalock–Taussig shunt utilizes a 3.5 or 4.0 mm polytetrafluoroethylene (PTFE) tube graft, and is now the procedure of choice. The shunt involves an end-to-side anastomosis of the tube graft to the subclavian or innominate artery and the ipsilateral branch PA. To prevent occlusion of the duct whilst performing the anastomosis, the shunt is placed on the side opposite the aortic arch, therefore usually the right. The shunt is most frequently constructed via a thoracotomy but with hemodynamic instability a median sternotomy and CPB may be required. The shunt usually provides adequate PBF for some months before proceeding to either a full correction for those with TOF or a cavopulmonary shunt in patients with a functional single ventricle such as tricuspid atresia or pulmonary atresia with intact ventricular septum.

Palliation to reduce pulmonary artery blood flow

As the pulmonary vascular resistance falls during and after the neonatal period, any cardiac defects, which result in a left-to-right shunt, will result in excessive PBF. Banding of the main PA may be indicated to reduce PBF. The most frequent indications for a PA band include the presence of multiple muscular VSD ('Swiss cheese' septum) or the presence of a VSD with an associated coarctation. In this setting the coarctation is repaired and the PA is banded through a left thoracotomy. Three to four months later, via a median sternotomy, the band is removed and the VSD closed. PA banding is also indicated in patients with a functional single ventricle and excessive PBF such as in those with tricuspid atresia, a large VSD and no pulmonary stenosis.

As a guide, the circumference of the band in millimeters should equal the weight of the child in kilograms plus 20, according to Truslers's rule. The band is further adjusted according to the PA pressure distal to the band, the arterial saturation values and the systemic pressure as the band is tightened. In the context of a functionally biventricular heart the band is tightened to achieve systemic saturation values in the low 90s. Banding tighter than this can result in suprasystemic RV pressures and right-to-left shunting. In patients with a functional single ventricle circulation the distal PA pressure should be reduced to one-third systemic pressure with an arterial saturation of about 75%.

More recently, PA banding has been used in patients with ventriculoarterial discordance to attempt to train the morphologic LV before switching it to the systemic circulation. This is relevant in those patients with transposition of the great arteries (TGA) who have developed systemic RV failure following an atrial switch (Mustard or Senning procedure) in preparation for an arterial switch operation and for those with congenitally corrected TGA in preparation for a double switch procedure. The band is tightened to achieve over 80% of the systemic pressure in the morphologic LV. The band may have to be gradually tightened at several separate procedures some months apart.

Palliation to improve intracardiac mixing

In CHDs which require a septal communication for mixing of the pulmonary and systemic blood, enlargement of a restrictive ASD can markedly improve cyanosis. This may be important in a number of situations including total anomalous pulmonary venous connection and tricuspid atresia. The restrictive ASD is enlarged by balloon atrial septostomy. This potentially life-saving procedure may be undertaken at cardiac catheterization, or less frequently under echocardiographic control. The most common indication for balloon atrial septostomy is the newborn with simple TGA. Atrial septal thickness increases with age and children beyond the neonatal period with a restrictive ASD require either a blade septostomy or surgical atrial septectomy.

Permanent palliation

It is not always possible to successfully septate the heart into two separate ventricles. Patients in this situation may be described as having a functional single ventricle. Usually one of the ventricles is hypoplastic and consequently too small to work effectively as the pumping chamber for either the pulmonary or systemic circulation. Less commonly, both ventricles are a good size but straddling of one of the atrioventricular valves across the ventricular septum prevents closure of the VSD. In certain situations the position of the VSD in relation to the great vessels may preclude septation. Palliation of patients with a functional single ventricle often involves more than one operation. The first of these is commonly carried out in the neonatal period. At about 6 months of age a cavopulmonary shunt is undertaken, and finally, around the age of 4–5 years a Fontan procedure is performed.

The small left ventricle

When the LV is small it can be difficult to decide whether it is big enough for biventricular repair. This is important because if biventricular repair is attempted in patients with a small LV the results will be poor. Furthermore, converting to a Norwood procedure after an attempted biventricular repair is almost always fatal. Various unfavorable risk factors for survival have been identified in patients with hypoplasia of the LV undergoing biventricular repair. The Rhodes score, for example, uses various factors to predict the outcome of children with critical aortic stenosis. Although there are no absolute measures applicable to all situations, these factors may be useful indicators of an LV which is too small for biventricular repair. The more important of these include an LV which is non-apex forming, mitral valve size <8 mm, aortic annulus size <6 mm, LV volume <20 ml/m^2, retrograde flow in the ascending aorta, the presence of endocardial fibroelastosis and an LV inflow diameter (distance from mitral valve annulus to apex) <25 mm.

Early palliation for patients with a functional single ventricle

When the RV is hypoplastic, as in tricuspid atresia or pulmonary atresia with intact ventricular septum, initially the LV provides both systemic and PBF. In the neonatal period, the commonest situation is cyanosis due to reduced PBF, and a modified Blalock–Taussig shunt is therefore undertaken. Less commonly, when PBF is increased, for example in certain patients with tricuspid atresia, a PA band is required. When the LV is hypoplastic, as in hypoplastic left heart syndrome, the RV provides both the systemic and PBF. Initial palliation, the stage I Norwood procedure involves augmentation of the aortic arch and relief of the coarctation with a patch, a Damus procedure (anastomosis of the divided end of the main PA to the ascending aorta), an atrial septectomy and a systemic to PA shunt (usually a PTFE tube graft from the innominate artery to right PA).

Cavopulmonary shunt

This is usually undertaken at about 6 months of age. It tends not to be undertaken earlier when the pulmonary vascular resistance is high because it directs, rather than pumps, systemic venous return into the pulmonary arteries. The SVC is divided low down near the RA and anastomosed to the upper surface of the right PA. A previous modified Blalock–Taussig shunt if present is ligated and divided. Any forward flow from the RV into the pulmonary arteries is usually interrupted by dividing and oversewing the main PA. In the context of pulmonary atresia with intact ventricular septum, when the RV is small rather than truly hypoplastic, a 'one and a half' ventricle repair may be possible. In this situation PBF is derived from both the cavopulmonary shunt and RV output. A cavopulmonary shunt reduces the volume load on the heart. It also prevents the development of pulmonary vascular disease as PBF is at low (systemic venous) pressure in contrast to the high (systemic arterial) pressure present with a modified Blalock–Taussig shunt. The term cavopulmonary shunt is synonymous with a bidirectional Glenn procedure or, in the context of hypoplastic left heart syndrome, a Stage II Norwood procedure.

Fontan/Stage III Norwood procedure
For a detailed description refer to Chapter 36.

Further reading

1. Trusler GA, Mustard WT. A method of banding the PA for large isolated ventricular septal defect with and without transposition of the great arteries. *Ann Thorac Surg* 1972; **13**: 351–5.
2. Rhodes LA, Colan SD, Perry SB, Jonas RA, Sanders SP. Predictors of survival in neonates with critical aortic stenosis. *Circulation* 1991; **84**: 2325–35.
3. Cohen MS, Rychik J. The small left ventricle: how small is too small for biventricular repair? *Semin Thorac Cardiovasc Surg Pediatr Card Surg Annu* 1999; **2**: 189–202.
4. Lemler MS, Scott WA, Leonard SR, Stromberg D, Ramaciotti C. Fenestration improves clinical outcome of the Fontan procedure: a prospective, randomized study. *Circulation* 2002; **105**: 207–12.
5. Gentles TL, Mayer JE Jr, Gauvreau K et al. Fontan operation in five hundred consecutive patients: factors influencing early and late outcome. *J Thorac Cardiovasc Surg* 1997; **114**: 376–91.

Related topics of interest

Index

Page numbers in *italics* indicate illustrations and tables

conventional coronary surgery 108–11
cords, valve 5
coronary angiography *see* angiography
coronary arteries *see* arteries, coronary
coronary artery bypass grafting (CABG)
    vs. angioplasty 131
    future prospects 132
    ischemic cardiomyopathy 221
    vs. PCI 131–2
    vs. PTCA with stenting 131–2
    see also off-pump CABG
coronary circulation *see* circulation, coronary
coronary sinus *13*
coronary veins *see* veins, coronary
correction vs. palliation, CHDs 317–20
Cox maze III procedure, AF 188, *189*
CPB *see* cardiopulmonary bypass
cross-clamp fibrillation (CCF), myocardial
    preservation 78–80
CT *see* computed tomography
Cumulative Summation (CUSUM), performance
    monitoring 97–8
CXR *see* chest X ray
cytokines, SIRS 63
cytomegalovirus infection (CMV) 240

Da Vinci® robotic system 124
DAM *see* dynamic aortomyoplasty
DCM *see* dynamic cardiomyoplasty
deep hypothermia with circulatory arrest (DHCA)
    70–2
depolarization, excitation-contraction coupling 21–2
DHCA *see* deep hypothermia with circulatory arrest
diuretics, postoperative complications 94
double outlet right ventricle (DORV) 293–6, *294*, *295*
    anatomic classification 293
    investigations 294
    pathophysiology 293
    surgical management 294–5
    surgical results 296
    VSD position 293
drugs
    antiarrhythmic *see* antiarrhythmic drugs
    postoperative complications 94
    see also pharmacology
dynamic aortomyoplasty (DAM) 233
dynamic cardiomyoplasty (DCM), skeletal muscle
    circulatory support 233

echocardiography 51–4
    aortic valve repair 155
    clinical applications 51–2
    IVUS 105
    modalities 51
    MS 52–3
    TAPVC 315
    TEE 155
    TTE 170–1
    valve disease 52–3

    see also imaging
EKG monitoring 24–6
embryonic stem cells (ESC), CCM 236–7
endarterectomy 110
endocarditis
    clinical presentation 170
    diagnosis 170–1
    etiology 169
    medical management 171
    pathophysiology 169–70
    TTE 170–1
    valve surgery 169–72
Endopath® robotic system 124
Endosaph® robotic system 124
endothelial cells, SIRS 64
ESC *see* embryonic stem cells
ethical considerations, xenografts, heart
    transplantation 246–7
excitation-contraction coupling 19–23
    action potential *20*, 20–3, *21*
    antiarrhythmic drugs 22, *23*
    clinical implications 22–3
    depolarization 21–2
    ion channel defects 22
    ion channels 19
    refractoriness 21
    see also arrhythmia; conduction system
extubation, intensive care 90–1

Factor XII, SIRS 63
Fallot tetralogy 273–5
fibrinolytics, pharmacology 42
fibroelastoma 196
Fontan circulation 276–81
    arrhythmia 277
    complications 276–7
    Fontan conversion 277–80
    historical evolution *278–9*
    pathway obstruction 277
    PLE 276
    pulmonary arteriovenous fistula formation 277
    thromboembolism 276
functional MR 223, 225
future prospects
    CABG 132
    PCI 132

gastrointestinal tract, CPB 64
geometric MR 223, 225
global vascular homeostasis 30, 33–6
glycoprotein (GP)IIb/IIIa inhibitors, pharmacology
    43
grafting, arterial *see* arterial grafting

heart failure
    artificial hearts 226–8
    CCM 235–8
    end-stage revascularization 219–22
    IABP 215–18

operative phase 73–6
postoperative phase 76
pre-operative phase 73
reperfusion phase 76
myocardial regeneration, CCM 237–8
myocardial revascularization 103–36
arterial grafting rationale/outcome 116–18
arterial grafting techniques 112–15
biological bypass 134–6
conventional coronary surgery 108–11
imaging, IHD 103–7
IMR 145
minimally invasive approaches 122–5
OPCAB 119–21
percutaneous coronary intervention 126–33
myocardium, CPB 64
myocytes, action potential 20, *20*
myopathic heart, cardiovascular homeostasis 33
myxoma 195–6

neutrophils, SIRS 63
Novacor LVAD, ventricular assist device 227
nuclear cardiology, imaging 49

off-pump CABG (OPCAB)
anesthetic aims 119–20
myocardial preservation 79–80
myocardial revascularization 119–21
patient selection 119
techniques 120
oliguria
intensive care 90
postoperative complications 93
OPCAB *see* off-pump CABG
organ dysfunction, SIRS 64–5
oval fossa *13*
oxygenation, poor, postoperative complications 93

PA/IVS *see* pulmonary atresia with intact ventricular
septum
pacemaker cells, action potential 20–1, *21*
palliation vs. correction, CHDs 317–20
papillary muscles, valve 5
patent ductus arteriosus (PDA) 262–5, *264*
anatomy 262
clinical features 263
diagnosis 263
management 263–5
natural history 262–3
physiology 262
PCI *see* percutaneous coronary intervention
PDA *see* patent ductus arteriosus
penetrating and branching bundles, conduction
system 13–14
penetrating cardiac trauma
diagnosis 208
pathophysiology 208
surgery 208–10
treatment 209–10

penetrating mediastinal trauma
diagnosis 202–3
pathophysiology 202
presentation 202
surgery 202–4
treatment 203–4
percutaneous coronary intervention (PCI)
acute myocardial infarction 128
adjunctive pharmacology 127
vs. CABG 131–2
complications 127
development 126
drug eluting stents 127–8
future prospects 132
intracoronary stents 126–7
myocardial revascularization 126–33
restenosis 127
vs. surgery 130–3
percutaneous transmyocardial revascularization
(PTMR) 135
performance monitoring 96–9
perfusion imaging, myocardial 106
pericardial disease
clinical assessment 191–2
complete pericardiectomy 193
diagnosis 191–2
etiology 191
investigations 192
morbidity 193
mortality 193
outcome 193–4
surgery 191–4
PET *see* positive emission tomography
pharmacology 40–4
adjunctive, PCI 127
angina 40
anti-platelet agents 41–4
anticoagulation 41–4
arrhythmia 40–1
aspirin 41–2
atrial fibrillation (AF) 40–1
clopidogrel 42
fibrinolytics 42
glycoprotein (GP)IIb/IIIa inhibitors 43
heart failure 40
heparin 42–3
hypertension 40
lipid-lowering therapy 41
ventricular arrhythmias 41
warfarin 43–4
plasma volume homeostasis 31, 33–6
PLE *see* protein-losing enteropathy
positive emission tomography (PET), myocardial
perfusion imaging 106
post-infarction ventricular septal rupture 137–9
postoperative complications 92–5
anticoagulation 94
arrhythmia 92–3
drugs 94